28605   362.1 MAL

Setting Priorities in Health Care

Setting Priorities in Health Care

Edited by
M. MALEK

University of St Andrews, Fife, Scotland

JOHN WILEY & SONS

Chichester . New York . Brisbane . Toronto . Singapore

Other Wiley Editorial Offices

John Wiley & Sons, Inc. 605 Third Avenue,
New York, NY 10158-0012, USA.

Jacaranda Wiley Ltd, 33 Park Road, Milton,
Queensland 4064, Australia

John Wiley & Sons (Canada) Ltd, 22
Worcester Road,Rexdale, Ontario M9W
1L1, Canada

John Wiley & Sons (SEA) Pte Ltd, 37 Jalan
Pemimpin #05-04, Block B, Union
Industrial Building, Singapore 2057

British Library Cataloguing in Publication Data

A catalogue record for this book is available from the British Library

ISBN 471 94394 0

Produced from camera-ready copy supplied by the Editor
Printed and bound in Great Britain by Antony Rowe Ltd, Chippenham, Wiltshire

Contents List

List of Contributors

André Ament

Department of Health Economics,
University of Limburg

Djona Avocksouma

Faculté de Médicine,
Université de Montréal

Beryl Badger

The Management Research Centre,
The University of Plymouth

Stephen Bailey

Department of Economics,
Glasgow Caledonian University

Louise Bell

Southend Health care NHS Trust,
Southend Hospital

Nick Bosanquet

St. Mary's Hospital Medical School,
University of London

Reva Berman Brown

Department of Accounting & Financial
Management,
University of Essex

Allan Bruce

Department of Law and Public Administration,
Glasgow Caledonian University

Ewart Carson

Department of Systems Science,
City University, London

Francois Champagne

Faculté de Médicine,
Université de Montréal

Ian Chaston

The Management Research Centre,
The University of Plymouth

Joanna Coast   *Health Care Evaluation Unit,*
                                University of Bristol

Bill Cobb   *Department of Public Health Medicine,*
                                Solihull Health Authority

André-Pierre   *Faculté de Médicine,*
Contandriopoulos   *Université de Montréal*

Rob Cooper   *Department of Public Health Medicine,*
                                Solihull Health Authority

Derek Cramp   *Department of Systems Science,*
                                City University, London

Jean-Louis Denis   *Faculté de Médicine,*
                                Université de Montréal

Jenny Donovan   *Health Care Evaluation Unit,*
                                University of Bristol

Stéphanie Ducrot   *Faculté de Médicine,*
                                Université de Montréal

Rhiannon Edwards   *Department of Public Health,*
                                University of Liverpool

Marc-André Fournier   *Faculté de Médicine,*
                                Université de Montréal

Stephen Frankel   *Health Care Evaluation Unit,*
                                University of Bristol

Nick Freemantle   *Centre for Health Economics,*
                                University of York

Rosie Geller   *Department of Public Health Medicine,*
                                Shropshire Health Authority

John Goddard   *School of Accounting Banking and Economics,*
                                University College of North Wales

Felicity Green   *Department of Epidemiology & Health Sciences,*
                                Manchester University

David Hambleton

Management Consultant,
Coopers & Lybrand

James Harrison

Aston Business School,
Aston University

Sandra Hill

Department of Management,
Glasgow Caledonian University

Allen Hutchinson

Department of Public Health,
University of Hull

Ann Langley

Faculté de Médicine,
Université de Montréal

Département des sciences administratives,
Université du Québec à Montréal

Anne Lemay

Faculté de Médicine,
Université de Montréal

Brenda Leese

Centre for Health Economics,
University of York

Daniel Lozeau

Département des sciences administratives,
Université du Québec à Montréal

Annabelle Mark

Middlesex University Business School,

Alan Maynard

Centre for Health Economics,
University of York

Sean McCartney

Department of Accounting & Financial
Management,
University of Essex

Elaine McColl

Centre for Health Services Research,
University of Newcastle

Kevin McKeown

Department of Epidemiology & Health Sciences,
Manchester University

John Newton

Centre for Health Services Research,
University of Newcastle

Charles Normand   *Department of Public Health and Policy,*
                                   London School of Hygiene and Tropical
                                   Medicine

Wija Oortwijn   *Department of Technology in Health Care,*
                                   University of Limburg

Julie Quinlan   *Cranfield School of Management,*
                                   Cranfield University

Sharon Scaggs   *Thameside Community Health care NHS Trust,*
                                   Basildon Hospital

James Seldon   *Division of Business, Computing &*
                                   Mathematics,
                                   The University College of the Cariboo

Khesh Sidhu   *Department of Public Health Medicine,*
                                   Solihull Health Authority

Ala Szczepura   *Warwick Business School,*
                                   University of Warwick

Manouche Tavakoli   *Department of Management,*
                                   University of St Andrews

Caroline Taylor   *Centre for Health Economics,*
                                   University of York

Hinddrik Vondeling   *Department of Epidemiology and Biostatistics,*
                                   Free University of Amsterdam

                                   Department of Health Economics,
                                   University of Limburg

Keith Ward   *Cranfield School of Management,*
                                   Cranfield University

Ian Watt   *Centre for Health Economics,*
                                   University of York

Sandy Whitelaw   *Dept of Epidemiology and Health Sciences,*
                                   Manchester University

Acknowledgements

I wish to thank all the participants in the Second Symposium in Health Care Strategy held at the University of St Andrews, Scotland, in March 1994.

Thanks are also due to my colleagues in the PharmacoEconomics Research Centres in both Dundee and St Andrews Universities.

Verity Waite of John Wiley and Sons was instrumental in producing the book and offering general advice. Deirdre Jones and Chris Evans deserve a very special mention for persevering with me throughout the entire project. Without their help this volume would not have been possible.

Mo Malek

Editor's Preface

In April 1993, when the *First International Conference on Strategic Issues in Health Care Management* was being held in St Andrews, *Setting Priorities in Health Care* was proposed as the main theme of the Second Conference. The participants, whether from North America or Africa, Latin America or Asia, were all too aware of the pressing demand for a proper debate on the issues related and/or arising from prioritisation of scarce health care resources. In Britain the issue of rationing and prioritisation emerged as early as 1950s in the academia and reflected in the political arena in 1960s when adoption of overt rationing was proposed as a means of containing the ever increasing cost of health care provision.[1] At the other side of the Atlantic there has been intense public discussion surrounding what has been termed as the Oregon Experiment.[2] In July 1987, Oregon legislators voted to stop funding selected organ transplants (at a cost of $65,000 to $250,000 a piece) and stated their preference to divert the money saved from 34 potential transplant patients to give *basic, preventative* health care to 1,600 children. In November of that year Coby Howard, a 7 year old boy suffering from leukaemia was refused to have a $100,000 bone-marrow transplant, and subsequently died. In Oregon and the rest of the United States this was the start of an emerging era in which these issues of (literally) life and death have been put on the agenda and linked to various other, equally emotive issues. Priority setting, or rationing, is also on the agenda for Britain, Sweden, France, Finland, Netherlands and the rest of Europe, although some may not like the choice of the word 'rationing'. There is no consensus about the need for or the best method of prioritising the limited health care resources. The papers in this volume, selected from more than 200 papers submitted for the conference and the one hundred or so which were finally selected for presentation at the conference, advance the debate on health care prioritisation in many ways. They have been selected precisely because they represent the diversity of the opinions and the multitude of the disciplines which claim to have a legitimate stake in this debate. They examine a wide range of ethical, methodological, technical and political issues that must be addressed by any serious researcher. Some of the papers directly address these issues, while others are concerned with the 'environmental context' against which these problems are debated. As it is the case with all conference volumes, the chapters stand on their own, and there are differences in the style, the coverage, as well as on the way the authors have addressed their subject area. The merit of the papers included in the volume lies in the fact that they have highlighted the unacceptability of the customary approach of avoiding explicit choice. Two hundred experts from 20 countries came together to share the experiences and exchange ideas, on a highly controversial subject which is going to be with us and affect us for the rest of our lives. This volume is dedicated to all of them for their positive outlook and optimistic attitude.

Mo Malek

REFERENCES

[1]\Powell, J.E. (1966), *A New Look at Medicine and Politics,* London, Pitman.

[2]Strosber, M.A. et al., (eds.) (1992), *Rationing America's Medical Care: The Oregon Plan and Beyond,* Washington, The Brookings Institution.

1 Prioritising Health Care - Dreams and Reality

ALAN MAYNARD

University of York

INTRODUCTION

There are two certainties in life: the scarcity of resources and death. In the health care industry the issue is not whether to prioritise but how i.e. what criteria should be used to decide who will be treated, who will live in pain and discomfort, and who will be left to die. The combined effects of technological developments, most of which are unevaluated, and the greying of the population, which creates increasing demand for unevaluated technologies in the hope that death can be delayed and the quality of survival improved, is inducing cost inflation in all health care systems. The paradox of health care systems has been that the expansion of insurance has paid for the development of cost increasing technologies and these technologies have expanded the demand both for insurance and Government intervention (Weisbrod (1991)).

Cost inflation together with an economic depression[1] inevitably, induces talk of a "health care crisis" and frenetic searches for a "quick fix" to ill-defined policy problems. The current "quick fix" is competition and markets but whatever the proposed solution to the current "crisis", it usually includes focus on issues other than prioritisation. The "market solution" virus, which is currently very virulent, focuses on better definition of the roles of purchaser and providers and the creation of contestability. The theory is that these arrangements will lead to greater efficiency and cost containment although the evidence to sustain such hypothesis is absent (Maynard (1993)).

Why has the development of market-like mechanisms (e.g. HMOs) and enhanced regulation (e.g. DRGs) in the United States and the continuous discussion of prioritisation and reorganisation of the NHS in the UK in the last 15 years, produced only limited developments to assist in the processes of prioritisation ?

---

[1]Which inevitably affects the denominator more swiftly than the numerator.

Setting Priorities in Health Care. Edited by M.Malek
© 1994 John Wiley & Sons Limited

At present it is practically impossible to describe the processes which determine the allocation of resources between competing patients (i.e. prioritisation): indeed, as Williams (1993) has argued, this is one of the priorities for health service research in the 1990s. Despite this ignorance difficult choices are made everyday and the public recognition of this has led to some efforts by researchers and policy makers to set priorities more openly.

In the last 10 years there has been continuous discussion of prioritisation but little advance in the development and use of explicit techniques to facilitate life and death choices. Four examples of attempts to prioritise are: age, the development of QALYs, the Oregon prioritisation work and the report of the Dunning Committee in the Netherlands. These are described in section 1.

In the next section each of these initiatives are evaluated with a focus on the inadequacy of knowledge about "what works". To remedy this ignorance and the lack of knowledge about how to change clinical behaviour (i.e. "teach old docs new tricks"), basic principles of good practice in research will need to be preached further and practised better as R&D activities become better targeted to produce knowledge-based clinical practice. These basic principles will be reiterated in section three together with evidence of failure to practice in desirable ways.

Evidence based health care is a major threat to the economic interests of producers. The producers of pharmaceuticals and equipment may lose markets. Clinicians and other health care personnel will have to learn evidence based practice by reading the literature and retraining or facing redundancy. Change in the flow of health care expenditure inevitably redistributes incomes and jobs and so produces resistance to change (Reinhardt (1982), Reinhardt (1993)). Is there any reason to believe that evidence based health care will evolve more rapidly in the late 1990s or are the dreams of rational processes of prioritisation likely to be frustrated by these familiar obstacles to change? The grounds for optimism and pessimism are presented in section 4 where it is argued that professional regulation (i.e. the adoption of a new Hippocratic oath) may be more efficient than market mechanisms and bureaucratic regulation and that progress in informing choices with knowledge and improving prioritisation will be slow..

THE PRACTICE OF PRIORITISATION

Introduction

In all health care systems there are rules which determine the allocation of health care resources (i.e. rationing or prioritisation). Often these rules are implicit: in the United States loss of employment leads to loss of insurance cover and the unemployed are "rationed out" of some types of care. Sometimes these rules are explicit: in the NHS the rules for rationing care for patients with chronic renal failure have been discussed in the literature and access is related to age, sex, marital status and absence of other medical conditions.

The open discussion and application of such rules tend to be the exception rather than the rule. The rule tends to be that different methods are put forward but they are rarely applied to the practice of rationing care. Four examples of this are prioritisation on the basis of age, of capacity to benefit (i.e. cost per quality adjusted life year or QALY), and of "social utility" (Oregon and the Netherlands).

Prioritisation by age

The American ethicist David Callahan (1987, 1990) argued that in order to "curb our insatiable appetite for longer life regardless of expense" it was necessary to ration fairly in a way which sets limits to care. He proposed that care should be focused on enhancing the quality of life, not necessarily extending life, with long term, low technology care. Callahan argues that rationing should not be determined by clinicians' views of patients' needs but on the basis of a flat age limit in the late 70s or early 80s. Once this age is achieved, the elderly should be deprived of health care.

Prioritisation by capacity to benefit

The concept of the quality adjusted life year (QALY) was devised in the late 1970s by the US office of Technology Assessment (OTA). The OTA wanted a single measure which combined the benefits of enhanced duration of life with enhanced quality of survival. The principle is that if the quality of life can be measured on a scale 0 (dead) to 1 ("perfect" health), the impact of different interventions can be charted (as in figure 1) and the QALYs produced by intervention A (e.g. a surgical intervention) compared to intervention B (e.g. a medical intervention).

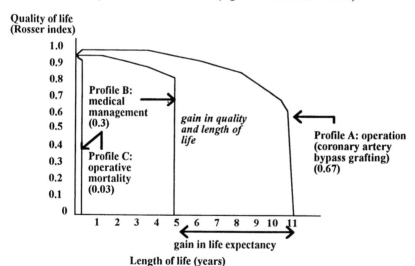

Figure 1. Expected Value of Quality and Length of Life Gained for Patients with Severe Angina and one Vessel Disease

Table 1. QUALITY ADJUSTED LIFE YEAR (QALY) OF COMPETING THERAPIES: SOME TENTATIVE ESTIMATES

	Cost/QALY (£ August 1990)
Cholesterol testing and diet therapy only (all adults, aged 40-69)	220
Neurosurgical intervention for head injury	240
GP advice to stop smoking	270
Neurosurgical intervention for subarachmoid haemorrhage	490
Anti-hypertensive therapy to prevent stroke (ages 45-64)	940
Pacemaker implantation	1100
Hip replacement	1180
Valve replacement for aortic stenosis	1140
Cholesterol testing and treatment	1480
CABG[1] (left main vessel disease, severe angina)	2090
Kidney transplant	4710
Breast cancer screening	5780
Heart transplantation	7840
Cholesterol testing and treatment (incrementally)	14,150
of all adults aged 25-39 years	17,260
Home haemodialysis	18,830
CABG[1] (1 vessel disease, moderate angina)	19,870
CAPD[2]	21,970
Hospital haemodialysis Erythropoietin treatment for anaemia in dialysis	54,380
patients (assuming a 10% reduction in mortality)	107,780
Neurosurgical interventions for malignant intracranial tumours	126,290
Erythropoietin treatment for anaemia in dialysis patients (assuming no increase in survival)	

1. CABG = coronary artery bypass graft
2. CAPD = continuous ambulatory peritoneal dialysis
Sources: Department of Health (1990), Pickard *et al.*, (1990), Teeling Smith, (1990), Williams (1985), Department of Health & Social Security (1986), Hutton *et al.*, (1990).

In Britain the seminal article using this approach was by Alan Williams (1985). He adopted the Rosser-Kind disability and distress matrix (Rosser, Kind and Williams (1982)) and used small groups of experts to identify how particular groups of patients move through the Rosser-Kind matrix before and after treatments. His results and others using a similar approach are shown (updated to 1990 prices) in table 1. (Maynard 1991).

A similar approach, using different quality of life measures and valuation techniques, has been used in North America (e.g., Goel & Detsky (1989)). In Britain the English Department of Health has gathered these data together and produced a QALY league table for nearly five hundred interventions. This league table has been presented at conferences (e.g. the 1993 Conference of the National Association of Health Authorities and Trusts) but has not yet been published.

Prioritisation by "social utility"

Two government agencies, one in Oregon and one in the Netherlands, have sought to create frameworks to rank health care interventions and facilitate the process of prioritisation.

In Oregon the State legislators, faced by cost inflation and incomplete health care cover for the poor in employment, outside the labour force and in Medicaid, set up a commission to rank available interventions, to cost them, and to use clinical and epidemiological data to advise the legislature where alternative budget allocations would produce "cut-offs" for interventions.

Table 2. Oregon Priorities 1993: the top 10.

Line 1	Diagnosis	Severe/moderate health injury: haematoma/edema with loss of consciousness
Line 2	Diagnosis	Insulin dependent diabetes mellitus
Line 3	Diagnosis	Peritonitis
Line 4	Diagnosis	Acute glomerulonephritis
Line 5	Diagnosis	Pheumothorax and haemothorax
Line 6	Diagnosis	Hernia with obstruction and/or gangrene
Line 7	Diagnosis	Addisons disease
Line 8	Diagnosis	Flail chest
Line 9	Diagnosis	Appendicitis
Line 10	Diagnosis	Ruptured spleen

Table 3. Oregon Priorities 1993: the bottom 10.

Line 735	Diagnosis	Benign neoplasm of external female genital organs
Line 736	Diagnosis	Benign neoplasm of external male genital organs
Line 737	Diagnosis	Xerosis
Line 738	Diagnosis	Sarcoidosis
Line 739	Diagnosis	Congenital cystic lung - severe
Line 740	Diagnosis	Ichthyosis
Line 741	Diagnosis	Lymphedema
Line 742	Diagnosis	Other aplastic anaemias
Line 743	Diagnosis	Tubal dysfunction and other causes of infertility
Line 744	Diagnosis	Heparatorenal syndrome
Line 745	Diagnosis	Spastic dysphonia

The Commission searched the literature, acquired advice from expert panels, consulted the community about their valuation of different health states in local "meetings with the people" and by telephone surveys which sought to elicit respondents' valuations of different health states, and debated publicly about the rankings. They produced several "league tables" in 1991-93 and some data from the

May 1993 listings are reported in tables 2 & 3[2]. For each item there is a diagnosis (with identified ICD 9 categories) and a treatment pair. The 1993 list has 745 pairs of lines in descending order of the Commission's judgement of effectiveness and hence, priority. All illnesses in the eligible population will be diagnosed but treatment will be provided only for those conditions which are above the budget line[3].

The Bush Administration refused to allow Oregon to implement this scheme. However the Clinton Administration has given Oregon a waiver from the Federal Medicaid legislation and it is planned that the scheme will be implemented in 1993-95 with full evaluation.

Whilst the Oregonians have tried to prioritise condition-treatment pairs by their effectiveness, the Dutch have only discussed the necessity to do it. (Government Committee on Choices in Health Care (!992)). The Commission was established to facilitate the definition of a basic package of health care. This aim was a product of both cost inflation and the Dekker reforms of the Dutch health care system which established a purchaser-provider split and the goal for the Government of limiting its coverage to proven package or 'core' of basic health care interventions. The proposed Dutch system for priorities involves "sieving" competing interventions at 4 levels. The first filter is to identify what is necessary and sieve out what is unnecessary. The Dutch distinguish three levels of necessary care: those which guarantee normal functioning of the individual, those which restore social functioning and those determined by disease severity. The ambiguity of these groupings is obvious.

The second sieve is to be used to reject those interventions which are ineffective. The Commission concluded that only those services which are "confirmed and documented" in terms of effectiveness should be included in the basic health care package. If this rule was followed the cost of health care everywhere would be cut magnificently !

The third sieve rejects those treatments which are inefficient e.g. those which have some effect but are very costly. The Committee proposed a cut-off level of cost-effectiveness below which interventions would be excluded from the basic package.

The final sieve rejects those interventions which are the responsibility of the individual. The Committee argued that there are limits to solidarity but were not explicit about how these limits would be defined.

The Oregon condition-treatment listing and the proposed principles set out by the Dunning Committee are both statements which reflect general values of "social utility" or "reasonableness" (in the case of Oregon).

---

[2]In the 1993 listing the Commission removed data generated by the phone survey and delayed all reference to quality of life because it violated the Americans with Disabilities Act.

[3]This was at item 568 in the (1992) previous 688 item listing.

A CRITIQUE OF THESE PROPOSED SYSTEMS OF PRIORITISATION

Introduction

The efforts to prioritise reported in the previous section have been subjected to intense criticism which has slowed both their development and implementation. What are these criticisms and are there common issues?

A critique of rationing by age

When Levinsky discussed Callahan's notion of rationing by age, he noted that if it had been proposed that health care entitlements be rationed on the basis of ethnicity or income there would have been uproar. The lack of uproar to the notion of rationing by age may reflect some social support for this type of approach.

However, this approach is fraught with difficulty (Maynard (1993(a)). Whilst there may be limits to the extent to which the fit young are prepared to redistribute to the ill elderly, the broad approach of Callahan has obvious difficulties:

- what age should be adopted for the cut-off and how should it be selected?
- is there to be the same age cut-off for men and women? Jeker (1991, 1992) argues that if the same age is used, this discriminates against women who, typically, live longer.
- people do not 'depreciate' in a uniform manner in relation to age and thus the capacity to benefit from care of the elderly is unequal.
- capacity to benefit will be related to the skills and techniques of surgeons and anaesthetists. For instance Davenport (1991) has shown that the post operative involvement of anaesthetists in the management of elderly patients improves outcomes and perhaps demonstrates that poor outcomes are the products not of the patients' ability to benefit, but of poor health care.

Brook and his colleagues have demonstrated that there is evidence of under and over utilisation of health care interventions on the elderly as well as evidence of misuse. They found evidence of substantial levels of inappropriate care: "Perhaps as much as one fifth to one quarter of acute hospital services or procedures were felt to be used for equivocal or inappropriate reasons, and two fifths to one half of medications studied were over-used in outpatients" (Brook *et al.,* (1990) p. 225). Furthermore they found underuse and overuse of ambulatory care and low cost technologies such as visits and preventive services.

Unthinking use of age as a rationing criterion can lead to elderly patients being deprived of care whose provision may be cost effective. Dudley and Burns (1992) surveyed age related policies for coronary care units (CCU) and thrombolytic therapy and found 20 per cent of CCUs and 40 per cent of consultants administering thrombolytic therapy had age related admission policies despite evidence that such interventions may be cost effective.

A critique of rationing by cost per QALY

The implication of the data in table one is that resources should be targeted at those interventions with a low cost per QALY. What caveats are to be recognised about this approach?

- are reported cost-QALY values marginal or average?
- what are the confidence intervals for these point estimates?
- how robust is the Rosser-Kind matrix? The York outcomes group found that the values in the original matrix, which were based on a non-random sample of 70 people, could not be replicated. Furthermore they concluded the disability and distress "descriptors" were inappropriate and different valuation methods produced different results. As a consequence they devised a new quality of life measure which they are now evaluating (Euro-qol Group (1990)). Thus there is much argument about whether the measures of a Q in QALY are robust, valid and replicable (Carr-Hill and Morris 1991).
- how "robust" are the clinical studies on which QALY estimates are based. This issue and other elements of "quality control" in the production of QALY estimates are dealt with unevenly and imperfectly (Drummond, Torrance and Mason (!993)).

However if a crude measure of patient capacity to benefit (QALY) per unit of cost is to be devised to inform choices and prioritisation this approach may be appropriate in principle even if it remains difficult to implement in practice.

A critique of rationing by social utility (Oregon and the Netherlands)

The initial thrust of the Oregon approach was to base it on cost and effectiveness data. The members of the Health Services Commission soon discovered that the knowledge base for their work was absent. As with all policy makers this came as something of a surprise because of the success of the medical profession in inducing the people erroneously to believe that their craft was scientific!

This discovery that the medical emperor had no clothes of knowledge led to the replacement of analysis with intuition. The use of clinical expert judgements is always dangerous as Feinstein argued:

> The agreement of experts has been the traditional source of all the errors through medical history.

Feinstein (1988)

Judgements may always be biased by expectations and beliefs which suit professional interests rather than reflect good trial data (Kaplan (1992)).

The Oregon priorities are determined by 'guesses' about effectiveness and social judgements about what the Commission calls "reasonableness" (which, for instance, makes it impossible to use disability and quality of life in prioritising (1993) list) and requires grouping of some categories regardless of risk and effectiveness (e.g. premature babies are aggregated regardless of term and birth weight) and ignore costs. To make choices properly the value of what is given up (the cost) has to be balanced against the value of what is gained (enhanced health status).

Another criticism made of the original Oregon approach was that the conditions were too aggregated. Eddy (1991) argues that ideally services should be narrowly defined so that each person who receives an intervention has the expectation of similar costs and benefits. The 1993 version of the Oregon list has tried to meet this criticism but appears to have dealt with it incompletely.

The work of the Oregon Health Service Commission was exemplary in that it sought to induce an explicit public debate about prioritisation and rationing. Unfortunately because of the injection of judgement and opinion about reasonableness it is not clear how the ranking was reached. However a ranking was reached thus challenging all to measure better and ensure that future lists are increasingly based on knowledge rather than guesses.

The Dutch Dunning Committee has discussed only the principles of rationing. No work has yet been done on the practice of prioritisation although there continues to be discussion of the definition of the basic benefits package there and in other health care systems.

TOWARDS EVIDENCE BASED HEALTH CARE

Introduction

There are two factors which combine to ensure that prioritisation cannot be based on evidence about the cost effectiveness of competing therapies. The first of these is that policy makers and practitioners are reluctant to take evaluation seriously. Research funders tend to argue that the creation of knowledge is expensive, ignoring the fact that the cost of ignorance is even greater.

The reluctance of the purchasers of R&D to finance it in insufficient volume is reinforced by the poor quality of practice in R&D. R&D practitioners know what we should do but we all seem deficient in turning principles into practice (Cochrane (1972))..

Clinical evaluation

John Bailar (1976, p. 117) argued "there may be a greater danger to public welfare from statistical dishonesty than from almost any other form of dishonesty". That is a bold assertion which regrettably may still be true. He put forward 12 laws of data analysis which continue to be ignored today (appendix 1). Perhaps the most important of these is law eight: more quacks practice statistics than medicine!

The principles to use in the rigorous evaluation of clinical trials, including their statistical virtues or lack of them, have been well articulated for over a decade (e.g. Sackett 1981 and 1984). Sackett advocated systematic appraisal of clinical trial data which simplified for the busy clinician required the addressing of six issues:

- did the study focus on what clinicians actually do?
- have the clinical actions studied been shown to do more harm than good?
- are the clinicians, patients and type of practice similar to yours?
- were the clinical actions measured in a clinically sensible fashion?
- were the clinical actions measured in a scientifically credible fashion?
- were both clinical and statistical significance considered.

He has written at length on these issues more recently (e.g. Sackett *et al.*, (1991), Oxman *et al.*, (1993) and Guyatt *et al.*, (1993)).

Despite the fact that such guides to good clinical evaluation have been available for many years, practice is still inadequate. Altman (1994) has argued that the "scandal of poor medical research" is caused by researchers driven by career needs to augment their curriculum vitae. Often researchers are ill-equipped for their work, nobody supervises them and, because of inadequate refereeing, bad papers are easy to publish. Despite the fact that these problems are well identified, the leadership of the medical profession does little to improve matters, ensuring that the creation of knowledge is impaired and research funds are squandered.

A nice review of the inadequacies of clinical trials in one area, non steroidal anti-inflammatory drugs (NSAIDs), is provided by Gotzsche (1989). He analysed overt and hidden biases in 196 double blind trials of NSAIDs by scoring the quality of their analysis against 8 criteria. He identified 22 factors that may increase the number and proportion of significant results favouring a new drug (table 4) and concluded that doubtful or invalid statements could be found in 76 per cent of the conclusions or abstracts and that bias consistently favoured the new drug in 81 of the 196 trials. Such conclusions are not an isolated event. For instance in a survey of manuscripts submitted to the British Medical Journal, Gardner *et al.*, (1986) concluded that the statistical analysis was poor in 31 of 45 clinical trial papers.

Obviously defects in the design and biases in the reporting of clinical trials means that meta-analysis has to be undertaken with great care. Gotzsche (1989) concluded that the deficits in the NSAID trials that he assessed were so gross that meta-analysis was impossible.

Table 4. Factors That May Increase the Number and the Proportion of Significant Results Favouring a New Drug

1.	Design bias
2.	Selection of patients dissatisfied with control drug
3.	Choice of dose
4.	Selection of indices
5.	Selective reporting among many variables
6.	Ineffective blinding
7.	Choice of Statistical methods or no statistics at all
8.	Handling of withdrawals
9.	Handling of missing data and other undertainties
10.	Change in measurement scale before analysis
11.	Choice of adjustment depending on result
12.	Uneven distribution of prognotic factors
13.	Wrong sampling unit for effect and side effects
14.	Wrong interpretation of within-group analyses
15.	Repeated testing on several groups or over time
16.	Subgroup analyses
17.	Selective reporting of $0.05 < p < 0.10$
18.	Omission of significant results favouring the control
19.	Wrong calculation
20.	One-sided tests
21.	Fraud
22.	Publication bias

Source: Gotzsche, (1989) p. 49.

Economic evaluation

Against this background of poor quality clinical research, economists have been advocating, with success, the use of their evaluative techniques. The number of studies in economic evaluation are growing expontentially (e.g. see Backhouse *et al.*, (1992)) and checklists to evaluate this work have existed for nearly two decades (e.g. see Williams (1974), in appendix two, and more recent lists, Drummond, Stoddart and Torrance (1987) and Maynard (1990)).

An important defect with economic evaluation is caused by the propensity of economists to take clinical data and use them uncritically. This can lead to the construction of ambitious economic modelling on the sands of poor clinical data (Freemantle and Maynard (1994)). Thus, whilst the costings may be nice, discounting done well and marginal data presented, economists, like their clinical colleagues, may be guilty of wasting scarce R&D resources and not facilitating as efficiently as they might the production of new knowledge. Further evidence about the defects of economic evaluation practice is nicely documented in Adams *et al.*, (1992) and Udvarhelyiet *et al.*, (1992).

Towards evidence based health care

The production of new clinical and economic knowledge is inefficient. However despite manifold deficiencies in these production processes new knowledge is emerging. That knowledge confirms the under and over use of expensive technologies. For instance a US-UK group evaluated, using an American and a British group of experts, the appropriateness of angiography and coronary artery by-pass surgery (CABGs) in Trent (Bernstein *et al.*, (1993). They concluded:

> Our study shows that inappropriate care, even in the face of waiting lists, is a significant problem in Trent. In particular, by the standards of the UK panel, one half of coronary angiographs were performed for equivocal or inappropriate reasons, and two fifths of CABGs were performed for similar reasons. Even by the more liberal US criteria, the ratings were 29% equivocal or inappropriate for coronary angiography and 33% equivocal or inappropriate for CABG.

(Bernstein, Kosecoff, Gray, Hampton and Brook Study (1993), p.8).

Brook (1994) has argued that it is essential to identify those procedures which are appropriate and carefully manage these into clinical practice. A literature on effectiveness is emerging (e.g. Coulter *et al.*, (1993). Song *et al.*, (1993) and Davey-Smith *et al.*, (1993)) which uses techniques such as meta-analysis to distil increased knowledge from many clinical trials. However the number and design of the available randomised clinical trials is inadequate and, as a result other methods of appraisal have to be used. These are unavoidable but weak mechanisms such as consensus conferences and their results must always be used with caution for as Abba Eban, the former Israeli foreign minister argued:

> consensus means that lots of people say collectively what nobody believes individually.

Abba Eban

Efforts to divine appropriateness and conjure up guidelines for clinical practice are to be welcomed. However this process must be seen as tentative and all involved in it must accept that guidelines will have to be flexible and be expected to change as knowledge increases. The wider application of checklists to evaluate the quality of data in organisations such as the Cochrane Centre and the Centre for Reviews and Dissemination will facilitate not only the production of practice guidelines but also the identification of gaps in research knowledge which must be removed by targeted investments of R&D resources.

However, research alone is inadequate. As Lomas (1993) has argued the related challenge is to change practice by teaching "old docs new tricks". Again knowledge, this time about the cost effectiveness of competing ways of changing behaviour, is very poor and careful evaluation of competing methods is needed. Clearly some organisations (e.g. the pharmaceutical industry) are very good at changing clinicians behaviour and lessons can, no doubt, be learned from such examples.

Because of the ignorance about what works and how behaviour can be changed cost effectively, practice is not knowledge based and any attempt to prioritise is likely to be frustrated and contentious. With a knowledge vacuum factional interests can shout loudly and convince decision makers by the volume of their rhetoric rather than be confused by facts !

THE OBSTACLES TO KNOWLEDGE BASED PRIORITISATION

Managing change

If knowledge was available about what works in health care it would engender major structural change which would be opposed by provider interests. The pharmaceutical industry's finances were directly affected by meta-analysis which shows that expensive SSRI are no more efficacious than cheap tricyclics in the treatment of depression (Song *et al.,* (1993)) and by similar work that demonstrates that lipid lowering cholesterol drugs should be targeted on high risk groups (Davey-Smith *et al.,* (1993)). ENT surgeons, only recently dissuaded from ineffective tonsil removal procedures, are now threatened by evidence that indicates that "glue ear" in most children is best treated, not with grommet insertion, but by watchful waiting (Effective Health Care (1992)). New surgical technologies, unevaluated of course, are leading to the dissemination of minimally invasive techniques which not only require retraining of practitioners but also seen to be inducing increased activity levels with mortality outcomes similar to old techniques. Effectiveness literature is showing that certain "mundane" interventions, such as the prophylactic use of antibiotics in caesarean procedures and the use of anti-coagulants in hip replacement procedures, save lives, improve the quality of life and save money.

Effectiveness knowledge will alter radically the distribution of income and employment in the health care market if practitioners can (all too slowly!) be persuaded to change their work practice. It is possible that change may best be induced not by crude and untested market and bureaucratic rules but by mechanisms such as professional ethics. A new Hippocratic oath based on an obligation to provide evidence based care to patients and informal policing of change by the profession may have such merit. A sense of duty may be more cost effective than both bureaucratic regulation and the forces of self interest and greed "gyrating" in the market place!. As Adam Smith argued:

> Those general rules of conduct when they have been fixed in our mind by habitual reflection, are of great use in correcting the misrepresentations of self-love concerning what is fit and proper to be done in our particular situation.............. The regard of those general rules of conduct, is what is properly called a sense of duty, a principle of greatest consequence in human life, and the only principle by which the bulk of mankind are capable of directing their actions.
>
> Smith (1790), chapter IV, para. 12
> chapter V, para 1, pages 160-162

Setting Priorities

In time evidence will inform priority setting and make it more robust than the present processes of "guestimation". Given the paucity of knowledge, greater sophistication in the computing of QALYs and the setting of priorities Oregon style will emerge slowly. The merit of such approaches is that they are explicit and challenge critics to do better and assist in the processes of development. To reject such approaches is "to throw out the baby with the bath water". These crude attempts to set priorities should be welcomed as a challenge to the covert, imprecise and inconsistent practice of prioritisation which exist in all health care systems today. In time proper measurement will lead not only to the clear identification of large (small area) variations in clinical practice but also to increasing knowledge of effectiveness and appropriateness. The dreams of simple solutions to prioritisation (such as QALYs or Oregon listing) are unlikely to evolve quickly. The processes of prioritisation will improve marginally but cumulatively over time .... and, after all, life is always marginal !

REFERENCES

Adams, M.E., McCall, N.T., Gray, D.T., Orza, M.J. and Chalmers, T.C. (1992). Economic analysis in randomised control trials, *Medical Care*, 30, 3, 231-243.

Altman, D.G. (1994). The scandal for poor medical research. *British Medical Journal*, 308, 283-4.

Backhouse, M.E., Backhouse, R.J. & Edey, S.A. (1992). Economic Evaluation Bibliography. *Health Economics*, Vol. 1, supplement.

Bailar, J.C. (1976), Bailar's laws of data analysis, *Clinical Pharmacological and Therapeutics*, 20:1, 113-119.

Bernstein, S.J., Kosecoff, J., Gray, D., Hampton, J.R. and Brook, R.H. (1993). The appropriateness of the use of cardiovascular procedures: British versus US perspectives, *International Journal of Technology Assessment in Health Care*, 9, 1, 3-10.

Brook, R.H., Kamberg, C.J., Mayer-Oakes, A., Beers, M.H., Raude, K. and Steiner, A. (1990). Appropriateness of acute medical care for the elderly: an analysis of the literature, *Health Policy*, 14, 225-42.

Brook, R.H. (1994).Appropriate: the next frontier. *British Medical Journal*, 308, 218-219.

Callahan, D. (1987). *Setting Limits: medical goals in an ageing society*, Simon and Schuster, New York.

Callahan, D. (1990). *What kind of life: the limits of medical progress*. Simond and Schuster, New York.

Carr-Hill, R.A. & Morris, J. (1991). Current practice in obtaining the "Q" in QALYs: a cautionary note. *British Medical Journal*, 303: 699-701.

Cochrane, A.L., (1972). *Effectiveness and Efficiency: rendom reflections on health services*, Nuffield Provincial Hospitals Trust, London.

Coulter, A., Klassen, A., McKensie, I.Z. and McPherson, K. (1993). Diagnostic dilation and curettage: is it used appropriately?, *British Medical Journal*, 306, 236-39.

Davey-Smith, G., Song, F. & Sheldon, T.W. (1993). Cholesterol Lowering and Mortality: The Importance of Considering Initial Level of Risk, *British Medical Journal*, 306, 1267-1373.

Drummond, M.F., Stoddard, G.L. & Torrance, G.W. (1987). Methods for the economic evaluation of health care programmes. Oxford: *Oxford University Press*.

Drummond, M.F., Torrance, G. and Mason, J. (1993). Cost Effectiveness League Tables: more harm than good? *Social Science and Medicine,* 37, 1, 33, 40.

Eddy, D.M. (1991). Oregon's Plan: should it be approved? *Journal of the American Medical Association,* 266, 17, 2439-2445.

EuroQol Group, (1990). Euroqol - a new facility for the measurement of health-related quality of life. *Health Policy,* 16, 199-208.

Feinstein, A. (1988). Fraud, Distortion, Delusion and Consensus: the problems of human and natural deception in epidemiology studies, *American Journal of Medicine,* 84, 475-478.

Freemantle, M. *et al.,* (1992). The Treatment of Persistent Glue Ear, *Effective Health Care,* Bulletin No. 4, Centre for Health Economics (York) - School of Public Health, (Leeds).

Freemantle, N. and Maynard, A. (1994). Something Rotten in the state of clinical and economic evaluations? *Health Economics,* 3, 2, editorial (forthcoming).

Gardner, M.J. Machin, D., and Campbell, M.J. (1986). Use of check lists in assessing the statistical content of medical studies, *British Journal of Medicine,* 292, 810-12.

Goel, V. and Detsky, A.S. (1989), A Cost Utility Analysis of Preoperative Total Parenteral nutrition, *International Journal of Assessment in Health Care,* 5, 183-195.

Gotzsche, P.C. (1989). Methodology and overt and hidden bias in reports of 196 double-blind trials of nonsteroidal anti-inflammatory drugs in rheumatoid arthritis. *Controlled Clin. Trials,* 10, 31-56.

Government Committee on Choice in Health Care (1992). *Choices in Health Care,* Dunning Report, Ministry of Welfare, Health and Cultural Affairs, Rijswilk, Netherlands.

Guyatt, G.H., Sackett, D.L., and Cook, C.J. (1993). Users guide to medical literature: II How to use an article about a therapy or prevention. *Journal of the American Medical Association,* 270, 21, 2598-601.

Jeker, N.S. (1991). Age based rationing and women, *Journal of the American Medical Association,* 266, 21, 3012-15.

Jeker, N.S. (1992). Age based rationing and women, *Journal of the American Medical Association,* letters, 267, 12.

Kaplan, R. (1992). A quality of life approach to health resource allocation, *In* Strosberg M.A., Wiener, J.M., Baker, R. & Fein, I.A. (eds.), *Rationing America's Health Care: the Oregon Plan and Beyond,* Brookings Institute, Washington D.C.

Levinsky, M.G. (1990). Age as a criterion of rationing care, *New England Journal of Medicine,* 322, 25, 1813-15.

Lomas, J., (1993). *Teaching Old (and not so old) Docs New Tricks: effective ways to implement research findings.* CHEPA Working Paper Series No. 93-4, McMaster University, Ontario.

Maynard, A. (1991). The design of future cost-benefit studies. *American Heart Journal,* 3, 2, 761-765.

Maynard, A. (1991). Developing the health care market. *Economic Journal,* 101 (408): 1277-1286.

Maynard, A. (1993(a)). Intergenerational solidarity in health care, in D. Hobman (ed.), *Uniting Generations: Studies in Conflict and Cooperation,* Age Concern, London.

Maynard, A. (1993(b)).   Competition in the UK National Health Service: Mission Impossible. *Health Policy,* 23, 193-204.

Oxman, A.D., Sackett, D.L. and Guyatt, G.M. (1993).   Users guide to medical literature: how to get started, Journal of the American Medical Association, 270, 17, 2093-95.

Reinhardt, U.E. (1982).   Table manners at the health care feast, in D. Yaggy and W.A. Anylan (eds.), *Financing Health Care: competition versus regulation,* Ballinger, Cambridge, Massachusetts.

Reinhardt, U.E. (1993).   Comment on the Jackson Hole Initiatives for a Twenty-first century American Health Care System. *Health Economics,* 2(1):

Rosser, R., Kind, P. & Williams, A. (1982).   Valuation of quality of life.   In Jones-Lee, M.W. (ed.).   *The Value of Life and Safety,* North Holland, Amsterdam.

Sackett, D. (1981).   How to read journals: why to read them and how to start reading them critically, *Canadian Medical Association Journal,* 124, 555-558.

Sackett, D. (1981).   How to read journals: to learn about a diagnostic test, *Canadian Medical Association Journal,* 124, 555-558.

Sackett, D. (1981).   How to read journals: to learn the clinical course and diagnosis of disease, *Canadian Medical Association Journal,* 124, 555-558.

Sackett, D. (1981).   How to read journals: to determine etiology or causion, *Canadian Medical Association Journal,* 124, 555-558.

Sackett, D. (1981).   How to read journals: to distinguish useful from useless or even harmful therapy, *Canadian Medical Association Journal,* 124, 555-558.

Sackett, D. (1981).   How to read journals: to learn about the quality of clinical care, *Canadian Medical Association Journal,* 124, 555-558.

Sackett, D.L., Haynes, B.R., Guyatt, G.H. & Tugwell, P. (1991).   *Clinical Epidemiology: As Basic Science for Clinical Medicine,* Little, Brown and Company, Boston, Massachusetts.

Smith, A. (1790, 1976). *A Theory of Moral Sentiments,* Oxford, Clarendon Press.

Song, F., Freemantle, M., Sheldon, T.W., House, A., Watson, P., Long, A. & Mason, J. (1993) Selective serotonin reuptake inhibitors: meta-analysis of efficacy and acceptability. *British Medical Journal,* 306, 683-7.

Udvarhelyi, I.S., Colditz, G.A., Rai, G.A., and Epstein, A.M. (1993).   Cost effectiveness and cost benefit analyses in medical literature: are the methods being used correctly? *Annals of Internal Medicine,* 116, 238-44.

Weisbrod, B. (1991).   The health care quadrilemma: an essay on technological change, quality of care, insurance and cost containment, *Journal of Economic Literature,* XXXIX, p. 523-52.

Williams, A. (1974).   The cost benefit approach, *British Medical Bulletin,* 30, 3, 252-6.

Williams, A. (1985).   Economics of coronary artery bypass grafting.   *British Medical Journal,* 249, 326-329.

Williams, A. (1993).   Priorities and research strategy in health economics for the 1990's, *Health Economics,* 2(4): 295-302.

APPENDIX 1: BAILAR'S LAWS OF DATA ANALYSIS

1. There are no "right" answers. There are always several explanations that more or less fit available data, but rarely any that fit perfectly.

2. Statistics is not the only route to wisdom. Decisions may be reached by reason and the role of statistics is to support reasoning. Statistical analysis is not a goal in itself.

3. Rare events do happen. Almost everything is a rare event.

4. Serendipity is a dirty word. Structure is the most important ingredient in scientific discovery.

5. It is easier to get involved than it is to extricate yourself from data analysis (i.e. it is like war, committees and marriage !).

6. No sample is ever big enough. Big enough for what ?

7. Statistical crime sometimes pays handsomely. The analyst knows where to find the skeletons of inappropriate practice because he buried them !

8. More quacks practice statistics than medicine, and they do wholesale damage!

9. Good work requires time.

10. No analysis is ever perfect. Perfection is beyond human reach and may not be needed.

11. Something is always wrong with the data. The best that can be hoped for is that the probability of accuracy in the analysis is high.

12. Logic rapidly becomes irrelevant when politics, emotion and crass self interest determine action (as with, for example, health care reform).

Source: Bailar (1976)

APPENDIX 2: WILLIAMS; CRITERIA TO EVALUATE ECONOMIC EVALUATIONS

1. What precisely is the question which the study was trying to answer?
2. What is the question that it has actually answered?
3. What are the assumed objectives of the activity studied?
4. By what measures are these represented?
5. How are they weighted?
6. Do they enable us to tell whether the objectives are being attained?
7. What range of options was considered?
8. What other options might there have been?
9. Were they rejected, or not considered, for good reasons?
10. Would their inclusion have been likely to change the results?
11. Is anyone who has not been considered in the analysis likely to be affected?
12. If so, why are they excluded?
13. Does the notion of cost go wider or deeper than the expenditure of the agency concerned?
14. If not, is it clear that these expenditure cover all the resources used and accurately represent their value if released for other uses?
15. If so, is the line drawn so as to include all potential beneficiaries and losers, and are resources costed at their value in their best alternative use?
16. Is the differential timing of the items in the streams of benefits and costs suitably taken care of (e.g. by discounting, and, if so, at what rate)?
17. Where there is uncertainty, or there are known margins of error, is it made clear how sensitive the outcome is to these elements?
18. Are the results, on balance, good enough for the job in hand?
19. Has anyone else done better?

Source: Williams (1974)

2 Setting Priorities - Science, Art or Politics

**KEVIN MCKEOWN[1], SANDY WHITELAW[2],
DAVID HAMBLETON[3] & FELICITY GREEN[2]**

[1] *East Lancashire Public Health & Intelligence Centre and Manchester University*
[2] *Manchester University*
[3] *Coopers & Lybrand*

INTRODUCTION - THE ORIENTATIONS OF THE WRITERS AND THE NATURE OF THE PROBLEM

It is somewhat unusual for specialists from the worlds of academia, the NHS. and management consultancy to sit down together to write a joint paper on a matter of intense current interest to theorists, managers and organisational specialists. It was not easy. This was not because of personality clashes or procedural disputes. The essential tension was between the academic's search for explanation and understanding and the manager's demand for an immediate, meaningful and practical plan for setting priorities more methodically and fairly than what is currently available. This tension between the intellectual search for explanation and the practical dash for a useful method could not be fully resolved, but its presence generated a paper which tries to pull together theory and practice, despite the gap which can often exists between the two.

One central initial point of agreement between all the authors is that there is a fundamental conceptual problem at the very heart of current priority setting processes which is not currently being addressed. Just as politicians have shied away from the complex task of health service prioritisation by decentralising decision making to local purchasers within the new internal market (Moore, 1993; Whitty & Jones, 1992), purchasers have sought to deal with these new pressures by searching for a cloak of scientific certainty (Smith, 1993; Klien, 1993). In essence, there has been a concerted push for the rapid development of a *technically* oriented solution which could provide a neutral, mathematical formula which would deliver a defendable and scientific list of priorities. For example, the QALYs debate, with its buried value system, has fuelled this pursuit of scientific certainty. However, it will be

Setting Priorities in Health Care. Edited by M. Malek
© John Wiley & Sons Ltd

argued in this paper that there is no absolute scientific end-point or perfect solution. There can be no Q.E.D.!

We suggest that a careful examination of the true nature of policy making and priority setting reveals that the search for scientific exactness is conceptually futile and practically ineffectual (Wittrock, 1991; Wagner *et al.*, 1991; Hunter, 1993) and current energies should be invested in approaches which focus on processes and the ways in which they are actively shaped by dominant ideologies, implicit market-oriented values and the political impact of key professions and pressure groups (Hirschon Weiss, 1991). In short, there is no value free solution to social problems via science; the approach set out in this paper highlights the socially constructed nature of science and suggests that 'values', philosophy and ideology, which are the 'hidden' driving forces behind priority setting approaches, need to be made explicit. Any other approach is dishonest and false. As Lassman (1989) points out:

> despite all denials and attempts to be 'value free' and to avoid discussion of the political implications of social sciences, political ideas and political judgements creep in through the back door

(Lassman 1989: 5)

If, therefore, the main thrust of this paper is that we should shift our focus from the illusion of scientific certainty to the reality of value ridden processes, it is important for us to set out the logic and purpose of our approach.

OUR STARTING POINT

From the start, we assume that no-one would seriously suggest that priority setting processes are completely free from values, and we estimate that few could fail to see that priorities are based on, and influenced by, some value system. Indeed, it seems beyond doubt that many key decisions on priorities are driven by extremely powerful values (Miliband, 1993). These initial points are taken for granted, and this paper attempts to go beyond these simple contentions towards a more critical and perceptive exploration of the complex nature of priority setting. The journey is intended to be intellectually honest and practically useful, and it will, at the very least, cover the following key issues:

- Why has priority setting suddenly raced up the NHS **agenda?**
- What perspectives, influences and values drive current priority setting practice? Is there a single set of **values at work**, or are there mixed, and at times conflicting, value systems operating in the process of priority setting?
- If there is **value conflict and confusion** within the priority setting system, can this be explained by the fact that many of these value systems are never made explicit? Is there not a tendency to acknowledge the more admirable and worthy ones, keeping hidden those that are more austere and unpopular?
- Is it not inevitable that a partial, incomplete and academically dishonest assessment of the nature and purpose of current priority setting within the NHS

will cause **intellectual confusion and practical problems,** particularly if there
are conflicting value systems at work?

- If this analysis is accepted, is it not possible to **move quickly away from a
search for correct economically-driven scientific solutions to our priority
setting problems towards the evolution of a priority setting process** which
more fully embraces the real conflicts and difficulties in current priority setting?
- What are the **implications for the new "Purchasers"** of health care?

We will pursue these issues along the following lines. We will set out our stall by
describing a priority setting methodology. This will lead directly to a consideration of
the nature of the process. Is priority setting primarily a technical exercise or do the
visible technicalities disguise a highly value laden process? In answering this question,
we will move towards an analysis of the fundamental social and political dynamics
which provide the context for any consideration of rational science in general or
attempts to prioritise the value of competing health services in particular.

Whilst drawing upon social theory, this exercise is not intended to be purely
academic. The tendency to critique approaches in a distanced and purely academic
fashion, and more importantly to suggest alternatives in a similarly detached way, is
unhelpful to the *actual promotion* of alternative values. Rather, we hope that the
proposed theoretical context will offer practitioners, who may want to advance our
ideas, a clear appreciation of the social and political circumstances and dynamics they
may face in doing so. This relative failure of practitioners to draw meaningfully upon
social and political theory is already well recognised. Harrison, Hunter & Pollitt note

> ideas of power come from the political literature. This is a highly relevant body of
> writing for an exploration of the environment within which the foreground processes
> of NHS decision making take place. On the whole, however, most health policy
> specialists have *not* made much use of this potential. Doctors and health service
> specialist tend not to be very familiar with political theory.

(Harrison, Hunter & Pollitt 1990: 13-14)

In summary, the paper attempts to provide a comprehensive package which both
suggests an alternative perspective to the dominant preference for rational models
and, by exploring the environment within which practitioners find themselves, offers a
starting point to those who need to negotiate change as well as the barriers to it.

PRIORITY SETTING - EXAMINING THE METHOD

At the very heart of this paper is an astonishingly simple proposition. Quite simply,
the new 'priority setting' ventures of the new NHS. 'purchasers' can only be saved
from public anger and academic disgust if they concentrate on the *quality* of their
priority setting processes rather than the *'scientific correctness'* of their final
decisions on priorities. There are no perfect solutions or right answers, so why
pretend? Purchasing plans set out clear agendas and priorities, but how on earth were
they arrived at? Even in the scientific heartland of mathematics, there can be no
marks for an answer conjured from thin air without a clear and logical demonstration

of the assumptions, methods and working. In short, it is *methodology* that is all important, and that is the case here.

Any meaningful and appropriate approach to priority setting must deal explicitly with the contradictions, confusions and conflicts which are to be set out in this paper. At the very least, the following seven critical stages should be included, and clearly laid out, in any NHS. priority setting methodology:

- Set out a clear **framework of principles** which should act as criteria against which developments should be judged - principles reflecting the original purpose of the NHS. not the current obsessions of economists.
- Start a programme to begin to assess systematically the local impact of the full range of current services and interventions, and establish a mechanism for automatically checking relevant published **research and local data** in relation to the effectiveness of interventions.
- Assess, carefully and honestly, the **room for manoeuvre** in relation to changing contracts, including a consideration of the impact of central directives, financial constraints and ring-fenced arrangements.
- Agree to invest in **community based needs assessment** - not as an Oregon-inspired way of off-loading the responsibility for priority setting, but as a method for listening to an important 'local voice' for too long ignored.
- Arrive at a vision of the **best balance of services - preventive, diagnostic, treatment, care, rehabilitation and terminal care** - knowing, and admitting, that there can be no RIGHT answer but only sensible, informed, explicit and openly shared judgements.
- **Sift the available data,** including epidemiological, economic and social data, **against the framework of values already agreed**.
- Agree priorities - and **publish the final decisions alongside your "workings"**. There can be no marks for the final decisions without a clear, explicit, comprehensive and totally honest statement of the assumptions, methods and values employed.

This is not, of course, a purely technical list. As Richard Titmuss argued, "There is no escape from value choices in the formation of social policy". Such is the case here and this is why we will now locate our argument in a broader framework which recognises a range of perspectives on the nature of the social and the research which occurs within it. We are proposing a fundamental shift in the values that have traditionally defined ways of enquiring into the 'real' world (Guba, 1990). The shift is reflected in three dimensions: the way we perceive 'reality' and what is 'knowable'; the relationship between this reality and us as inquirers; and subsequently, the methods required to uncover this reality. Using these, we can locate the above principles in a broad 'paradigm' - by which we mean a basic set of beliefs that guide what enquiry is pursued and in what ways - which in turn can be located against a dissatisfaction with other paradigms.

Our initial dissatisfaction with rational and scientific values can perhaps be more accurately described as a dissatisfaction with positivist and post-positivist paradigms. These are essentially driven by a desire and expectation that we are able, or given enough effort, will be able to discover 'how things *really* are' or 'how things *really* work'. The assumption is that there is something real to be measured and some tangible end point to be reached. Most importantly, there is an assumption that this can be done in a detached and objective fashion by 'purchasers'. In many ways, this scenario is seen as seeking a simple and all embracing formula which will drive priority setting, and it is essentially 'apolitical' in that it operates within what are perceived to be common and value-free principles. In summary, priority setting has adopted an image which is 'formal' in nature (Gurnah & Scott, 1992) in two ways. First of all, it uses methods which suggest certainty and secondly, it condenses enterprise and exploration down to a set of methodological procedures.

This false view is firmly rejected. Rather, we would like to locate our views within a 'critical' or 'constructivist' framework, which adopts a different perspective fundamentally at odds with the position just outlined. Above all, our new view of the world is sceptical of the existence of any absolute or objective truth. As such the search for one is seen as largely futile. There is also a recognition of the impossibility of researchers being in any way detached or impartial in their perception. In other words, values and ideologies are recognised as an indisputable part of research which inevitably colours one's view. From this perspective, the notion of objective priority setting becomes essentially unrealisable. Indeed, writers in this area would argue that formal research processes are heavily value laden and that their *apparent* neutrality is merely a facade for the continuance of traditional power structures based on, for example, gender, class, ethnicity, and of greatest importance to our present concerns, professional grouping (Rossides, 1978). Hence we have two highly contrasting perspectives that define approaches to any enquiry. We would now like to relate these views to the specific issue of NHS priority setting.

THE IMPACT OF SCIENTIFIC THINKING

At the outset, we suggested that whilst practitioners may have empathy with our views, the application of them to current priority setting situations may be significantly more problematic. This section seeks to describe and understand the context within which attempts may be made to pursue values that deviate from the scientific norm.

Our first task is to provide a backdrop against which to identify and understand the values that currently shape priority setting processes. Primarily, we need to tease out the characteristics of formal scientific values, identifying where they have come from and highlighting how and why they have come to contribute to the decision making process.

The nature and form of early NHS structures and processes have been extensively described elsewhere (Small, 1988; Klien, 1989). The traditional planning framework can be visualised as being based upon the values arising from two systems: the broad and overt political values of equity, access and universality consistent with a strongly moral socialist 'vision'; and in a more applied and largely hidden fashion, the values of clinicians. In both cases, they display, in very different respects, a high degree of formality. Firstly, socialist visions arose from highly structured and scientific Marxist ideals. As a product of planned social engineering, these values suggested that large-scale improvements in well being could be achieved at a population level. At an individual level, the work of clinicians offered similar certainty. They suggested that medical intervention would implicitly and unquestionably improve health status. Both are ideological in that they possess strong values and are 'certain' in their outlook. They are also hegemonic in that they have values that, at the time, few would argue against. They thus appeared to be universal and apolitical. This latter point is of greatest significance. It indicates that, despite the existence of powerful values, their taken for granted status made them hidden and thus difficult to access, examine or question.

Subsequent developments have undoubtedly altered the nature of these values. In many ways one could argue that there has been a move away from the certainty implied in these early visions towards a questioning of the fundamental acceptability and practical efficacy of both Marxist social engineering (Marsland, 1993) and clinical intervention (McKeown, 1979). In this sense, their hegemonic status has been, to a greater or lesser extent, broken and subsequently their values have been brought to the surface and critically questioned. Thus, we are currently seeing the questioning of these traditionally accepted positions on welfare and medicine, and there is the subsequent emergence of a *range* of *competing* values. Based on a critique of the claimed 'neutrality' of dominant values, this process has allowed viewpoints which are sceptical of the motives and claims of socialist politicians and biomedical practitioners - see for example, Foucault (1970) & (1975). In this context of the breakdown of consensus and common values, competing agents are contesting for ownership of the resultant 'space' (Skinner, 1990). This has notionally allowed a debate on what *should be* considered as preferred values in shaping health care priority setting and in particular, the forwarding of 'alternative' strategies that had previously been politically insignificant.

This analysis goes some way towards explaining the apparent existence of an increasing range of competing value systems in contemporary NHS planning. Depending on one's views on the role of state welfare and the medical profession, this unearthing of values will have different degrees of acceptability. However, it would suggest that in principle, there has been partial fulfilment of a desire to see a move away from formal and accepted means of enquiry and adjudication.

In this context, the fact that explicit priority setting is now on the agenda would suggest the rejection of traditional formal planning mechanisms and practices. We have seen over the past 15 years an increasing tendency for traditional modes of health care to be brought into question and notionally, the creation of a free market in health care provision would suggest that based on pure market choice, alternative perspectives could be forwarded. Some may interpret and utilise this opening up of debate as a fundamental shift in perspective, creating space into which alternative value systems can find favour. In our desire to promote values and practices which do not conform to a rational scientific image, this opportunity has been seen as positive, with for example, the advent of the principle of needs assessment, the primacy of local voices and the adoption of consumer views.

However, it is our opinion that this scenario should not be seen as a real shift and thus acceptable in terms of our desire to promote alternative processes of enquiry. Our major contention is that an *image* of critical and enlightened revision within the NHS has been promoted, whilst traditional and narrow ways of operating have been maintained. The formal ethos of rigour and absolute truth is, *in practical terms,* still predominant.

EXPLANATION AND UNDERSTANDING

A range of explanations may be possible for this tendency. At one extreme, global and detached values are easy to maintain whilst there is no obligation to enact them, while for those in power, there has been a radical shift towards concentrating on the public presentation of policy rather than the difficulties of implementation. In short, there is a tendency for political *action and substance* to be obscured by a more powerful desire to create a favourable *representation* of action (Lyotard, 1984). Implicit in the recent criticisms of the Public Sector Charters and the Health of the Nation is a warning of this shift of attention from implementation to image. But why are idealistic values entertained at all? Two explanations stand out. At a positive level, there is clearly much to be gained from being associated with generally indisputable and favourable concepts, particularly if image is so important. In more defensive terms, the ability to embrace potentially conflicting values, ostensibly quelling them without having to practically act upon them is a subtle means of control. Marcuse (1964) calls this a form of 'repressive tolerance'. This confirms our earlier suggestion of a relatively narrow set of rational and scientific values being maintained within an apparently attractive relativist context.

Another force towards the maintenance of formalism are the new values that have been introduced into planning mechanisms over the past 20 years. These can be seen as the related forces of managerialism and the concern of cost containment. From 1983's Griffiths Report, efforts to bring managerial rigor to the NHS have continually been stressed. Whilst accepting that some have seen this movement as potentially introducing 'virtuous' or 'moral' ethics into planning (Cox, 1992) the predominant nature of general management has been 'technical' (Antony, 1986); 'lacking virtue' (MacIntyre, 1981) or even 'Stalinist' (Ham, 1994). The essence of these views are that general management has been introduced to fulfil a narrow rational and technical role. Similarly, the role of purchasing as a superficial and technical activity has been recognised by Hunter (1991).

Such profound forces are clearly important in considering the existence of rational values in priority setting. In trying to understand and relate to them, an understanding of the relationship between policy by image and managerialism is important. We have already suggested that there exists an image of policy making moving away from traditional rational modes of priority setting towards a more flexible basis. The introduction of the above forces - policy by image and the managerial concerns for economy go some way towards explaining this process in more detail. Most importantly, it suggests that we should be sceptical of initiatives that suggest a move away from the traditional basis for planning. In accepting the image of a more flexible approach to priority setting, what has perhaps been overlooked is firstly the superficial nature of these changes and secondly the existence of other powerful values systems which exist alongside them or actually pre-determine them. Thus, the process of opening up debate which is central to a less formal approach converges with a quite separate political dimension and accompanying value systems. As such discourses on client participation, the need to consider alternative modes of health care delivery and the value of lay perspectives on health either mix with or are determined by other 'parent' discourses such as the promotion of self responsibility, the drive towards effectiveness and efficiency in health care and the 'deregulation' of health professionals (Parker, 1992). In other words, the reason why formal values continue to be prominent despite the critical environment lies in the formal nature of the latter values and the type of formal activities needed to bring them about. For example, we can link the discourse of economic rigour to the diversification of provision. The latter may be seen as a move away from the formalism of professionally provided medical care and as such 'progressive'. However if one sees the parent discourse as economic rigor, the true values continue to be rational and scientific - only they are expressed through a less direct and formal medium.

So, what are the implications of a relativist debate occurring within a context that still displays a high degree of formality and rationality? What happens when one form of logic is seen to compete against another *within a set of shared formal assumptions?* The answer is that there will be an overwhelming desire to adopt scientific language and concepts - even amongst those who are unhappy with the fundamental concept. The debate will thus focus on the need to compare the 'effectiveness' of essentially different types of activity - for example health promotion versus clinical medical practice. The ability to make straight comparisons may be too readily assumed. The most important feature of this relationship is that *the whole process occurs on the basis that there is some absolute end point of 'true' rationality.*

In these circumstances, emergent and relatively weak discourses do not try to step out of the existing scientific paradigm but try to operate *within it.* This clearly reflects a pragmatic recognition of the strength of traditional power bases and the difficulty of successfully supplanting existing values and practices. So, what emerges is unrelenting pressure to work within paradigms which may be fundamentally oppositional. The search for absolute truth must go on even though the searchers know that it cannot be found. Relativism exists, but within clear rational boundaries. Our central contention is therefore is that this narrow form of relativism, which could be called 'rationally oriented relativism', restricts consideration of values that fall outside the limits of scientific assumption.

The inability to make progress within this framework means that, to some extent, we may need to leave behind these assumptions and operate *outside* the rational scientific paradigm. These thoughts lead us on to our final two questions; why do rational values within scientific paradigms prevail and how can we explain the apparent conflict of values as reflected by the vision/practice split? What has perhaps been overlooked is the existence of several values systems which existing alongside each other. As the debate on the limits of science has been developed, it has converged with a quite separate political debate underpinned with an appropriate, accompanying value system. The contrast is a sharp one. On the one hand, there has been a discourse on client participation, the need to consider alternative modes of health care delivery and the value of lay perspectives on health, while on the other, there have been arguments around the promotion of self responsibility (Naidoo, 1986), the drive towards effectiveness and efficiency in health care (Mihill, 1993), and deregulation within health professional (Cooper, 1991). The latter agenda has been particularly persuasive.

IMPLICATIONS FOR PURCHASERS

There is no direct and automatic connection between academic explanation and managerial action. Yet, the analysis set out here does have implications for those locked into the new purchasing structures of the NHS.. With a radical shake-up of the organisation of purchasing agencies being proposed by government, there is no better time to be clear about the nature, purpose and pitfalls of priority setting. In truth, many new 'purchasers' may rightly claim that they already appreciate the complexities and pressures of their new purchasing responsibilities. That is not in question here. What is very much in question is the fact that 'purchasers' may not fully appreciate, nor want to acknowledge, the incremental, highly political and pseudo-scientific nature of priority setting. There is no room for scientific pretence no matter how strong the perceived pressure for the right decisions. Priority setting is neither pure science nor clever art nor wicked politics. It is a highly political process where values, science, data and argument collide. The case being made here is for a radical shift on three fronts. First of all, the process of priority setting needs to be reviewed, with the emphasis placed on laying bare the real social and political processes at work. Secondly, there needs to be a permanent warning against all those who claim to have right answers to offer, be they economists or scientists. Thirdly, if community-based health needs assessment is to be the cornerstone of the new purchasing activity, there must be a much more honest dialogue about the nature, purpose and potential of purchasing.

There are no right answers which science will conveniently provide. Supposedly scientific answers can be critiqued in relation to their technical weakness (Carr-Hill and Morris, 1991) and their ability to mask philosophical debates on for example, the primacy of either the values of equity or utilitarianism (Smee, 1992). This uncomfortable fact confronts all 'purchasers'. It needs to be more honestly embraced and more explicitly and consistently communicated. It is surely better to own up now than to be found out in the not too distant future. There is a new journey to be made. Like the budding mathematician who meticulously shows his assumptions, workings and methods, we may even get more marks in the end!

REFERENCES

Anthony P.D. (1986) *The Foundation of Management* Tavistock.

Carr-Hill RA., Morris J. (1991) Current practice in obtaining the 'Q' in QALYS: a cautionary note *British Medical Journal* 303, 699-700.

Cooper J. (1991) The future of social work: a pragmatic view Loney M. (ed.) *The State or the Market: politics and welfare in contemporary Britain* , Sage, 58-69.

Cox D. (1992) Crisis and Opportunity in Health Service Management, Loveridge R. & Starkey K. *Continuity and Crisis in the NHS* OU Press, 23-42.

Foucault M. (1970) *The Order of Things* Tavistock.

Foucault M. (1975) *The Birth of the Clinic* Random House.

Guba E. (1990) *The Paradigm Dialog* Sage.

Gurnah A. & Scott A. (1992) *The Uncertain Science: criticisms of sociological formalism* Routledge.

Ham C. (1994) Search for a vision *The Guardian* 19-1-94, 16-17.

Harrison S., Hunter D. & Pollitt C. (1990) *The Dynamics of British Health Policy,* Unwin.

Hirschon Weiss C. (1991) Policy Research: data, ideas or arguments? in Wagner P., Hirschon Weiss C., Wittrock B. & Wollmann H. Social Sciences and Modern States *Cambridge University Press.*

Hunter D. (1991) The Pain of Going Public *Health Service Journal* 29-8-91, 20.

Hunter D. (1993) Social Research and Health Policy in the Aftermath of the NHS Reforms in Popay J. & Williams G. (eds.) Social Research and Public Health Salford Paper in Sociology

Klein R. (1989) *The Politics of the NHS* Longman, London.

Klien R. (1993) Dimensions of rationing: who should do what?, *British Medical Journal* 307, 309-11.

Lassman P. (1989) *Politics and Social Theory* Routledge.

Lyotard J.F. (1984) *The Postmodern Condition: A Report on Knowledge* Manchester University Press.

MacIntyre A. (1981) *After Virtue* University of Notre Dame Press.

McKeown T. (1979) *The Role of Medicine*, Blackwell.

Marcuse H. (1964) *One Dimensional Man* . Routledge.

Marsland D. (1992) The Roots and Consequences of Paternalist Collectivism: Beveridge and his Influence *Social Policy and Administration* Vol. 26 (2) 144-150

Miliband D. (1993) Neutral markets not free from the taint of political involvement *The Guardian* 12-4-93, 21.

Mihill C. (1993) NHS policy changes put patients at risk *The Guardian* 7-11-93, 6.

Moore W. (1993) Rationing the Blame *Health Service Journal* , 18-3-93, 16.

Niadoo J. (1986) Limits to Individualism, Rodmell S. & Watt A. (eds.) *The Politics of Health Education* RKP, 17-37

Parker I. (1992) *Discourse Dynamics* Routledge.

Rossides D.W. (1978) *The History and Nature of Sociological Theory* Houghton Mifflin.

Skinner Q. (1990) *The Return of Grand Theory in the Human Sciences* Cambridge University Press

Small N. (1988) *Politics and Planning in the National Health Service* OU Press.

Smee C. (1992) How might measures of quality of life be useful to me as a health economist? Hopkins A. (ed.) Measures of Quality of Life *Royal College of Physicians of London* 15-28.

Smith R. (1993) Conference agrees on need to ration but not on how *British Medical Journal* 306, 737.

Whitty P. & Jones I. (1992) Public health heresy: a challenge to the purchasing orthodoxy *British Medical Journal* 304, 1039-41.

Wagner P., Wittrock B. & Wollmann H. (1991) Social science and the modern state: policy knowledge and political institutions in Western Europe and the United States in Wagner P., Hirschon Weiss C., Wittrock B. & Wollmann H. Social Sciences and Modern States *Cambridge University Press.*

Wittrock B. (1991) Social knowledge and public policy: eight models of interaction in Western Europe and the United States in Wagner P., Hirschon Weiss C., Wittrock B. & Wollmann H. Social Sciences and Modern States *Cambridge University Press.*

3 Public Preferences in Priority Setting - Unresolved Issues

JENNY DONOVAN & JOANNA COAST

University of Bristol

INTRODUCTION

Health authorities are being increasingly encouraged to elicit public views about the content of health care (Department of Health, 1992; NHS Management Executive, 1992). Documents have been commissioned to offer guidance concerning appropriate research methods (Sykes *et al.*, 1992b; Sykes *et al.*, 1992c; Sykes *et al.*, 1992a). Many health authorities have forged ahead, undertaking research to assess public preferences using any or a combination of methodologies including quantitative surveys, interviews, public meetings, focus groups, rapid appraisal and community initiatives. In this way, many serious and contentious issues can be avoided in the rush to consider methodological and logistical details. Issues such as whether or not public preferences should or should not be included in priority setting; how 'the public' should be defined, and whose views should be incorporated; whether preferences can or should be aggregated, and if so, how this should be achieved; what sort of views, attitudes or beliefs should be elicited under the umbrella term of 'preferences'; and how preferences, once determined, can or should be incorporated into the priority setting exercise, seem to have escaped detailed debate. This chapter summarises the methodological information available to health authorities who want to obtain public preferences. It then attempts to open up the debate on some of the unresolved issues which threaten to hinder the collection of public preferences and also to consign public consultation to an empty academic cul de sac, where public views can have little impact upon the decisions that are made concerning health care priorities.

HOW TO OBTAIN PUBLIC PREFERENCES

There are a number of methodologies that can be utilised on their own or in combination by health authorities in order to obtain public views and preferences.

Setting Priorities in Health Care. Edited by M. Malek
© 1994 John Wiley & Sons

The choice of methodology will depend largely upon the aims of the exercise, and particularly the individuals or groups from whom the preferences are being collected. Methodologies can be quantitative, qualitative, or a combination of the two. The most commonly used methodologies for obtaining public preferences include:

Surveys of public opinion

Perhaps the most commonly used methodology is the quantitative survey which has the aim of obtaining information from individuals that can be aggregated to provide data about the whole population, or specific groups within it. Data are obtained in order to generalise about groups following statistical analyses. Surveys can include whole populations, such as the census, or a sample of identified individuals selected at random from a published list, such as the electoral roll or FHSA register; or chosen from lists according to a pattern or quota.

Surveys are characterised by their systematic measurement of variables, obtained from standardised questions. Careful piloting is required if new questions are devised or if complex issues are to be tackled. The use of a survey necessitates that decisions are taken about the content of the survey before it commences. Quantitative surveys cannot be adjusted afterwards, and there is a limit to the complexity of information that can be analysed statistically after data collection.

Surveys can be administered in different ways, depending on the complexity and length of the questionnaire. Postal questionnaires have been used to obtain local opinions and priorities for example in New Zealand (National Advisory Committee on Core Health and Disability Support Services, 1992) and Coventry (CASPE, 1991). Utilities based on a rating scale have also been obtained by postal questionnaire (The EuroQol Group, 1990). An interviewer-administered survey was used in Cardiff (Vetter *et al.*, 1989). Questionnaire surveys may also be administered over the telephone with the advantage that they can be quick, avoid the expense of interviewers travelling to meet respondents, and can be linked to computer systems. They may, however, be biased because of the distribution of telephones in the population, or the method of obtaining numbers. A telephone survey was used to obtain utilities for particular health states in the Oregon experiment (Oregon Health Services Commission, 1991).

Quantitative surveys can be used to measure change over time, usually by administering the same basic questionnaire to the same individuals over a given time period, such as six months or one year - a longitudinal study (Sykes *et al.*, 1992c). Surveys may also be repeated at intervals among similar but independent samples - a tracking survey (Sykes *et al.*, 1992c).

Quantitative surveys are thus common and, in many cases, useful for obtaining information from large groups of people. This information is, however, by the nature of the survey and its administration, likely to be somewhat simple and may be superficial. The quality and validity of the results of surveys inevitably rely heavily on the quality of the questionnaire design and methodology. Many surveys suffer from inadequate planning, weak methodology and poor question design.

Qualitative methods

Qualitative research offers several methods which can be used either as an alternative to quantitative surveys, or in combination with them. The aim of qualitative research is primarily to understand as thoroughly as possible the beliefs and experiences of the group of individuals being studied. Qualitative methods can be used, for example, in the exploration of sensitive issues and deeply-held beliefs, including views about, and reasons for, expressed health care priorities. They are most appropriate when information is required about the meanings of, and reasons for, behaviours, when issues are not amenable to quantification, or where disadvantaged or 'silent' individuals or groups require sensitive and/or flexible approaches.

There are two major methods of research which are commonly used and essentially qualitative:

Participant observation

Participant observation requires that the researcher observes what is going on whilst participating in activities. In the fullest sense, a complete participant carries out the research unbeknown to others by becoming totally immersed in the activities of the group. At the other end of the scale, the researcher observes in a much more detached way what is going on. Data are collected by the researcher, either by making comprehensive notes or by tape recording events.

In-depth interviews

In-depth interviews involve the researcher in talking to individuals (or sometimes groups) about a wide variety of issues surrounding the topic under investigation. In some cases, informants (interviewees) are seen only once (Eyles and Donovan, 1990), although it is more common for the researcher to build up a relationship with informants over time and with a number of interviews (Cornwell, 1984; Donovan, 1986).

Interviews are rarely short, because of the need to build up a relationship and rapport with the informant. The researcher usually prepares a checklist of topics to be covered by each informant, but the wording of questions and their order of delivery is determined by the progress of the interview. It is usual to tape-record all the interviews with all the informants so that everything spoken, including the tone and inflection, is available for analysis. All the taped material has to be transcribed, and, as this is time-consuming, there are practical limits to the number of interviews that can be undertaken and analysed. There are also substantive reasons why the numbers are and should be limited. It is not the aim of qualitative research to indicate the quantities of variables within groups of the population - this is more properly the concern of quantified surveys (see above). The aim of in-depth interviews is to explore and describe in detail the perceptions and experiences of particular individuals or groups *from their points of view,* to try to understand the perspectives of the individuals or groups being interviewed, to explore the reasons for behaviours, and the beliefs that underpin actions, none of which are easily accessible in a structured survey.

The analysis of in-depth interviews (and participant observation) requires lengthy and painstaking scrutiny of transcriptions and field notes. Results are typically presented in detail, in the form of lengthy descriptions of the research setting, and the perceptions and experiences of the informants, alongside theoretical insights.

In-depth interviewing techniques are likely to be of great relevance to the assessment of public preferences in priority setting. Many of the issues concerned with priorities are sensitive or require thought and/or discussion before an opinion can be reached, and these can be much more easily and successfully collected by interviews rather than structured surveys. Further, while surveys may collect information about pre-determined categories of preferences or priorities, in-depth interviews can allow the exploration of the reasons for these expressions. So far, interviews have been used in the Wirral and West Dorset (NHS Management Executive, 1992).

Other methods

Other methods of obtaining public preferences include public meetings, focus groups, health for a, rapid appraisal, community initiatives, patient satisfaction surveys, telephone hotlines/helplines and the use of local voluntary groups.

Public meetings may be specially convened, focusing on particular aspects of priority setting (e.g. City and Hackney Health Authority (Tomlin, 1992), Oregon (Oregon Health Services Commission, 1991), Bromsgrove and Redditch Health Authority (NHS Management Executive, 1992)). They can also comprise meetings with local organisations, such as local employers (e.g. Vermont (Bowling, 1992)). The meetings usually aim to elicit the priorities for health care held by individuals in a locality (Tomlin, 1992; Oregon Health Services Commission, 1991). There are a number of problems associated with public meetings. They are likely to be subject to volunteer bias, in that it may be only the most informed, or the most concerned, or members of society with the greatest incentives and/or fewest constraints who attend the meetings and it is likely that the preferences of individuals attending and speaking at meetings will differ considerably from those of the "general" public. A further problem is that there is no distinct and validated methodology for obtaining views at a public meeting. A number of different processes may be used, including questionnaires (Tomlin, 1992), or frequency of mention of particular values (Oregon Health Services Commission, 1991). Public meetings may be particularly appropriate at the early stages in priority setting where issues can be raised without necessarily following a particular priority setting model. They can also be used to discuss specific (usually emotive) issues such as the option of closing a local facility.

Focus groups are specially convened groups of local people which usually meet to discuss a particular issue in some detail. Group members may be drawn randomly from the local population or, more typically, from a particular section of the community. They have been used in Coventry (NHS Management Executive, 1992) and in North Derbyshire (NHS Management Executive, 1992; Department of Research and Information, 1992). Focus groups can be used to devise questionnaires (Department of Research and Information, 1992). Health fora are similar but tend to meet on a more regular basis. Health fora are usually locality-based groups drawn from a cross-section of the community, and aim to foster a two-way dialogue between health authorities and local communities (NHS Management Executive, 1992). To date, health fora have been used in Bromsgrove and Redditch, Great Yarmouth and Waveney, and Wirral FHSA (NHS Management Executive, 1992).

The rapid appraisal method was developed by Ong *et al.*, and uses a combination of public fora and interview survey methods (Bowling, 1992). The aim of rapid appraisal is to gain insight into a community's own perspective on its priority needs, to translate these findings into managerial action, and to establish an on-going relationship between service commissioners, providers and local communities (Sykes *et al.*, 1992c). An important aspect of rapid appraisal is the reliance on community 'representatives' and leaders, such as councillors, teachers, corner shop owners. The selection of representatives may be crucial to the results of the exercise. In some cases, the choice of representatives can appear to be rather arbitrary.

The aim of a community initiative is to develop "locality based approaches to purchasing which involve developing direct links with local people, building up a profile of local needs and agreeing an action plan for meeting those needs with local people" (NHS Management Executive, 1992, p.10). West Dorset health authority has established a community initiative assisted by facilitators, comprising fora and one-to-one interviews, called the planned approach to community health (PATCH) (NHS Management Executive, 1992; Ham, 1992). Locality purchasing has also been undertaken in Bath, East Sussex, North Yorkshire, South East London and Stockport (Ham, 1992). In Stockport, six health strategy managers are each responsible for sectors of around 50,000 people (Ham, 1992).

Although patient satisfaction surveys are one of the most common methods of seeking patient views about the health service, they take into account only the opinions of recent patients. While this has some advantage in that recent patients have a direct experience of treatment in the National Health Service, they are clearly a biased group. It is also the case that many patient satisfaction surveys are established without due consideration for sampling and questionnaire development and that they tend to tackle only superficial issues such as waiting times, decor and food. Such surveys are unlikely to be useful in priority setting.

Telephone hotlines may produce a rapid response to an emotive appeal, but that response is unlikely to be representative of the public, and of limited use in priority setting. Local voluntary groups can provide very detailed information on topics concerned with their own special interests (NHS Management Executive, 1992), but again, the information obtained may differ substantially from information obtained from the local population.

There are, then, very many methodological techniques that may be used to obtain public preferences for use in priority setting and a 'cookbook' of methods is now available (Sykes *et al.*, 1992c). The methodology chosen by health authorities will be crucial in determining the quality of evidence achieved, but it should not be the only or overriding consideration.

OBTAINING PUBLIC PREFERENCES - A REASONABLE OPTION?

Although there is a great deal of advice for purchasing authorities about methodological details, it remains that there are a number of crucial issues which need to be addressed before priority setting commences and a methodology is chosen. Principal amongst these is whether or not the public should be involved at all in priority setting. With increasing health care costs and restrained budgets, health authorities are facing difficult decisions concerning health care delivery, in that it may not be possible to provide care for all cases in all circumstances. In the absence of good quality data concerning the effectiveness of interventions, it is suggested that the public should help in making these decisions. The argument follows the course that since the public pays for and uses the health service, why should it not have a say in priority setting?

Where decisions are not controversial, it is likely that the views of the public could be incorporated without difficulty, but in many cases, decisions are controversial, even unpalatable. There is a serious question as to whether the public could or should be forced to make unpalatable judgements, such as between the old and young, deserving and not. Inevitably, such decisions tap prejudices and preconceptions, and people's views are shaped by the media and by the mode of presentation. It is also unclear as to how acceptable members of the public will find being involved in explicit priority-setting. Further, forcing the public to make such decisions allows health authorities to abrogate their responsibilities. It can be argued that health authorities were created to ensure the efficient and effective delivery of health care, and to make informed judgements about these, on behalf of the public.

The question of whether or not the public should be consulted about setting priorities in health care raises the further question of the reason *why* the views of the public should be included. If the issues were not difficult and unpleasant, it seems unlikely that the public would have been invited to contribute. The NHS survived until the 1980s without any attempt to include the views of the public, except through parliamentary candidates (via legislation) or the Community Health Councils (CHCs). Health authorities are being strongly encouraged by the government to introduce public consultation, but it is difficult to assess the degree of seriousness with which they may be willing to incorporate public preferences which might differ from their own. Health policy will continue to be made at a national level, with target-led programmes such as the Health of the Nation. At a local scale, public preferences may directly contradict national policy. It is not clear what health authorities should or would do then - argue for national policies, or implement local preferences?

WHOSE PREFERENCES - WHAT IS/WHO ARE 'THE PUBLIC'?

If the question of whether public preferences should be included in priority setting is answered affirmatively, the question of *whose* preferences should be incorporated into priority setting becomes crucial. Exhortations to health authorities to consider the views of 'the public' or 'local people' conceal a plethora of issues concerning who should or could be included or consulted. Inevitably, the inclusion or exclusion of some groups or individuals can have significant effects on the content and tone of the opinions expressed. A variety of forms of 'the public' can be identified, ranging from the total population (or a sample of it), to specified community representatives (such as councillors, GPs, shop owners), or consumers (patients). It is clear that some individuals and groups will have strong and particular views about health services. These include those involved in health care provision, such as doctors, paramedics; purchasers; representatives or groups with a special interest in a disease or service, such as charities; patients or users/consumers; and politicians. The influence of each of these groups or individuals can vary according to the particular issue and their position in relation to the decision-maker. Individual consultants, for example, can sway public opinion by identifying and publicising a case with great emotional impact (so-called 'shroud-wavers'), and potentially, shroud wavers could triumph over those seeking dull but incrementally effective treatments. Other groups with particular interests include pressure groups, patients, commercial interests (such as drug companies), and the media (in informing generally and publicising specific issues).

Balancing the views of different individuals and groups is a complex matter. It may be that health authorities incline towards listening to the views of those who most closely represent their own views, or they may choose to rely on agents who should act in the best interests of the overall population or of patients. Public health physicians, for example, could be seen to have an overall view of the health of 'the public', and, by implication, to know what health programmes should or should not be in the interest of local or national populations. In fact, they may express the preferences and priorities that reflect their training in traditional medicine, and, as many public health physicians are involved in purchasing, they may consciously or inadvertently reflect the policies of purchasers in their attempts to obtain 'public' preferences, perhaps through their selection of particular individuals or groups to 'represent' the public, or by excluding those who might offer an alternative viewpoint from that of purchasers.

Others who might have a claim to represent the public include Community Health Councils (CHCs) and elected leaders. CHCs often claim to be people's or patients' representatives, but members are not elected but appointed by local authorities, local voluntary groups and the Regional Health Authority, and so are not likely to be representative in any statistical or intuitive sense. Even elected leaders, such as councillors or MPs, are unlikely to have been elected on their views about the health service, let alone its priorities. They are also likely to express the views of their party on health issues, and, even with wide consultation, will not be able to express the opinions of all their constituents.

The 'public' may also be selected at random from published lists. Although this may introduce bias as all published lists have flaws and omissions, the resultant sample, if drawn correctly, should be representative of a local population. It has been suggested, however, that this population should not include those who have recently suffered from a condition involved in the priority setting exercise (Hadorn, 1991).

The issue of who defines the part of the public that will be included in the priority setting exercise thus becomes crucial as this decision may influence the outcome of the exercise. Health authorities obtaining public preferences will need to be explicit about their reasons for including or excluding certain groups or individuals if they wish to avoid being accused of 'fixing' the result.

SHOULD PREFERENCES BE AGGREGATED?

During the priority setting exercise, it is likely that there will be divergent opinions. Averaging these opinions may produce a view that removes extreme or idiosyncratic opinions. In some cases this may be desirable, but it may also lead to an unnecessary 'flattening out' of public opinion. Health and illness are complex matters and people imbue them with a wide range of beliefs and emotions which may fluctuate and even conflict, depending on the issue under consideration (see, for example Cornwell, 1984; Donovan, 1986; Eyles and Donovan, 1990; Calnan, 1987). Averaging out the views that people express, for example about different health states, may remove from the priority setting exercise those things that explain why people act in the ways they do (see Donovan *et al.*, 1993).

Economists, in particular, have concentrated on the difficulties associated with making social choices based on individual preferences. Ordinal preferences can be combined in a method akin to voting: if more individuals prefer increased community care (A) to increased acute care (B) then increased community care may be suggested as a priority. There are, however, problems associated with the use of such voting schemes. For example, if the choice is increased to three options, it becomes possible that any of the three alternatives could then be chosen, depending on how they are presented. This problem is known as the paradox of voting and is a specific example of a more general problem, known as Arrow's Impossibility Theorem (Arrow, 1963) which shows that there is no perfect way to make social choices or to "aggregate" individual preferences to obtain a single social preference (Varian, 1990).

There are further difficulties associated with the interpersonal comparison of individual cardinal utilities, such as those obtained to identify the strength of preference for different health states. Economists are divided on the issue of interpersonal comparison of utility. Classical expected utility theory rejects the notion that it is scientifically meaningful to compare individual preferences (Mansfield, 1985; Hadorn, 1991; Mooney and Olsen, 1991). A number of economists such as Torrance *et al.*, (1982), however, insist that comparison of preferences is essential, and that, in any case, such comparisons are common practice in social decision making (Harsanyi, 1975; Harsanyi, 1955; Torrance *et al.*, 1982).

There are, then, considerable problems associated with the whole question of the aggregation of preferences expressed by individuals, and there is no theoretically perfect way in which preferences can be aggregated. For the practical purposes of priority setting in health care, however, aggregation of preferences is unavoidable, but attention must be given to the appropriateness of the method of aggregation because it is likely to affect the results that are obtained. The ultimate aim should be to choose a method of aggregation which does not obscure the information obtained from the public.

OBTAINING PUBLIC PREFERENCES - WHAT SHOULD BE INCORPORATED?

Public preferences can incorporate a wide range of attributes, including beliefs, utilities, choices, attitudes, priorities, complaints and views. These may be general or specific, and may be obtained from a number of different individuals and or groups via a range of methodologies. Health authorities will need to be careful that they are aware of the sort of preferences that they are actually collecting, and that they make these clear both to those whom they approach and to those making use of the priorities developed. The sorts of public preferences that may be collected range from the very specific views of particular individuals (such as complaining patients), to the lay beliefs of local people.

Complaints

At the simplest level, health authorities may want to make use of the criticisms that individual patients make of services. Such criticisms may include formal and informal complaints, usually directed at particular service providers or organisational matters by disgruntled patients. Such complaints may be a useful trigger to change, but they are likely to be extreme and the 'tip of the iceberg' in terms of general patient views. Any reliance on complaints alone would ignore the views of the majority of the population, both sick and well, and would be difficult to use in isolation for the purpose of setting priorities.

Utilities

Individual preferences can be incorporated into the priority setting process in a somewhat indirect way by obtaining information about the utilities (preferences) that individuals hold for particular health states. These utilities must be cardinal, in that the size of the utility difference between two health states will reflect the difference in preference for the two states. There are four main methods: rating scale, standard gamble, time trade-off, and magnitude estimation (Drummond *et al.*, 1987; Torrance, 1986; Williams and Kind, 1992; Rosser and Kind, 1978). Each method involves somewhat hypothetical exercises in which individuals are asked to assign values to particular health states, in some cases directly and in others by more indirect routes.

An advantage of using utilities is that the method can involve the public without requiring them to have extensive knowledge of medicine or the health service. But the method does not give individuals the opportunity to express their preference for one service over another directly, and may require individuals to make judgements that they find very difficult. It is also not possible to determine how well the results of such exercises reflect people's real attitudes and values, nor how they might be affected by personal experience.

Beliefs, attitudes and views

Attitudes and views about priorities can be collected from individuals and groups by questionnaires, public meetings and interviews. These may include wide ranging attitudes, such as the preference for acute rather than chronic care; or more explicit priorities, for example that those with a history of alcohol abuse should or should not receive certain treatments. It is difficult, however, to see how such attitudes could be incorporated easily into priority setting unless the issues are very clearly defined before the attitudes are elicited. While the approach of asking members of the local population directly about their attitudes towards explicit priorities may seem to be the most obvious method of obtaining local preferences, there are particular problems. Those questioned may, for example, lack specific knowledge about particular conditions or treatments, and the amount of information they are given is likely to affect their response. It is also the case that discovering people's explicit priorities is only part of the story. The reasons for their attitudes are likely to remain hidden from questionnaire derived priorities, and so health authorities may be faced with sets of possibly conflicting priorities, and with no information about how these have arisen, or how they might be explained or changed.

A much wider view of public preferences would take into account the lay beliefs of local people. These beliefs include common sense, but also incorporate the theories and explanations that ordinary people develop to cope with everyday life, and particularly events that disrupt it, including illness. Lay beliefs underpin views and attitudes as well as much health related behaviour. There is a small but increasing body of academic research devoted to lay beliefs. While much of this has focused on particular groups or medical settings (see, for example Cowie, 1976; Locker, 1983; Anderson and Bury, 1988; Donovan, 1986), there has been a move towards studying members of the general population (see, for example Cornwell, 1984; Calnan, 1987; Eyles and Donovan, 1990). This work has shown that lay beliefs have developed over many years of experience. They may include 'folk' remedies, often handed down through generations and developed through trial and error. Beliefs can include scientific theories, such as the concepts of viruses and modes of infection, as well as common sense ideas. People are able to hold different sets of beliefs in different circumstances, and while lay beliefs are usually internally consistent, they can be conflicting. People may, for example, express clearly the notion that smoking is injurious to health, while also declaring their need to smoke to calm nerves or even to help a chesty cough (Eyles and Donovan, 1990).

Eliciting lay beliefs is not easy. The uncovering of deeply held beliefs takes time, and usually requires a researcher to interview a small number of respondents in great detail, often on more than one occasion. Large scale investigations of lay beliefs are thus unlikely to be undertaken by health authorities as part of the priority setting exercise. It is the case, however, that an understanding of lay beliefs can help to explain particular attitudes and behaviours of individuals and groups. Health authorities may want to take an interest in these beliefs *per se*, or more particularly where unexpected views emerge from other sources, such as surveys or public meetings.

THE INCORPORATION OF PUBLIC PREFERENCES - WHEN AND AT WHAT LEVEL?

The degree to which public preferences (however defined) will be incorporated into priority setting is not clear. Health authorities are exhorted to make the health service more responsive to the needs, views and preferences of local people, and to involve local people in needs assessment, purchasing choices and setting priorities (NHS Management Executive, 1992). The question of when and to what degree these views should be incorporated does not seem to have been given much consideration.

There are various theoretical models which aim to set priorities according to specific objectives and which can incorporate public preferences. The choice of any particular model, however, implies that the purchasing authority has already made certain value judgements concerning public preferences.

Purchasing authorities wanting to set explicit priorities on the basis of public preferences have a number of options. They may, for example, make no attempt to define criteria before establishing the methodology for obtaining public preferences. They may begin the exercise by asking whether members of the public would like to be involved in the process of priority setting. Alternatively, they may make prior decisions about criteria by which the public preferences are to be elicited, such as focusing on particular conditions or aspects of health care or population/patient groups, or timing the exercise so that it follows a local health promotion campaign. Such factors are likely to influence the sorts of results that are obtained. Health authorities will need to be explicit about the value judgements that lie beneath these decisions.

A further problem which may arise is a diversity between the views of the public and purchasing authorities. The public may express a desire for something that a purchasing authority felt to be completely unacceptable (e.g. no treatment of individuals aged over 70). It is not clear then whether the purchasing authority should follow the public preferences obtained and implement them, or ignore them on the basis that they are 'wrong.'

Health authorities wishing to use public preferences also need to decide whether and at what level the public should become involved in the decision making process. A further decision must be made about the extent to which public preferences should inform decision making, and the ways in which information about public preferences can be combined with other important information about effectiveness, equity and efficiency. These are difficult issues but need to be tackled if public preferences are to be seen to be incorporated into priority setting, and not just part of a public relations initiative.

CONCLUSION

There are thus very many unresolved issues in the area of obtaining public preferences for priority setting: Should the public be involved in decisions about priorities? Who should be consulted? What should they be asked? When should they be involved? How should they be consulted? Why should they be included? What should be done with the information? None of these questions has an easy answer, although many health authorities have chosen to focus their attention onto the 'how' question, particularly methodological and logistical issues concerned with obtaining public preferences.   Often, this interest has deflected attention away from more difficult issues.

Opening up the can of issues concerned with the setting of priorities, however, releases a number of unpleasant worms. There is talk of rationing, of haves and have nots, the deserving and the undeserving. Groups become singled out for having treatment withheld: those deemed incapable of benefit, such as the infirm, elderly or disabled. It would not then be an enormous step to single out other disadvantaged groups, such as the unemployed, or the 'intentionally' sick (alcoholics, the obese), or the current public enemy, single parents, for reduced levels of treatment.

A major question remains about whether or not preferences for priorities should be obtained from the public. To say that the public should *not* be included suggests that the public should be excluded from the decision-making process; that those with medical training or administrative experience should continue as they have since the NHS began, to implement implicit and unspoken priorities. Such a view is difficult to defend.   Obtaining public views is not, however, a simple matter. There are many aspects that can be included, ranging from very general views about priorities to choices between specific treatments, and these can be collected in many ways, as views, attitudes, complaints, utilities and so on. The method of presentation of information can also clearly affect the views obtained. Asked to choose between cases or categories of patients, members of the public will inevitably be swayed by emotional considerations and personal experience.

The question of *how* public preferences should be elicited and measured is also crucial.   The methodological details are relatively easy to debate: there are many different techniques and approaches, although no single methodology can be advocated. Once obtained, however, there is the question of what health authorities should do with these public preferences.   It is not clear, for example, how willing health authorities really are to uncover the views and opinions of the public, and, if they do obtain them, whether or not they will change existing services when public preferences contradict their own or national policies.

These issues are emotive and easily over drawn, but making priorities explicit and incorporating public preferences may not result in answers to the difficult issues of reducing expenditure and making the health service more effective and efficient. Making explicit the need for setting priorities (and thus rationing) also represents a significant change in the fundamental underpinnings of the NHS, taking away the automatic right of all citizens to health care according to need. Incorporating the views of the public into decision-making about priorities is not a simple matter. The involvement of the public, if this is the real aim of current policy, will require a great deal more thought about a number of thorny and complex (even contradictory) issues. Without active debate, it is likely that, even if public preferences are collected with methodological rigour and innovation, they will remain part of an empty academic or public relations exercise, contributing little, if anything, to decision-making about the setting of explicit priorities in health care.

REFERENCES

Anderson, R. and Bury, M. (1988), *Living with chronic illness*, Unwin Hyman, London.

Arrow, K.J. (1963), *Social choice and individual values*, Wiley, New York.

Bowling, A. (1992), Setting priorities in health: the Oregon experiment (part 1), *Nursing Standard*, 6(37), 29-32.

Calnan, M. (1987), *Health and illness*, Tavistock, London.

CASPE, (1991), *Coventry Health Authority survey of future provision of services*, CASPE Ltd, London.

Cornwell, J. (1984), *Hard earned lives: accounts of health and illness from East London*, Tavistock, London.

Cowie, B. (1976), The cardiac patient's perception of his heart attack, *Soc Sci Med*, 10, 87-96.

Department of Health, (1992), *The patient's charter*, HMSO, London.

Department of Research and Information, (1992), *"What kind of maternity care do you want?" Results of a priority search survey of 721 women living in North Derbyshire, November-December 1991*, North Derbyshire Health Authority, Chesterfield.

Donovan, J.L. (1986), *We don't buy sickness, it just comes*, Gower, Aldershot.

Donovan, J.L., Frankel, S.J. and Eyles, J.E. (1993), Assessing the need for health status measures, *J Epid & Comm Health*, 47, 158-162.

Drummond, M.F., Stoddart, G.L. and Torrance, G.W. (1987), *Methods for the Economic Evaluation of Health Care Programmes*, Oxford university press, Oxford.

Eyles, J. and Donovan, J.L. (1990), *The social effects of health policy: experiences of health and health care in contemporary Britain*, Gower, London.

Hadorn, D.C. (1991), The role of public values in setting health care priorities, *Soc Sci Med*, 32(7), 773-781.

Ham, C. (1992), Local Heroes, *Health Service Journal*, 19 Nov, 20-21.

Harsanyi, J.C. (1955), Cardinal welfare, individualistic ethics, and interpersonal comparisons of utility, *J Pol Econ*, 63, 309-321.

Harsanyi, J.C. (1975), Nonlinear social welfare functions. Do welfare economists have a special exemption from Bayesian rationality? *Theory and Decision*, 6, 311-332.

Locker, D. (1983), *Disability and disadvantage*, Tavistock, London.

Mansfield, E. (1985), Microeconomics. Theory and applications, *Welfare Economics*, W. W. Norton and Company, New York, 458-488.

Mooney, G. and Olsen, J.A. (1991), QALYs: where next? McGuire, A., Fenn, P. and Mayhew, K. (eds.)*Providing health care: the economics of alternative systems of finance and delivery*, Oxford University Press, Oxford, 120-140.

National Advisory Committee on Core Health and Disability Support Services, (1992), *The best of health. Deciding on the health services we value most*, Department of Health, Wellington.

NHS Management Executive, (1992), *Local voices. The views of local people in purchasing for health*, Department of Health, London.

Oregon Health Services Commission, (1991), *Prioritization of Health Services. A report to the Governor and Legislature*, Oregon Health Services Commission,

Rosser, R. and Kind, P. (1978), A scale of valuations of states of illness: is there a social consensus? *Int J Epidemiol*, 7(4), 347-358.

Sykes, W., Collins, M., Hunter, D.J., Popay, J. and Williams, G. (1992a), *Listening to local voices. A guide to research methods. Volume III. The research process*, Nuffield Institute for Health Services Studies, Leeds and The Public Health Research and Resource Centre, Salford.

Sykes, W., Collins, M., Hunter, D.J., Popay, J. and Williams, G. (1992b), *Listening to local voices. A guide to research methods. Volume I. Summary of Main Issues*, Nuffield Institute for Health Services Studies, Leeds, and The Public Health Research and Resource Centre, Salford.

Sykes, W., Collins, M., Hunter, D.J., Popay, J. and Williams, G. (1992c), *Listening to local voices. A guide to research methods. Volume II. An introduction to available research methods*, Nuffield Institute for Health Services Studies, Leeds, and The Public Health Research and Resource Centre, Salford.

The EuroQol Group, (1990), EuroQol© - a new facility for the measurement of health-related quality of life, *Health Policy*, 16(3), 199-208.

Tomlin, Z. (1992), Their treatment in your hands, *The Guardian*, 29 April.

Torrance, G.W., Boyle, M.H. and Horwood, S.P. (1982), Application of multi-attribute utility theory to measure social preferences for health states, *Operations Research*, 30(6), 1043-1069.

Torrance, G.W. (1986), Measurement of health state utilities for economic appraisal: a review, *J Health Econ*, 5, 1-30.

Varian, H.R. (1990), Welfare, *Intermediate microeconomics. A modern approach*, W.W. Norton and Company, New York, 524-536.

Vetter, N., Lewis, P., Farrow, S. and Charny, M. (1989), Who would you choose to save? *Health Service Journal*, 99, 976-977.

Williams, A. and Kind, P. (1992), The present state of play about QALYs, Hopkins, A. (ed.)*Measures of the quality of life*, Royal College of Physicians, London, 21-34.

4 Dimensions of Quality and Prioritization

IAN WATT & NICK FREEMANTLE

University of York

INTRODUCTION

Quality is a concept which has an elusive, partly subjective nature which varies slightly depending on its context. The Oxford English Dictionary defines quality in terms of a "degree of excellence" which although concise does not overcome the problem of subjectivity.

With respect to health care, some definitions attach a rather narrow meaning to quality. As Black has pointed out, this is particularly common in the USA (Black, 1990). In such narrow definitions concern is normally restricted to the scientific-technical ability of health workers and the humanity with which care is delivered. Whilst both these dimensions are important, particularly for an individual, they do not reflect other concerns which from a population perspective at least, can be argued to be equally as relevant to the quality of health care. For example, the acceptance of a narrow definition could lead to a situation where health services although excellent technically and delivered in a caring way, were also ineffective, inefficient, inequitable, and inadequate to meet a population's need.

In taking account of such dangers, wider definitions exist which identify several components of quality. Donabedian states that quality can be identified in terms of the work of the caring professional (Donabedian, 1988); this can be further subdivided into technical and interpersonal dimensions. In addition, he identifies quality of the amenities of care and consumer satisfaction. Maxwell has proposed six dimensions of quality which need to be considered in assessing any health service (Maxwell, 1984). These are:

- Access to the service
- Relevance to need (appropriate for a specific population)
- Effectiveness (for individual outcome)
- Equity

Setting Priorities in Health Care. Edited by M. Malek
© 1994 John Wiley & Sons Ltd

- Social acceptability
- Efficiency and economy

It is rarely possible to maximize all the principal dimensions of quality in a broad definition such as Maxwell's. Normally choices or trade offs have to be made and a decision made on the optimum balance of quality dimensions in any given health care setting. Such trade offs are seldom based on objective evidence and mostly reflect political and managerial agendas with little direct involvement of other parties such as the public. Thus one of the consequences of adopting a wider definition of quality is that it emphasises the political nature of health care. This paper goes onto examine these issues further and illustrates the discussion by considering the health care received by rural populations in the UK.

Health Care in Rural Areas

In considering the health and health care of rural populations, a difficulty is posed by the lack of an agreed definition of the word "rural". Commonly, a rural area is defined by the low density of the population; other definitions have attempted to combine the different elements of rurality into a single index. However it has been argued that due to the multidimensional nature of the concept of "rurality" (e.g. cultural differences, employment patterns, geographical isolation), a universally accepted measure may be difficult to achieve (Muscovice, 1989).

If the OPCS definition of rural is used, in effect settlements of up to 1000 persons, the population of rural England is given as 4,329,092; if settlements up to 5000 persons are included then it increases to 7,479,380 (Rural Development Commission, 1989). Despite such numbers, official practice in the UK often pays little attention to the problems of rural areas. Whilst the health and health care of rural populations are seen as specific concerns in many developed and developing countries, concern over Britain's health service has focused mainly on the problems of urban areas (Watt *et al.*, 1993).

Further difficulty is posed by the often wide spectrum of people who make up a rural community, ranging from those who have lived and worked in the countryside all their lives, to individuals who may have recently moved and commute to urban centres for their work. There is often considerable variation in the influence of the rural environment on these disparate groups. For example, the two car commuter family are likely to experience less difficulty in accessing health services than the elderly widow who lives alone and is dependent on public transport (Bentham, 1986). Although their experiences may become more similar in cases which require urgent medical attention, such as the use of thrombolytic therapy following myocardial infarction. Socio-cultural factors are also influenced by the rural environment, and reflecting this, the perceptions of some groups of their health needs have been found, at least partly, to be influenced by remoteness (Bloor *et al.*, 1978).

Health in Rural Populations

A recent review concluded that whilst in very general terms, the majority of evidence points to there being greater morbidity in urban than rural areas, there is little to indicate if this pattern is true for all rural populations and that levels of morbidity and mortality in rural areas are higher than commonly believed (Watt *et al.*, in press). Measures of deprivation indicate that some people in rural communities may be experiencing levels of social disadvantage comparable to that in the worst inner city areas (Townsend, 1979). Homelessness is reported to be growing faster in rural areas than in towns (Lambert *et al.*, 1992) and declining rural employment is demonstrated by the fall in agricultural jobs from 758,000 to 663,000 between 1978 and 1988, with forecasts suggesting that a further 60,000 to 100,000 farming jobs will disappear in the 1990s (Guardian, 1992).

The Quality of Health Care in Rural Populations

As service provision becomes increasingly centralised, the concept of access may be argued to be the dimension of quality most influenced by rurality. Evidence shows that distance from a health care facility is negatively related to utilisation rates (Haynes and Bentham, 1982; Parkin, 1979; Haynes and Bentham, 1979). Although data from primary care suggests that this relationship is not as strong as the differences in consultation rates associated with age sex or social class (Ritchie *et al.*, 1981). The term often given to the phenomenon is "distance decay". In general, a consultation rate lower than expected may be taken to indicate some hindrance to access, although access may not offer the sole explanation. The effects of distance may be explained, at least partially for example, by variations in morbidity, although this is ruled out in some studies (Haynes and Bentham, 1982). What is not clear from the relevant studies, is the degree to which decreased use of health care with increasing distance represents unmet need, rather than a reduction of utilisation surplus to need.

Although evidence is scant, barriers to access may have significant effects on health outcomes. A recent study of the presentation of colorectal cancer in France (Launoy, 1992) showed that a lower proportion of rural populations were treated in specialised health centres than urban populations and a higher percentage were diagnosed at a later stage, especially in women. In addition, among women, a rural environment appeared to confer a worse prognosis.

High quality health care in rural and urban areas requires adequate funding. Most of the available evidence indicates that the direct costs of providing services in rural areas tend to be higher than in urban areas because of (Wollett, 1990):

- the lack of economies of scale
- additional travel costs
- additional telecommunication costs
- high level of unproductive time
- the extended time-scale and slow pace of development work

- the extra costs of providing mobile and outreach services
- the extra costs of accessing training and other support

Therefore resource allocation based on capitation can disadvantage rural areas. When actual service costs are less in rural areas than urban, it may reflect low levels of provision rather than low need or low unit costs. For example, sparsely populated areas have a slightly higher proportion of over 75 year olds than densely populated, yet densely populated areas provide far higher levels of home help and "meals on wheels" contact per head (Prince, 1988).

The NHS does not seem to have a consistent policy about whether to explicitly take rurality into account when allocating resources (Watt and Sheldon, 1993). Scotland and Wales use a sparsity weighting when allocating resources to community health care, but not the Department of Health or English health authorities despite the fact that England has many large rural areas. Rurality is however taken into account throughout the UK when funding general practice but not at all in allocating resources for hospital services.

Priorities in Rural Areas

The ways in which health care is delivered in rural areas reflects the priority given, either explicitly or implicitly, to differing dimensions of quality. For example, one interpretation of the increasing centralisation of much of British health care is that efficiency would seem to receive a higher priority than concerns over access and equity.

Since the 1960s District General Hospitals (DGHs) have been the main source of British hospital care (Ministry of Health, 1962; Central Hospitals Services Council, 1969), a policy which has seen hospital services become increasingly centralised and urban based (Lievesley and Maynard, 1992). The policy has not been without its critics (Draper, 1986), especially in rural areas (Llewelyn Jones, 1987), where such services were traditionally provided by locally accessible hospitals, often referred to as GP or cottage hospitals, but now commonly called community hospitals.

The arguments against provision of community hospitals have centred partially on concerns over their effectiveness with respect to their lack of specialised facilities. This ignores the fact that, for many in-patients and out-patients, highly specialised services are not required. The major argument for centralisation however, is based on efficiency and the perceived economies of scale offered by DGHs (Russell *et al.*, 1978). This argument is partial; if overall social costs, and not just costs to the NHS are considered, decentralising services such as out-patient clinics may be cost-effective. In support of this argument, the Office of Health Economics has suggested that "there is, in economic terms, no justification for assuming that the patient's time is expendable and that he must always bear the inconvenience of seeking medical attention." (Office of Health Economics, 1970.)

A cost-benefit analysis undertaken in Carlisle (Russell *et al.*, 1978) evaluated a proposed transfer of out-patient clinics from a DGH to a community hospital in a rural community. Of the estimated 43,000 out-patient consultations occurring annually in the DGH, it was thought feasible to transfer 4,700 to the rural hospital. It was believed the transfer would generate as many as 2,000 additional attendances. The analysis suggested that, although the transfer was likely to increase NHS expenditure, this was outweighed by benefits to patients and the rest of society. The fewer the number of additional attendances generated, the smaller the increase in NHS spending, and the stronger the case became for transfer if considering only health service costs.

In addition to the implications for access, the financial incentives offered by centralisation also have an effect on equity. When considering overall costs of hospital services, it is helpful to consider how the cost of hospital travel affects different groups within rural communities. The costs of accessing centralised services, in terms of money, time and effort, do not fall equally on all the groups that make up rural communities. Transport to hospital in a rural area is particularly difficult for individuals who do not have access to a car, especially in the light of declining rural bus services. By the beginning of the 1980s, 10% of households in rural areas had a bus service consisting of less than one bus per weekday (Department of Transport, 1983). A recent report from Trent Regional Health Authority stated that in some places it is still not possible to attend an out-patient appointment in a DGH and return home the same day if relying on public transport (Trent RHA, 1991). Even in households with a car, equal levels of personal mobility cannot be assumed to apply to all members. Mosely found 34% of adults in one-car households did not have a license and that men made most use of the car, mainly for work (Department of Transport, 1983).

The groups identified by research as being most likely to be deprived in terms of personal mobility include: the elderly, women with pre-school children, low income groups, the disabled and adolescents (Department of Transport, 1983; Bentham and Haynes, 1986; Reid and Todd, 1989); all groups most likely to have a greater need for health care (Bentham and Haynes, 1986).

Furthermore, distance would seem to be an important determinant of at least two types of cost. The financial costs of travel, by whatever mode, are directly related to distance, and the costs of time spent travelling are usually also influenced by distance. Time has costs in terms of activities forgone such as paid work, child care and leisure activities. In rural areas, journeys to centralised hospital services are often difficult, and many hours can be spent travelling to and from an appointment. However, the costs, both financially and in terms of time, are usually less when travelling by private car than by public transport, a point which favours the wealthier members of a community who usually have easier access to private transport. In terms of activities forgone, whereas professional people would usually be given paid leave to attend a hospital appointment, it is less likely that manual workers would receive such benefits. The Welsh Consumer Council survey for example, found that two out of five mothers taking a child to clinic appointments lost pay as a result (Welsh Consumer Council, 1988).

The overall effect of this is to support the view that it is the poor and those people with low levels of personal mobility in rural communities (two groups which largely overlap) who face the greatest costs in accessing centralised hospital services. Thus a strategy which some commentators have referred to as "come and get it" (Gibson *et al.*, 1985) whereby those who need the health service most should be expected to come first to the queue and to stay longest in it may not be equitable, since the costs of physically getting to the queue will not be equal.

DISCUSSION

The reasons for the priority afforded to individual quality dimensions in the arena of rural health care only partially reflect explicit policy. Historically, official practice in British society has often paid little attention to the problems of rural areas. Shaw for example has noted that:

> All of the early post-war planning initiatives were based on an urban viewpoint and even the planning of recreation, introduced by the National Parks Act 1949, was geared to the needs of city dwellers

(Shaw, 1979)

More recently, the problems of inner cities have been recognised and attracted many specifically funded projects such as the Department of the Environment's "City Challenge" (Department of the Environment, 1992).

A major reason put forward as to why problems in rural areas receive little attention, is that the rural sphere is rife with popular imagery and stereotypes. Some authors have stated that rural society has been subject to a process of cultural colonization in that the dominant images have been formulated by middle class urban dwellers and projected on to the countryside (Cater and Jones, 1989). Newby identifies two interlocking images which together under pin the romanticized and sentimental urban biased definition of the countryside (Newby, 1977). The first is the "Good Old Days" syndrome:

> One of the best examples can be seen in the works of Cobbett. In his critique of industrialism he used the opportunity to conjure up a rural arcadia peopled by merrie rustics and sturdy beef-eating yeomanry. The repressions and privations of old England were forgotten in a welter of nostalgia for the mythical lost paternalistic community

The second image, actually a corollary of the first, is that of the "Good Life" or "Rural Idyll", the feeling that despite change and modernisation the countryside still retains "sufficient of its ancient virtues to stand as a symbol of all that is best in the English character".

Although this historical perspective may in part explain the quality of care received by rural populations. Other considerations also apply. One of the ideals on which the National Health Service was founded was that of providing a uniform standard of care for all, to ensure, as Bevan said in 1945, "that an equally good service is available everywhere" (Bevan, 1945). Further support for Bevan's ideal was given by the 1974 Resource Allocation Working Party who described their terms of reference as (DHSS, 1976):

> to reduce progressively, and as far as feasible, the disparities between the different parts of the country in terms of the opportunity for access to health care of people at equal risk

As already indicated, evidence exists, that this ideal has not been met, notably summarised in Tudor Hart's "inverse care law" (Hart, 1971). The relatively low priority given to access in much of the health care available to rural areas would also seem to contradict Bevan. It is interesting to note that no commitment to access similar to that of Bevan's is to be found in the recently restated key objectives of the NHS (Department of Health, 1993). Although this may be an oversight, it may equally represent a move to make health policy more explicitly consistent with present practice.

Managerial agendas are another influence on the quality of care in rural areas. In interviews held with senior health service managers in Yorkshire, all perceived efficiency and effectiveness to be the most important dimensions of quality (Watt, 1992). Whilst all those interviewed identified access as a problem in rural areas, none of them chose it as the most significant aspect of high quality health care. All agreed that financial pressures were such that an increasingly centralised service would have to be provided. Although the majority of managers interviewed thought that the NHS should consider costs faced by patients and society in accessing health care, this was only felt to be feasible if the prevailing financial circumstances were favourable. This strong financial agenda of managers has been demonstrated elsewhere (Pollitt *et al.*, 1991; Freemantle *et al.*, 1993).

Although doctors have had a major effect on UK health policy, their importance in shaping the quality of care received by rural populations appears to be less than political and managerial influences. Nevertheless, examples of the priorities of clinicians influencing the quality of rural health care can be found. For instance, branch surgeries may increase access to general practice, although the recent tendency has been for them to be closed down (Haynes, 1987). A survey of branch surgeries in rural parts of Norfolk found that, despite often being poorly equipped, they seemed to improve the access to primary care for many, especially for people who would normally be expected to have a high demand for medical care such as the elderly (Fearn *et al.*, 1984). Unfortunately branch surgeries tend to be unpopular with GPs because of the poor level of care they feel they are able to provide in them (McAvoy, 1984). It is not clear whether this perceived poor quality of care affects outcome in any way, or is compensated for by improved access. Another reason for the unpopularity of branch surgeries with some GPs is that they find them inconvenient to work in, especially since they have not been shown to reduce GP workload (Bentham and Haynes, 1992). Few examples exist of situation where public pressure has been able to influence GPs sufficiently to reverse decisions to close branch surgeries.

Of all relevant parties the public appear to have the least influence on the trade-offs made between the different dimensions of quality. Compared to many countries the rural lobby is poorly developed in the UK. In response to an approach from ACRE, the national association of England's 38 Rural Community Councils, the Department of Health reply included the following (Fennel, 1992):

> It is perhaps inevitable that there will be instances of conflict between local groups in rural areas who wish to retain some much supported local health facility, and a health authority which would prefer to rationalise services to achieve not only greater efficiency but higher standards for everyone. I am sure that most country dwellers accept the need to travel greater distances to health facilities than is necessary for those who live in a town, as part of country life.
>
> You may find it interesting to note that Ministers in this Department are more frequently lobbied on aspects of "urban deprivation" than its alleged rural counterpart.

The low level of involvement of the rural population in decisions concerning the quality of their health care may also reflect differences in perceptions of need that have been demonstrated between rural and urban populations. People with similar health status do not have similar perceptions because of differences in health beliefs, illness behaviour, social networks, willingness or ability to pay for a service and other social and economic processes. Although the nature of the relationship would benefit from further study, distance from health services also appears to have a direct effect on people's perception of need (Bloor *et al.*, 1978).

CONCLUSION

As indicated in the introduction, quality in the provision of health care is a multi dimensional concept and it may not be possible to maximise all facets. The provision of high quality care requires trade-offs to be made and differing priorities to be given to individual quality dimensions. The health care of rural populations provides a good illustration of how the quality of care received reflects the values of a number of different parties. In rural areas these trade-offs mostly reflect political and managerial agendas, with little involvement of health care professionals and even less of the public.

For the most part, the priorities and values underlying the trade-offs represent implicit decisions rather than explicit policy. So far, the recent reforms in the NHS and the introduction of purchaser/provider separation would seem to have done little to bring about more explicit decision making (Freemantle *et al.*, 1993). Certainly, clear and unambiguous statements about the provision of health care in rural areas are at a premium. The effect of this is to make open debate of the issues difficult and hinder some of the relevant actors from expressing their views. The recently restated key objectives of the NHS include a commitment to "secure continuous improvement in the quality of patient care". If this is to be more than a platitude the multi-dimensional nature of quality needs to be explicitly recognised by policy makers. This in turn will allow all interested parties to take part in a more informed debate than at present about the priority to be given to individual dimensions of quality in a particular health care setting. Such debate has important consequences for the health at both an individual and population level. For example, the administration of thrombolytic therapy following myocardial infarction can markedly reduce the risk of death. However, such benefits are dependent on the treatment being given early after the onset of symptoms (Cobbe, 1994). If the priorities of the NHS mean that rural patients are to be excluded from the potential benefits of such treatment then they should be made aware, and given an opportunity to contest the underlying policies if they so wish.

REFERENCES

Bentham, G., and Haynes, R. (1992), Evaluation of a Mobile Branch Surgery in a Rural Area, *Social Science and Medicine*, 34 (1), 97-102.

Bentham, C.G., and Haynes, R. (1986), A Raw Deal in Remoter Areas? *Family Practitioner Services*, 13 (5), 84-87.

Bevan, A. (1945), *Memorandum by the Minister of Health to the Cabinet, 5 October 1945*, Public Record Office, CAB 129/3.

Black, N. (1992), Quality Assurance of Medical Care, *Journal of Public Health Medicine*, 12 (2), 97-104.

Bloor, M., Horobin G., Taylor, R., and Williams, R. (1978), *Island Health Care: Access to Primary Services in the Western Isles*, Occasional Paper No 3, Institute of Medical Sociology, University of Aberdeen, Aberdeen.

Cater, J., and Jones, T. (1989), *Social Geography: An Introduction to Contemporary Issues*, Edward Arnold, London.

Central Hospital Services Council (1969), *The Functions of District General Hospital*, Bonham Carter Report, HMSO, London.

Cobbe, S.M. (1994), Thrombolysis in myocardial infarction, *British Medical Journal*, 308, 216-217.

Department of the Environment (1992), *City Challenge: Action for Cities-Bidding Guidance 1993-94*, DoE, London.

Department of Transport (1983), *National Travel Survey 1978/9 Report*, HMSO, London.

Department of Health (1993), *Managing the New NHS*, NHS Management Executive, October, Leeds.

DHSS (1976), *Sharing Resources for Health in England*, Report of the Resource Allocation Working Party, HMSO, London.

Donabedian, A. (1988), The Quality of Care. How it Can be Assessed?, *Journal of the American Medical Association*, 260, 1743-1748.

Draper, P. (1986), Why Not Plan for Locally Based Out-patient Services?, *Health and Social Services Journal*, 96, 108-109.

Fearn, R., Haynes, R.M., and Bentham, C.G. (1984), Role of Branch Surgeries in a Rural Area, *Journal of the Royal College of General Practitioners*, 34, 488-491.

Fennell, J. (1992), *Rural Health Care*, Acre Conference Guide, ACRE, Cirencester.

Freemantle, N., Watt I.S., Mason J. (1993), Developments in the purchasing process in the NHS: towards an explicit politics of rationing, *Public Administration*, 71, 535-548.

Gibson, D.M., Goodin, R.E., and LeGrand, J. (1985), Come and Get It: Distributional Biases in Social Service Delivery Systems, *Policy and Politics*, 13 (2), 109-125.

Hart, J.T. (1971), The Inverse Care Law, *Lancet*, i, 405-412.

Haynes, R. (1987), *The Geography of Health Services in Britain*, Croom-Helm, London.

Haynes, R.M., and Bentham, C.G. (1979), Accessibility and the Use of Hospitals in Rural Areas, *Area*, 11, 186-191.

Haynes, R., and Bentham, G. (1982), The Effects of Accessibility on GP Consultations; Out-patient Attendances and In-patient Admissions in Norfolk, England, *Social Science and Medicine*, 16, 561-569.

Lambert, C., Jeffers, S., Burton, P., Bramley, G. (1992), *Homelessness in Rural Areas*, Rural Development Commission, Salisbury.

Launoy, G., Le Coutour, X., Gignoux, M., Pottier, D., and Dugleux, G. (1992), Influence of Rural Environment on Diagnosis, Treatment and Prognosis of Colorectal Cancer, *Journal of Epidemiology and Community Health*, 46, 365-367.

Lievesley, K., Maynard, W. (1992), *1991 Survey of Rural Services*, Rural Development Commission, London.

Llewelyn Jones, H. (1987), *Do District General Hospitals Meet Rural Needs?: A Study of the Community Hospital Experience*, MA dissertation, Nuffield Centre for Health Services Studies, University of Leeds, Leeds.

Maxwell, R. (1984), Perspectives in NHS Management, *British Medical Journal*, 288, 1470-1472.

McAvoy, B.R. (1984), Trials and Tribulations of Closing Branch Surgeries, *Update*, 50-58.

Ministry of Health (1962), *A Hospital Plan for England and Wales*, Cmnd 1604, HMSO, London.

Moscovice, I.S. (1989), Rural Hospitals: A Literature Synthesis and Health Services Research Agenda, *Health Services Research*, 23 (6), 891-930.

Newby, H. (1977), *The Deferential Worker*, Penguin, Harmondsworth.

Office of Health Economics (1970), *Building for Health*, OHE, London.

Parkin, D. (1979), Distance as an Influence on Demand in General Practice, *Journal of Epidemiology and Community Health*, 33, 96-99.

Pollitt, C., Harrison, S., Hunter, D.J., and Marnoch, G. (1991), General Management in the NHS: The Initial Impact, *Public Administration*, 69, 61-83.

Prince, D. (1988), Local Government Comparative Statistics, *County Councils Gazette*, May.

Reid, N., and Todd, C. (1989), Travel to Hospital: Accessibility of Outpatient Services in Rural Communities, *Health Services Management*, 85 (3), 129-133.

Ritchie, J., Jacoby, A., and Bone, M. (1981), *Access to Primary Care*, HMSO, London.

Rural Development Commission (1989), *Rural Research Note No 2: The Changing Population of Rural England*, RDC, London.

Russell, I.T., Reid, N.G., Philips, P.R., Glass, N.J., and Akehurst, R.L., (1978), The Transfer of Out-patient Clinics to Rural Hospitals: A Feasibility Study and Cost Benefit Analysis, in Anderson, J. (ed.), *Medical Informatics Europe 1978 - Proceedings of the 1st Congress of the European Federation for Informatics*, Springer-Verlag, New York.

Shaw, J.M. (ed.) (1979), *Rural Deprivation and Planning*, Geo Books, Norwich.

The Guardian (1992), *When shepherds give up on their flocks*, The Guardian, January 7, London.

Townsend, P. (1979), *Poverty in the UK*, Penguin, Harmondsworth.

Trent Regional Health Authority (1991), *Grasping the Nettle: Working Party on Health Care to Rural Populations*, Trent RHA, Nottingham.

Watt, I.S., and Sheldon, T. (1993), Rurality and Resource Allocation in the UK, *Health Policy*, 26, 19-27.

Watt, I.S. (1992), Perceptions of Quality: The Rural Dimension, *Journal of Management in Medicine'*, 6 (4), 30-35.

Watt, I.S., Franks, A., Sheldon, T. (in press), Rural Health and Health Care in the UK: Better or Worse? *Journal of Epidemiology and Community Health*.

Watt, I.S., Franks, A., Sheldon, A. (1993), Rural Health and Health Care - unjustifiably neglected, *British Medical Journal*, 306, 1358-1359.

Welsh Consumer Council (1988), *Getting to Outpatient Clinics: Report of a Survey of Elderly People, Mothers and Child Escorts Attending Outpatient Appointments*, Welsh Consumer Council, Cardiff.

Wollett, S. (1990), *Counting the Rural Cost: The Case for a Rural Premium*, National Council for Voluntary Organisations, London.

5 An Economic Perspective of the Salisbury Waiting List Points Scheme

RHIANNON TUDOR EDWARDS

University of Liverpool

INTRODUCTION

At the 1993 NHS Management Executive Waiting Times conference, it was clear that the waiting list initiative is still heavily focused on requiring provider units to meet waiting time targets, reducing inpatient waiting times to their minimum through pace setter initiatives to clear backlogs, thereby maximising throughput.

There was however considerable excitement over an attempt by Salisbury District Hospital to look beyond short term waiting time goals, to address the question of how patients on an inpatient waiting list should be prioritised.

This paper sets out to describe the Salisbury waiting list points scheme, and consider its implications for explicit rationing within the NHS. The issue of the quantification of clinical freedom is raised, and likely issues regarding clinical consensus over the relative priority of different patients, and potential for delegation of prioritisation are discussed in the light of the experience of previous attempts at the establishment and implementation of eligibility criteria for the management of waiting lists.

Finally, the paper compares the criteria used within the Salisbury points scheme with those that would apply under a strictly efficient waiting list policy of health gain maximisation. It concludes by suggesting the need for QALY information to be collected alongside the Salisbury points scheme.

THE SALISBURY WAITING LIST POINTS SCHEME

A waiting list prioritisation points scheme is currently being tested at Salisbury District Hospital. The scheme was initiated with the goal of making more explicit the criteria that consultants use to manage and schedule their inpatient waiting lists,

Setting Priorities in Health Care. Edited by M. Malek
© 1994 John Wiley & Sons

and to facilitate factors other than time waited to determine a patients place on a waiting list (Lack and Fletcher, 1993).

In an interview with the *Mail on Sunday* Chris Mould, Chief Executive of the Salisbury Hospital explained the underlying philosophy of the scheme:

> It is all about treating each NHS patient as an individual....Waiting lists have always been a political hot potato. This is an attempt to try to deal with people more fairly, based on their degree of pain and personal circumstances. We are trying to make some sense of an unsophisticated system which gives priority to people simply because of the time they have been waiting, while those who are in greater pain are forced to take their turn

Under this scheme, each patient on an inpatient waiting list is given 0 - 4 points in each of the following categories:

- progress of disease
- pain
- disability or dependence on others
- loss of usual occupation (job, house work, school)
- time waiting

Points are then squared to emphasise differences and summed to give a score out of a possible 80 points

The criteria chosen were arrived at through discussion between local consultants and GPs in the Wessex area. They are based on criteria originally suggested by Culyer and Cullis who proposed the need for an admissions index for the management of NHS waiting lists, (Culyer and Cullis, 1976). The criteria originally suggested by Culyer and Cullis were as follows and clearly provide the basis for those used in the Salisbury scheme.

- clinical deterioration
- health status
- social productivity
- other social factors
- time on list

The following examples of how the scheme would work were given to the press, (The Mail on Sunday, 5th September 1993)

Example 1

A pensioner with progressive hip disease in constant but controlled pain who is unable to walk and has been on a waiting list for 6 months

progress of disease	2
pain or distress	3
disability or dependence	4
loss of occupation	3
time waiting	2
priority rating	42

Example 2

A child with tonsillitis, or adenoidal problem, who experiences occasional sore throat and sleepless nights, loss of school days, who has been on a waiting list three months,

progress of disease	2
pain or distress	2
disability or dependence	0
loss of occupation	3
time waiting	1
priority rating	18

Example 3

A woman needing hysterectomy, because of fibroids that have been causing heavy bleeding, who has been on a waiting list for six months,

progress of disease	2
pain or distress	3
disability or dependence	2
loss of occupation	3
time waiting	2
priority rating	30

Example 4

A pensioner needing cataract operation, with limited sight, who has been on a waiting list for six months,

progress of disease	1
pain or distress	3
disability or dependence	3
loss of occupation	4
time waiting	2
priority rating	39

The scheme was developed by Dr Alistair Lack, a consultant anaesthetist at the hospital and is now being marketed by Delian Medical Systems Ltd.

IS THIS THE BEGINNING OF EXPLICIT RATIONING IN THE NHS?

Points schemes such as the Salisbury scheme for the management of NHS waiting lists, represent explicit rationing in an attempt to reconcile a limited supply of health care with demand.   Rather than their adoption being seen as the introduction of rationing, it is probably more appropriate to think of them as an initiative to make informal, covert rationing, which has occurred since the inception of the NHS, more formal, explicit and publicly accountable.

An analysis of formal and informal rationing mechanisms in health is the subject of a paper published by the Institute of Health Policy Studies, discussed in (Higgins and Ruddle, 1991).

Examples of informal rationing mechanisms are offered (Higgins and Ruddle, 1991)

- rationing by delay
- rationing by dilution of quality of services
- rationing by deterrence
- rationing by ignorance
- termination or withdrawal of services

It is possible to find many examples of how these various forms of informal rationing have occurred in the NHS, before the reforms, and how they are likely to occur in the future reformed NHS.

Before the NHS reforms, rationing in the NHS largely occurred through deterrence and delay. Patients gained access through their GP and had to face a long wait for certain common non urgent conditions.

The structure and incentive schemes of the reformed NHS, in particular with regard to the internal market for health care, will mean that in the future health care will be rationed, again through deterrence, with fund holding GPs having a greater incentive to discourage patients seeking health care services from the secondary sector for which fundholders may have to pay.   More importantly, health care services may be rationed through their termination or withdrawal, for example where purchasers refuse to fund extra contractual referrals or providers cease to treat patients once a cost and volume contract has been completed in a financial year

> If hospitals are judged by waiting time or waiting list lengths, they will have an incentive to decline to add patients to their waiting lists where contract numbers have already been fulfilled (Mullen, 1993, p.63)

In comparison, formal rationing systems, such as points schemes for the management of waiting lists appear more appealing.

> Formal rationing would include the use of queues or waiting lists, charging for services, the allocation of resources to priority classes of need and the application of eligibility rules. In theory, formal rationing should lead to uniformity of treatment

for similar people in similar circumstances and it is open to public scrutiny and debate" (Higgins and Ruddle, 1991, p. 19)

It is this concept of introducing eligibility criteria so that people in similar circumstances receive similar access that provides support for explicit waiting list points schemes. This concept has a distinguished heritage, it is Aristotle's concept of equal treatment of equals and unequal treatment of unequals.

The need to set priorities, and in some way restrict access through eligibility criteria is increasingly widely accepted. It is the nature of eligibility criteria, their philosophical basis, and more pragmatically, who is to set them, that will lead to a diverse spectrum of opinion.

RESOURCE USE INFORMATION

Alongside the Salisbury waiting list points scheme is being developed a system of classifying patients into groups according to their resource use requirements. These iso-resource groups IRGs, are aimed to improve information on resource use within a hospital, facilitate better scheduling of staff, in theatre and on wards, and most importantly, ensure that the hospital can accurately project the resource requirements associated with contracts negotiated with purchasers. The system is not designed to be prospective, or tailored for tracking individual patients for reimbursement purposes, (Lack *et al.*, 1993).

Patient information is collated as follows, (Lack and Fletcher, 1993)

Diagnosis:	Hip Pain
Intended Treatment:	Left Total Hip Replacement
IRG Code:	W37.1E
RUBRIC:	Total Hip Replacement
Pre-Op. Stay:	1 day
Post-Op. Stay:	8 days
Theatre Time:	60 minutes (includes anaesthetic time)
High Cost Items:	£ 350 prosthesis

It is intended to include nursing skill mix and other items such as drugs and diagnostic tests into the profiles. This system facilitates the analysis of waiting lists alphabetically, by purchaser, by Iso-Resource Group, or by time waited, and offers a much needed opportunity for more sophisticated analysis of the resource use implications of any given waiting list for NHS care.

QUANTITATIVE CLINICAL FREEDOM

Before the NHS reforms, NHS waiting lists were the property of hospital based consultants who would decide who to treat and in what order. The creation of the NHS internal market and separation of purchaser and provider raised questions as to the "ownership" of waiting lists. Purchasers hold responsibility to meet the health care needs of their population, some of whom are on NHS waiting lists, while hospital based consultants now face a responsibility to meet contracts on behalf of their provider unit, while trying to continue to exercise their clinical freedom in managing their waiting lists.

The Salisbury waiting list points scheme, the initiative of a consultant anaesthetist may be viewed as an attempt to claim back clinical freedom, albeit in a new auditable, quantitative form, from the managers responsible for negotiating contracts with purchasers.

At a hospital level, operation of a universal waiting list points scheme in all clinical specialties must require some degree of consensus between doctors as to the relative priority of different patients waiting for different conditions treated by different clinical specialties. In the case of the eligibility criteria set up at Salisbury, this will mean consensus about spread of disease in a particular patient, pain or distress, disability and dependence on others, and family employment circumstances.

Another important issue is whether consultants have the time to prioritise patients, or whether this task might be delegated.

CAN DOCTORS REACH CONSENSUS IN PRIORITY SETTING?

An example of a purely clinical approach to prioritising patients on a waiting list is provided by (Naylor *et al.*, 1990) who attempted to construct clinical guidelines for the urgency of patients with angiographically proven coronary disease needing revascularisation procedures. A panel of cardiac specialists were asked to rate 436 hypothetical case histories, on a seven point scale based on a maximum acceptable waiting time for surgery, where 1 indicates emergency surgery and 7 represents an acceptable delay of up to 6 months. Panellists responses were used to establish triage guidelines. Three factors were felt to be the main determinants of urgency. These were, severity and stability of symptoms of angina, coronary anatomy from angiographic diagnostic studies, and results of noninvasive tests for the risk of ischaemia (Naylor, 1990). Only for 1 percent of cases there was agreement by at least 12 out of 16 specialists. When the 7 point scale was divided into 3 main categories of (1) urgent revascularisation, (2) place on a waiting list and (3) no agreement, consensus was agreed for 60 percent of cases by at least 12 out of 16 specialists.

The issue here is whether consultants within a clinical specialty can reach agreement on the progression or spread of a disease or condition, let alone on the pain suffered by a patient or his or her social circumstances. Inter specialty consensus on the relative priority of patients treated in different clinical specialties is likely to be more difficult to achieve.

CAN DOCTORS DELEGATE THE PRIORITISATION OF PATIENTS ON A WAITING LIST?

Operation of a sophisticated waiting list points scheme will inevitably involve more paperwork or time in front of a computer for consultants. Could this job of assigning points for different eligibility criteria be delegated to a nurse or to clerical staff, through for example the use of questionnaires to be completed by patients giving information on their pain, disability, dependence on others and the impact of their condition on their day to day activities and employment circumstances.

Brattberg 1988 describes an experiment in a Pain Clinic in a Department of Anaesthesia at Sandvikken Hospital in Sweden, to prioritise patients waiting on a waiting list for treatment. The author carried out a survey asking pain clinics throughout Sweden whether they operated any prioritisation scheme in the management of their waiting list. Schemes were found to be rare, so the scheme described by Brattberg was innovative, particularly in trying to find out the implications of a departmental secretary and nurse ranking patients according to specific criteria, with the help of a questionnaire completed by the patient describing their pain.

The criteria used in this case for prioritisation on the waiting list were:

* acute severe pain
* cancer pain
* Herpes Zosta Neuralgia
* inpatients
* young rehabilitable patients

The rankings of the secretary and nurse were compared to those of the doctor, based on a consultation with the patient but without access to the questionnaire completed by the patient. The secretary and nurse generally overestimated the urgency of patients, underestimating, in comparison with the doctor's ranking, in only 12 out of 142 patients. Of these, only in one case was this deemed to increase risk. Battberg concluded that the disadvantages of slightly increased risk in patient management, associated with delegated ranking should be compared with the outcome where there was no patient prioritisation scheme in operation, and the benefits of delegating down this duty from the doctor.

WILL POINTS FOR PAIN MEAN GREATER EFFICIENCY?

Application of an economic definition of "efficiency" to health care would mean the implementation of health care policy that maximised health gains per £ spent. On egalitarian grounds it may be argued that this would be a fair or equitable public health care policy, prioritising the treatment of those patients who could benefit most from the resources available to the health care sector.

The Salisbury waiting list points scheme has set eligibility criteria which take into account conventional clinical measures of urgency, i.e. progression or rate of spread of disease, and suffering of the patient i.e. pain or anxiety. Added to these are more holistic factors that reflect quality of life, such as disability and dependence on others, and social and economic factors such as loss of family occupation or employment.

What the points scheme does not do, is explicitly link a patients priority position on a waiting list to his or her expected health gains from the treatment. However it is stated that consultants have a professional responsibility not to place patients on the waiting list who are unlikely ever to reach the front of the queue, and that all treatments must be beneficial, but "how" beneficial?, and how beneficial relative to those that could be gained by other patients on the waiting list, or on waiting lists in other clinical specialties?

Although the Salisbury waiting list management initiative is making a valuable contribution to collection of resource use information through its Iso-Resource Grouping system, this information is in no way related to the priority a patient receives on a waiting list. There is therefore, in the present points scheme no linkage between health gain and resources used.

One possible method of ranking patients on a waiting list in order of their health gains per £ spent would be to calculate their expected Quality Adjusted Life Years (QALYs) to be gained per £ spent or per unit of resource.

In his presentation to the Harrogate conference, Dr Lack the author of the Salisbury waiting list points scheme was dismissive of Quality Adjusted Life Years as they in the past have been based on Rosser's Classification of Illness, with only two dimensions, disability and distress.

At a practical level, the major criticism of QALYs raised by Dr Lack was that it was difficult or impossible to score patients as has traditionally been done, on a generic, non disease specific health related quality of life measure such as Rosser's Classification of Illness, or more recently the EuroQoL questionnaire.

Surely, it is equally difficult to score patients on a 0 - 4 basis on subjective criteria such as pain, disability, dependence on others or loss of occupation.

HOW WOULD AN EFFICIENT WAITING LIST POINTS SCHEME WORK?

An efficient waiting list policy, aiming to maximise health gain from available resources, might complement a general health care policy of giving priority to treatments and health care services that offer the greatest health care benefit per unit of resource, whether this be expressed in terms of £'s spent or in terms of more physical units such as bed days.

At an inter-specialty level this would doubtless lead to the redistribution of resources, e.g. bed capacity between clinical specialties, and would be the approach favoured by egalitarian proponents of health gain maximisation.

Figure 1 shows how patients would be drawn from the waiting list, in order of their expected QALY gain per bed day from treatment. In Figure 1 the vertical axis shows total health gain per bed day (QALYs), and the horizontal axis shows resource capacity (Beds). The vertical line C1 shows capacity in the current time period, e.g. month. The downward sloping total health gain per bed day curve shows the order in which patients will be treated. Patients to the left of C1 are treated in the current time period, patients to the right of C1 must wait and take their chance in the next time period. If resource capacity is expanded, e.g. through a shift from C1 to C2, then more patients may be treated in the current time period, and treatment extended to patients expecting a smaller total health gain per bed day from treatment.

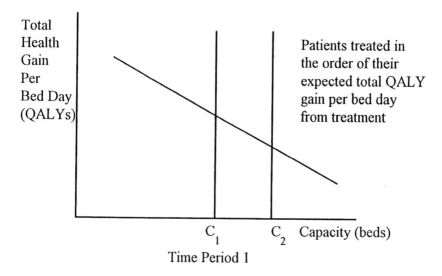

Figure 1. Efficient Waiting List Management Policy

If this waiting list policy were carried out at the clinical specialty level, resources could be distributed between clinical departments so as to equate the total health gain per bed day of the marginal patient treated per time period in each clinical specialty. This would mean that patients would have the same opportunity of being treated, given their expected total health gain per bed day from treatment, regardless of the nature of their condition and clinical specialty from whom treatment was received.

Although this efficient waiting list management policy of maximising health gain per bed day has strength in offering equal access to health care for equal need if need (is defined as ability to benefit from treatment), it is brutally explicit and likely to leave some patients with more minor conditions never being treated.

If society were to decide on a health gain maximisation policy then it is possible to visualise purchasers instead of setting cost and volume contracts with provider units, instead negotiating QALY gain per bed day levels - where thresholds for treatment depend on the level of funding.

A health gain per unit of resource maxmisation based waiting list points scheme would fail to take into account factors such as time already waited, family and employment circumstances, and would only indirectly take account of factors related to quality of life, i.e. those incorporated into the health state descriptors used in QALY calculation.

There is no doubt that major questions about our ability to measure health gain in terms of QALYs or any other unit, lie in the way of the serious consideration of such an efficient policy - but surely such questions surround the measurement of medical priority and social deservingness, and they are already being implemented on an experimental basis in Salisbury.

AN OPPORTUNITY FOR RESEARCH - COMPARING POINTS FOR PAIN WITH POINTS FOR HEALTH GAIN

This paper does not seek to advocate a purely efficient QALY gain per unit of resource based waiting list points scheme as an alternative to the Salisbury points scheme. Instead the aim of this paper has been to describe the Salisbury scheme, and welcome its arrival at an experimental level, and applaud its architects for their recognition of the need to move the waiting list debate beyond waiting time targets. Salisbury offers an opportunity for careful observation over time of the implications of operating a points scheme based on specific eligibility criteria. It is hoped that the staff at Salisbury will be willing to participate in a joint research project to collect QALY data alongside the existing points scheme, in order to identify how efficient the scheme is, in terms of getting high QALY gain per unit of resource patients to the front of the queue. If it is doing this, then a scheme based on criteria that are mainly of a clinical and social rather than economic nature may inadvertently lead to a more efficient use of health care resources. If the points scheme in its present form is leaving some high QALY gain per unit of resource patients languishing at the back of the queue, there is something to be learned about what might be an acceptable trade-off between health gain per unit of resource, and factors judged to determine deservingness of priority on a queue, such as dependence on others, loss of usual activity or time already waited.

ACKNOWLEDGEMENTS

I would like to thank Dr A. Lack for his correspondence, Professor Alan Williams for his continued interest in my work, and my RNIB Readers.

REFERENCES

Brattberg, G. Priority Setting with Regard to Placement on Waiting List to a Pain Clinic: The Feasibility of a Delegated Ranking Procedure, Scandinavian Journal of Social Medicine, Vol. 16, p. 173 - 179, 1988

CORMS, Clinical Office and Resource Management system Delian Medical Systems Limited, 0844 274 111

Culyer A.J. and Cullis, J.G. Some Economics of Hospital Waiting Lists, Journal of Social Policy, Vol. 5, No. 3, pp. 239 - 264, 1976

The Mail on Sunday, Points for Pain, 5th September, 1993

Higgins, J. and Ruddle, S. Waiting for a Better Alternative, Health Service Journal, 11th July, 1991

Lack A. and Fletcher, S. Surgical Waiting List analysis, Discussion Paper, 1993

Lack A. Fletcher, S. Fletcher J. A Method of assessing Priority on Surgical Waiting Lists Discussion Paper, 1993

Mullen, P. Waiting Lists and the NHS Review: Reality and Myths, HSMC Research Report 29, 1993

Naylor C.D., Baigrie, R.S., Goldman, B.S. and Basinski, A. Assessment of Priority for Coronary Revascularisation Procedures, Lancet, p. 1070, 5th May, 1990

6 Rationing and Waiting List Management - Some Efficiency and Equity Considerations

JOHN GODDARD[1] & MANOUCHE TAVAKOLI[2]

[1]University College of North Wales
[2]University of St Andrews

INTRODUCTION

Waiting lists have been a pervasive feature of the British health care system since the creation of the National Health Service (NHS) in 1948. Despite a progressive increase in the proportion of UK Gross National Product spent on the NHS from under 4% in 1949 to over 6% in 1987 (Cullis, 1993) and despite numerous 'initiatives' aimed at tackling the waiting list 'problem', both the number of patients on waiting lists and the average duration of wait for certain categories of non-urgent treatment have also tended to increase during the post-war period. The creation of an internal market and the separation of the functions of health care purchasers and providers as a result of the NHS reforms of April 1991 has drawn renewed attention towards the waiting list phenomenon, and created expectations that as a by-product of market-led gains in NHS efficiency, waiting times might be expected to fall (Freemantle et al, 1993; Harrison et al, 1990).

In the theoretical literature, the waiting list has been viewed (less pejoratively than in much of the political discussion) as a rationing device which functions in situations where the price mechanism fails or is inoperative, as is the case in the NHS where treatment remains (predominantly) free at the point of delivery (Lindsay and Feigenbaum, 1984; Cullis and Jones, 1985, 1986; Frankel, 1993). According to Lindsay and Feigenbaum, queues grow until the point is reached at which the expected wait reduces the value of treatment for some complainants to such an extent that they decide not to seek treatment. Willingness to wait implicitly rations access to treatment, so that the level of demand is brought into equality with the available supply. However, as pointed out by Gravelle (1990) among others, the waiting list is likely to represent an inefficient means of determining access to

Setting Priorities in Health Care. Edited by M. Malek
© 1994 John Wiley & Sons Ltd

treatment, because the time spent waiting represents a 'dead-weight' loss, imposing costs on the individual complainant which are not compensated by gains anywhere else in the system.

The present paper adopts this theoretical interpretation of the waiting list methods of managing the queue for hospital treatment. It combines a model of the determination of demand (which is the same in principle as the one proposed by Lindsay and Feigenbaum, 1984) with a queuing model which determines the level of treatment supplied and the average duration of wait (see West, 1993 for a general discussion of the applicability of queuing models to the analysis of NHS waiting lists). Our purpose is to show how three different queue management regimes lead to differing outcomes in terms of treatment levels and waiting times, and to consider the equity and efficiency implications of each one. In broad terms, the three queue management regimes are: (i) calling complainants for treatment strictly on a 'first-come first-served' basis; (ii) affording some priority to the more ill complainants in such a way that waiting times are determined (in some sense) equitably, in inverse proportion to the seriousness of each complainant's condition; and (iii) affording very high priority to the more ill complainants and imposing waits upon the less seriously ill which are so long that the latter are likely to be deterred from seeking treatment at all. The theoretical model suggests that on efficiency criteria, regime (iii) may be attractive because it minimises queuing congestion and waiting times for those complainants who do obtain (and who most need) treatment; however, regime (iii) also raises serious concerns about equity in respect of those complainants who are effectively excluded from treatment.

Our concern in this paper is with the efficient utilisation of a fixed pool of resources assumed to be designated for the treatment of one (unspecified but non-urgent) clinical condition, and especially with the efficient management of the queue of complainants seeking access to this pool of resources.

Therefore we do not address wider issues of public choice such as the question of the overall level of funding which should be provided to the NHS, or questions of resource allocation between competing functions within the service. Our scope is far more modest than this, and while our approach is purely theoretical, we hope that the paper does provide a framework which can help to shed light on issues of efficiency and equity which also arise in less abstract terms whenever practical decisions concerning the management of waiting lists are taken.

The rest of the paper is structured as follows. Section 2 sets out the assumptions and technical specification of the supply and demand sides of the queuing model. Section 3 presents the equilibrium solutions to the model under the three queue management regimes, and discusses their efficiency and equity properties. Some numerical simulations of the model's properties under various assumptions are also presented. Section 4 uses the model to investigate the implications of two hypothetical changes of policy regime: firstly, the announcement of a guaranteed maximum duration of wait; and secondly, the introduction of explicit rationing of the numbers permitted to join the queue to seek treatment. Finally, section 5 concludes.

THE QUEUING MODEL

We begin by investigating the relationship between the rate at which complainants enter the queue and the average duration of wait. At this stage, we are not concerned with what determines the rate of entry (which is considered later in section 2); neither do we consider what determines the order in which complainants in the queue receive treatment (which is discussed in section 3). For the purposes of the analysis, we assume that sufferers from some complaint queue to be admitted to a hospital which has a constant pool of k beds available for treatment of the complaint. We define e to be the average daily *entry rate* (the average number of complainants who enter the queue each day) and μ to be the average daily *discharge rate* for an individual occupied bed (the average number of complainants who are discharged from hospital each day from each occupied bed). μ is simply the reciprocal of the average duration of hospital stay; e.g. if the latter is 4 days, then the average daily discharge rate per bed is $1/4 = 0.25$.

We define j to be the total number of complainants in the *queuing system* at any time. A complainant is in the queuing system when he/she is either in the queue itself, or in hospital receiving treatment. We can then define d_j to be the average daily discharge rate for all k beds (whether occupied or not) when there are j complainants in the queuing system. The average daily discharge rate for all k beds depends on j because the latter determines whether or not some beds are unoccupied. In principle at least, it is possible that at certain times the queue is empty and some beds are unoccupied, in which case the average daily discharge rate for the k beds as a whole is lower than at times when all beds are occupied. In fact, we can specify d_j quite easily as follows. When $j \leq k$ there are sufficient beds for all complainants currently seeking treatment, so the queue is empty and the average daily discharge rate is the number of occupied beds (j) multiplied by the discharge rate per occupied bed (μ). When $j > k$, there are insufficient beds, so all k beds are occupied, (j-k) complainants are in the queue, and applying the same formula as before, the average daily discharge rate is $k\mu$. In short,

$$d_j = j\mu \quad \text{for} \quad 0 \leq j \leq k; \qquad d_j = k\mu \quad \text{for} \quad j > k.$$

A significant feature of NHS waiting lists is that at any time they include a proportion of complainants who, after joining the queue but before being called for treatment, find or decide that they no longer require treatment; this may be due to movement away from the area, admission to hospital for some more serious complaint, a decision to seek private treatment, recovery or even death (see Donaldson et al, 1984). Sometimes it only becomes apparent that such withdrawals have occurred when the complainant is called for treatment and fails to turn up. For the purposes of our model we shall assume that the *average daily withdrawal rate* for each complainant (i.e. the probability that a complainant withdraws on any particular day) is ω for all complainants in the queue. Defining w_j to be the total daily withdrawal rate when there are j complainants in the system, w_j is zero when $j \leq k$

and the queue is empty, and w_j is found by multiplying the individual withdrawal rate (ω) by the number in the queue (j-k) when j > k. In short,

$$w_j = 0 \quad \text{for} \quad 0 \le j \le k; \qquad w_j = (j-k)\omega \quad \text{for} \quad j > k.$$

As defined above, e, μ and ω represent *average* entry, discharge and withdrawal rates; however, from day to day it is possible for the actual entry rate to be higher or lower than e, for individual complainants to require shorter or longer stays in hospital than the mean duration of stay used to calculate μ, and for the number of withdrawals to be greater or less than would be expected given ω and the current size of the queue. Random daily fluctuations in the entry, discharge and withdrawal rates cause random fluctuations in the size of the queue and in the number of complainants in the queuing system[1]. In order to solve the queuing model mathematically, it is useful to define p_j to be the *proportion* of time for which there are exactly j complainants in the queuing system; p_j can also be interpreted as the *probability* that at any specific time there are exactly j complainants in the system.

Using these definitions, it is possible (see Appendix) to derive mathematical expressions for p_j for all values of j, in terms of the demand side and supply side parameters (respectively e and ω, and μ and k). These are as follows:

$$p_0 = \cfrac{1}{1 + \sum_{j=1}^{\infty} \prod_{h=1}^{j} \left(\cfrac{e}{d_h + w_h} \right)}$$

$$p_j = \prod_{h=1}^{j} \left(\frac{e}{d_h + w_h} \right) p_0 \quad \text{for } j=1,...\infty$$

It is then possible to obtain an expression for the *mean expected duration of wait* for an 'average' complainant whose expected wait is the length of time it would be expected to take for all those already in the queue at the time of his/her entry either to be treated or to withdraw (so if 'overtaking' in the queue is allowed, an 'average' complainant is one who is 'overtaken' the same number of times as he/she 'overtakes' others). Let t_j be the expected duration of wait for an 'average' complainant who enters the queue when there are j other complainants already in the system. If j < k, the new entrant is admitted to hospital immediately and there is no wait, so t_j=0. If

---

[1] In a recent paper, Livny *et al* (1993) present some simulations of the properties of queueing models with non-random (i.e. autocorrelated) rates of entry and exit. Although it seems probable that time series data on NHS entry, discharge and withdrawals would reveal evidence of autocorrelation, we have not allowed for this in the present analysis.

$j \geq k$, the new entrant will get a bed as soon as there have been $(j-k+1)$ discharges or withdrawals. In this case, the expressions for t_j (which are derived in the Appendix) are as follows:

$$t_j = 0 \text{ for } 0 \leq j < k; \qquad t_j = (1/\omega)\{\ln[(j-k)\omega+k\mu]-\ln(k\mu)\} + (1/k\mu) \text{ for } j \geq k.$$

The mean discharge rate $\bar{d}$, the mean withdrawal rate $\bar{w}$, and the mean expected duration of wait $\bar{t}$, can then be evaluated as follows:

$$\bar{d} = \sum_{j=k+1}^{\infty} p_j d_j \qquad\qquad \bar{w} = \sum_{j=k+1}^{\infty} p_j w_j \qquad\qquad \bar{t} = \sum_{j=k+1}^{\infty} p_j t_j$$

Table 1. Effect on $\bar{d}$, $\bar{w}$ and $\bar{t}$ for changes in e

e (entry rate)	$\bar{d}$ (discharge rate)	$\bar{w}$ (withdrawal rate)	$\bar{t}$ (mean expected duration of wait)
1.00	1.00	0.00	0.0
1.50	1.50	0.00	0.1
2.00	2.00	0.00	0.8
2.10	2.10	0.00	1.0
2.20	2.20	0.00	1.9
2.30	2.29	0.01	3.3
2.40	2.39	0.01	6.3
2.50	2.46	0.04	15.2
2.60	2.50	0.10	40.4
2.70	2.50	0.20	77.2
2.80	2.50	0.30	113.5
2.90	2.50	0.40	148.6
3.00	2.50	0.50	182.5

Assumed parameter values: $\mu = 0.25$, $k = 10$, $\omega = 0.001$.

Table 1 shows the relationship between these variables with an illustrative set of values for the parameters μ, k and ω as follows: $\mu=0.25$, $k=10$ and $\omega=0.001$. Table 1 shows that for entry rates which are substantially below the system's capacity (an average discharge rate of 2.5) most complainants are treated with little or no wait; even with e=2.4 (96% of capacity), the mean expected duration of wait is only 6.3 days. However, as the entry rate approaches and then exceeds 2.5, the size of the queue and mean expected wait increase rapidly, and withdrawals play an increasingly important role in ensuring equality between the numbers gaining access to treatment and the system's capacity. With e=2.6, the system is already operating at full capacity ($\bar{d}=2.5$), and the mean expected wait must be sufficiently long (40.4 days) to create a withdrawal rate of 0.1 (the difference between e and $\bar{d}$). Any further increases in the entry rate must raise the mean expected wait sufficiently so that the withdrawal rate rises in line with the entry rate, in order to maintain equality between the average numbers entering and leaving the system (either through discharge or withdrawal) per period (see Worthington, 1987 for some more extensive numerical simulations of the properties of queuing models applied to the NHS, although without explicit inclusion of a withdrawal rate parameter).

So far we have assumed that the rate of entry to the queue e, is exogenously determined. We are now ready to remove this assumption and examine a mechanism whereby e is itself determined, at least in part, by conditions in the queue. The mechanism is the same as that proposed in Lindsay and Feigenbaum (1984) which we now describe briefly. Lindsay and Feigenbaum argue that for complaints which do not deteriorate over time or which only deteriorate slowly, the present value to the complainant of hospital treatment is negatively related to the expected duration of wait: firstly, because the complaint may improve over time without hospitalisation, either with or without other forms of treatment (such as drugs); and secondly, because on standard time preference assumptions, the value of treatment diminishes as the period of deferral increases.

The decision to seek treatment and join the queue is assumed to impose an initial cost, including both pecuniary and non-pecuniary costs of obtaining an initial diagnosis in order to secure a referral. Following Lindsay and Feigenbaum we assume that this cost is entirely up front, and ignore any costs arising over time from being on the waiting list (see Propper, 1990). The complainant seeks treatment if the present value of treatment exceeds the initial cost. Since the former tends to zero as the expected wait increases, for each complainant who would accept treatment if it were available immediately, there is some value for the expected wait above which the present value falls below the initial cost. If the expected wait exceeds this value, the complainant does not seek NHS treatment, choosing either private care (an option explicitly incorporated into the Lindsay and Feigenbaum framework by Cullis and Jones, 1986) or to remain untreated.

We can formalise the argument as follows. We assume that illness imposes a daily utility cost of i upon the complainant; i varies between complainants in proportion to the seriousness of each one's condition. Utility costs arising from illness in the future are discounted back to the present at a rate of g, which reflects both the rate at which the illness is expected to deteriorate or improve over time if hospital treatment is not obtained, and the discount rate employed in evaluating the present value of future suffering. For simplicity we assume that g is the same for all complainants, and that $g > 0$ (i.e. without hospital treatment the condition either improves, or deteriorates at a rate which is less than the discount rate being employed).

The decision to seek treatment is assumed to impose a utility cost of c upon each complainant, which reflects the cost and inconvenience of visiting the hospital for an appointment with the consultant, and which varies between complainants. Treatment, when received, is assumed to be completely effective causing the complainant's symptoms to disappear and the utility cost from illness to fall to zero. On these assumptions, expressions for the present value of the utility cost arising from illness for each complainant are:

$$\int_{\tau=0}^{\infty} i \exp(-gt) \, d\tau = (i/g) \qquad \text{if treatment is not sought, and}$$

$$c + \int_{\tau=0}^{t} i \exp(-gt) \, d\tau = c + (i/g)(1 - \exp(-gt)) \qquad \text{if treatment is sought,}$$

where t represents the complainant's expected duration of wait.

Treatment will be sought by all complainants for whom the first expression is greater than the second. It can easily be shown that this is the case for all complainants for whom $i > cg \exp(gt)$. For any given value of t, this condition determines how many complainants would seek treatment with an expected wait of t, and therefore determines the value of e. It also ensures that as waiting times increase, e falls, because with longer waiting times fewer complainants have values of i sufficiently high to satisfy this condition for seeking treatment. For simplicity, in the diagrammatic analyses and the numerical simulations which follow, we assume that the relationship between t and e is linear; i.e. we can write e = a-bt, where a and b are positive constants.

SOLUTIONS TO THE QUEUING MODEL UNDER THREE QUEUE MANAGEMENT REGIMES

In this section we solve the queuing model by combining the supply side and demand side analyses of section 2 so as to determine the equilibrium values for the entry, discharge and withdrawal rates and the mean expected duration of wait. In order to do so, it is necessary to consider the management of the queue; i.e. the criteria which are used to determine the order in which complainants currently in the queue are called for treatment. This is important because it determines the number of complainants who perceive it to be worthwhile to join the queue, and it therefore affects the equilibrium which the queuing system achieves. We now consider the implications of three theoretical queue management regimes, which are as follows:

1. *'First-come First-served' (FCFS)*. Complainants are treated strictly in the order in which they initially join the queue; i.e. once in the queue no 'overtaking' is permitted, so no priority is given to complainants who are more seriously ill.
2. *'Equality of Suffering' (EOS)*. Priority is given to the more seriously ill complainants, with the waiting time for each complainant determined in such a way as to ensure equality between the total discounted utility cost arising from illness of every complainant who seeks and obtains treatment.
3. *'Marginal Contribution to Aggregate Wait' (MCAW)*. Priority is given to the more seriously ill complainants, with the waiting time for each complainant determined by the marginal contribution which that complainant makes to the aggregate wait for the entire cohort seeking treatment, when the complainants are ranked in order of the seriousness of their conditions.

Queue management regime 1: 'First-come First-served' (FCFS)

Figure 1 illustrates the determination of equilibrium when complainants are treated strictly in the order in which they join the queue. We start with the function $\bar{t}\,(e)$, which shows for any entry rate represented on the horizontal axis (e.g. OD), the corresponding value of $\bar{t}$ generated by the queuing model on the vertical axis (OA). Reading back from this value of $\bar{t}$ via the curve $\bar{d}(\bar{t})$ to the horizontal axis allows us to represent the corresponding discharge rate (OC) on the horizontal axis. The horizontal distance between the discharge rate and the original entry rate represents the withdrawal rate (CD).

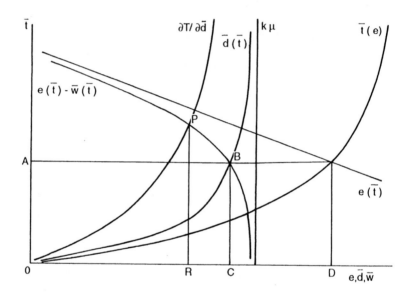

Figure 1

Based on the analysis of the decision whether to seek treatment, the function $e(\bar{t})$ shows, for any value of $\bar{t}$ represented on the vertical axis (e.g. OA), the corresponding entry rate (OD) if the expected wait for all complainants joining the queue is $\bar{t}$. For this entry rate, we can use the queuing model to determine the corresponding withdrawal rate as before (CD). The function $e(\bar{t})-\overline{w}(\bar{t})$, obtained by deducting this withdrawal rate from the corresponding entry rate (and read from the vertical to the horizontal axis) then represents the rate of entry of complainants who will not withdraw before being called for treatment (OC); i.e. the rate of entry of complainants who will eventually be treated.

If complainants are treated *FCFS*, all complainants experience the same expected duration of wait, which must be such as to ensure equality between the rates at which complainants enter and leave the queuing system; i.e. we must have $e=\overline{d}+\overline{w}$. In Figure 1 this occurs at point B, at the intersection of $e(\overline{t})-\overline{w}(\overline{t})$ with $\overline{d}(\overline{t})$. Therefore the equilibrium solution is $\overline{t}$=OA, $\overline{d}$=OC, $\overline{w}$=CD and e=OD.

Two significant disadvantages are associated with *FCFS*; these are addressed by the two alternative queue management regimes discussed below. The first disadvantage is that although the expected wait is the same for all complainants, this wait imposes different costs on different complainants because some are more seriously ill than others. Therefore *FCFS* is (in this sense) inequitable because it penalises the more seriously ill complainants.

Secondly, *FCFS* leads to over-utilisation of the pool of beds, and therefore over-consumption of treatment. This is because the least seriously ill complainants who seek treatment contribute to some extent to the overall level of queuing congestion, and therefore contribute to the length of wait which is experienced by all complainants. It can be shown that the waiting cost thereby imposed upon the more seriously ill complainants exceeds the benefit from treatment obtained by these less seriously ill complainants. In terms of overall welfare, it would therefore be better if these less seriously ill complainants did not seek treatment so that the queue is kept shorter for the more seriously ill complainants. *FCFS* is therefore inefficient in this respect.

In Figure 1, the function $(\partial T/\partial \overline{d})$ represents the addition to the *total* time spent waiting by *all* treated complainants ($T=\overline{d}\,\overline{t}$) for each unit increase in the discharge (i.e. treatment) rate. As $\overline{d}$ increases and approaches $k\mu$, the average duration of wait starts to increase, implying that each additional treated complainant makes a marginal contribution to the aggregate wait equal to his/her own wait *plus* the additional wait he/she imposes on all the other complainants by adding to the general level of queuing congestion. Therefore $(\partial T/\partial \overline{d})$ lies above and is more steeply sloped than $d(\overline{t})$. If we imagine progressively increasing the discharge rate by treating complainants in descending order of the seriousness of their illness, then for any increase in the discharge rate beyond OR, the marginal complainant's contribution to the aggregate wait $(\partial T/\partial \overline{d})$ exceeds the value of treatment to the complainant (measured by the time the complainant would be prepared to wait, and read from the function $e(\overline{t})-\overline{w}(\overline{t})$. This means that aggregate welfare would be increased if the RC least seriously ill of the OC complainants who *do* join the queue and receive treatment could be persuaded not to do so. Some reduction in the numbers seeking and obtaining treatment, and a corresponding reduction in congestion and waiting times, would be more efficient. In numerical terms, because $\overline{d}(\overline{t})$ is very steeply sloped when it is close to $k\mu$, only a relatively small reduction in the discharge (treatment) rate is likely to be needed to secure a large reduction in waiting times. In practice RC is likely to represent only a very small proportion of OC, and the system does not have to be operating very far below its maximum capacity for the queues to diminish substantially or virtually disappear. However, the preceding analysis shows that *FCFS* does not bring about this more efficient level of treatment[2] .

Queue management regime 2: 'Equality of Suffering' (EOS)

Figure 2 illustrates the determination of equilibrium when complainants are moved through the queue in such a way as to ensure that the total discounted utility cost of illness for each complainant who eventually obtains treatment is the same for all such complainants. In order to achieve this, the expected duration of wait must clearly be shorter for the more seriously ill. For any value of $\bar{t}$ which can be represented on the vertical axis of Figure 2 (e.g. OE), if we read down to the horizontal axis via the curve $e(\bar{t})$-$\bar{w}(\bar{t})$ we can determine the total number of complainants who would seek and eventually receive treatment (OK) if they all had an expected wait of $\bar{t}$ =OE. OE also represents the length of time which the most marginal (least seriously ill) of these OK complainants would be prepared to wait.

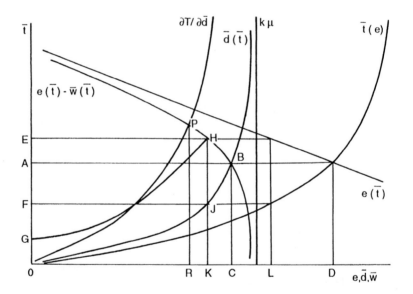

Figure 2

[2]The argument is analogous to that put forward in Walters' (1961) classic paper on traffic congestion. The limit to the number of cars on the road is reached when the private costs of congestion equal the private benefits of car useage to the most marginal driver. However, the social cost of the congestion which the most marginal drivers create for all other drivers exceeds the marginal drivers' private benefits. Therefore aggregate welfare would be increased if the most marginal drivers could be dissuaded from running a car.

If we reduce the expected wait for the more seriously ill of these OK complainants while maintaining an expected wait of OE for the most marginal (least seriously ill) complainant (and promising an even longer wait for any still less ill complainant who might be thinking of joining the queue), the total number who seek and eventually receive treatment remains unchanged at OK. Therefore, if we position these OK complainants in descending order of the seriousness of their illness from left to right along the horizontal axis, we can construct a curve GH which shows the expected wait which would give each complainant a total discounted utility cost equal to the total cost incurred by the most marginal complainant when the latter has an expected wait of OE. The total wait experienced by all OK complainants is then measured by the area under this curve, OGHK.

Finally, how do we know that the points shown in Figure 2 represent the *equilibrium* under this queue management regime? The answer is that they are the only set of points which satisfy the condition that the *total* time spent waiting by the group which seeks and receives treatment measured by summing the expected wait of each individual, OGHK, is consistent with the same total as measured by multiplying the *average* duration of wait (OF, $= \bar{t}$ at which $\bar{d}(\bar{t})$=OK) by the discharge rate (OK), OFJK.

The curve GH is a theoretical construct whose precise shape and position depend on the unknown parameters of each complainant's utility function (i, c and g). Williams' (1985, 1988) proposals for the estimation of Quality Adjusted Life-Years (QALYs) represents one approach by which benefits of treatment in different cases might be quantified (and compared with costs). In practice, it seems likely that most hospitals adopt a less systematic approach and perhaps attempt to find some approximation to our curve GH, by managing the queue in such a way as to strike what is perceived to be an equitable balance between the need to give priority to the most seriously ill complainants, and the desire that the less seriously ill should not be required to wait indefinitely. Most hospitals at the very least operate a three point scale of urgency (immediate, urgent and non-urgent), and it seems likely that judgements are routinely made about degrees of urgency within these bands (West, 1993). For the purposes of the numerical simulations of the queuing model which follow later in the paper, we (arbitrarily) assume that our hospital operates along a linear approximation to GH, with a ratio between the shortest and longest waits of treated complainants of 1:10. If the average duration of wait for this group is (for example) 100 days, this implies a minimum and maximum expected wait of 18.2 and 181.8 days respectively for the most urgent and least urgent cases.

By relating the duration of wait to the seriousness of illness, some of the less seriously ill complainants who seek treatment under *FCFS* are dissuaded from doing so under *EOS*. The demand for treatment falls (OL<OD), and in theory so too does the discharge rate (OK<OC) (although in practice the difference between OK and OC may be negligibly small if JB is located on the near-vertical section of $\bar{d}(\bar{t})$ close to kμ). Queuing congestion is eased as a result of the reduction in demand, so the average duration of wait falls (OF<OA). *EOS* is the most equitable of the three queue management regimes; furthermore, an efficiency gain is achieved by comparison with

the *FCFS* equilibrium. However, efficiency is not maximised because there is still over-utilisation of resources and over-consumption of treatment of RK. As before, the costs imposed on the more seriously ill by the congestion created by the most marginal complainants treated under *EOS* still outweigh the benefits received by the latter.

Queue management regime 3: 'Marginal Contribution to Aggregate Wait' (MCAW)

Under *MCAW* the more seriously ill complainants are allowed to move through the queue more rapidly (and the less seriously ill less rapidly) than under *EOS*. Even higher priority is given to the most ill, with the result that the less ill must wait longer. In the theoretical model, the speed at which each complainant is moved through the queue is determined by the marginal contribution which that complainant would make to the aggregate wait for all complainants who eventually receive treatment, if the number of complainants obtaining treatment were progressively increased one at a time in descending order of seriousness of illness. For those complainants who obtain treatment, the waiting times can be read from the curve $(\partial T/\partial \overline{d})$, and the most marginal complainant who joins the queue under this regime is determined at the intersection of $(\partial T/\partial \overline{d})$ with $e(\overline{t})-\overline{w}(\overline{t})$ (point P in Figure 3). The shape of $(\partial T/\partial \overline{d})$ is such that the most seriously ill receive treatment almost immediately (their marginal contribution to the aggregate wait is negligible because if they were the only ones treated, the system would be operating well below capacity and the queue would be virtually empty). However, beyond a certain point, the marginal contribution of each additional complainant to the aggregate wait increases rapidly (because if more complainants were treated the system would start to approach capacity and queues would start to build up). Under this queue management regime, the more marginal complainants are made to bear the entire cost of the extra queuing congestion they cause; this being so, the limit to the number of complainants who join the queue and eventually receive treatment is reached sooner than under the other two regimes, at OR. The average wait is ON, with the total wait equivalently measured either by OPR or by ONQR.

In practice, the *MCAW* regime involves offering a minimal wait to the most seriously ill complainants, and a wait to the less seriously ill which is so long that most of the latter perceive that it is not worthwhile for them to seek treatment. By deterring the less seriously ill in this way, the number of complainants who *do* seek treatment is restricted to a level with which the system can cope without significant queues building up. Queuing congestion is minimised, and the benefits to the more seriously ill from a shorter wait exceed the costs to the less seriously ill who would receive treatment under *FCFS* or *EOS*, but who are not treated under *MCAW*.

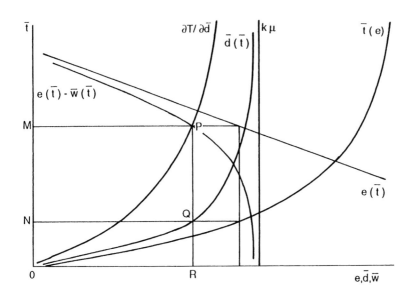

Figure 3

MCAW has the attractive efficiency property of avoiding over-utilisation of resources and over-consumption of treatment; however, it is a less equitable regime than *EOS* in the sense that total suffering (measured by the total discounted utility cost) is greater for the less seriously ill complainants (who bear most of the aggregate wait) than for the more seriously ill (who are treated almost immediately). Table 2 presents a comparison of the properties of the equilibria attained under the three queue management regimes we have considered.

Table 2. Equilibrium properties under three queue management regimes(refer Figures 1-3)

Equilibrium property	Queue management regime				
	FCFS		*EOS*		*MCAW*
Discharge rate (numbers treated)	OC	>	OK	>	OR
Over-consumption of treatment (by comparison with welfare maximising level)	RC	>	RK	>	zero
Average duration of wait	OA	>	OF	>	ON
Expected wait for most seriously ill complainant treated	OA	>	OG	>	zero
Expected wait for least seriously ill complainant treated	OA	<	OE	<	OM
Total discounted utility cost for most seriously ill complainant treated	high		medium		low
Total discounted utility cost for least seriously ill complainant treated	low		medium		high

We now investigate the sensitivity of the equilibrium solutions obtained under the three queue management regimes by means of some numerical simulations of the queuing model. These are based on the following parameter values: $\mu=0.25$, $k=10$ and $\omega=0.001$. Two sets of entry function parameters are used: in set (i), a=4.57 and b=0.01; and in set (ii), a=3.68 and b=0.005. The two sets of values are chosen so as to produce an identical mean expected duration of wait of 100 days under the *EOS* regime. Set (i) represents an entry function which is relatively sensitive to expected duration of wait (if the expected wait for all complainants were to increase from 100 days to 200 days, the number of complainants seeking treatment would decline by 28%); set (ii) represents an entry function which is less so (the same increase in wait produces a decline in the number seeking treatment of 19%)[3] . The simulation results which follow are of course entirely dependent on these parameter values (which we have chosen arbitrarily), but although they have not been tested or validated empirically, they do provide some impression of the sensitivity of the solutions to the theoretical model to supply and demand side changes of varying magnitudes.

Table 3. Solutions under three queue management regimes with two alternative entry functions

	(i) Entry function wait-sensitive			(ii) entry function wait-insensitive		
	FCFS	*EOS*	*MCAW*	*FCFS*	*EOS*	*MCAW*
e (entry rate)	2.95	2.77	2.44	2.92	2.77	2.45
$\overline{w}$ (withdrawal rate)	0.45	0.27	0.03	0.42	0.27	0.02
$\overline{d}$ (discharge rate)	2.50	2.50	2.41	2.50	2.50	2.43
$\overline{t}$ (mean expected duration of wait)	163	100	8	153	100	9

Parameter values: $\mu=0.25$, $k=10$, $\omega=0.001$ and (i) a=4.57, b=0.01   (ii) a=3.68, b=0.005

Table 3 shows the full set of equilibrium values under the three queue management regimes for the two sets of entry function parameters. Using the EOS regime as the basis for comparison, a change from *EOS* to *FCFS* would increase the average wait from 100 to 163 days under the more wait-sensitive entry function; in both cases, the system effectively operates at full capacity ($\overline{d}=k\mu=2.50$) so the difference between the numbers treated under *EOS* and *FCFS* is negligible. On the other hand, a change from *EOS* to *MCAW* would reduce the average wait to only 8 days, necessitating a small reduction in the discharge rate to 2.41 (96% of capacity). If the entry function is less wait-sensitive, the differences between the three regimes are slightly less

---

[3]In a relatively old paper, Frost (1980) found evidence of an elasticity of demand with respect to waiting time slightly greater than unity; i.e. considerably higher than the relatively conservative values we have preferred to employ here.

pronounced, with average waits of 153, 100 and 9 days under *FCFS*, *EOS* and *MCAW* respectively.

Table 4. Effect on $\bar{t}$ of changes in capacity under three queue management regimes

(i) entry function wait-sensitive

	Capacity (as a % of level assumed in table 3)								
	70	80	90	100	110	120	130	140	150
FCFS	235	211	186	163	140	119	99	79	59
EOS	141	126	113	100	85	74	62	50	38
MCAW	11	10	9	8	7	6	5	5	4

(ii) entry function wait-insensitive

	Capacity (as a % of level assumed in table 3)								
	70	80	90	100	110	120	130	140	150
FCFS	275	233	191	153	118	84	52	23	6
EOS	177	150	125	100	78	56	35	16	5
MCAW	14	12	11	9	7	6	5	3	2

Parameter values: $\mu=0.25$, $k=10$, $\omega=0.001$ and (i) $a=4.57$, $b=0.01$ (ii) $a=3.68$, $b=0.005$

Table 5. Effect on $\bar{t}$ of changes in demand under three queue management regimes

(i) entry function wait-sensitive

	Demand (as % of level assumed in table 3)								
	50	60	70	80	90	100	110	120	130
FCFS	2	30	73	109	138	163	184	202	218
EOS	2	20	47	67	86	100	111	122	131
MCAW	1	4	5	7	8	8	9	9	9

(ii) entry function wait-insensitive

	Demand (as a % of level assumed in table 3)								
	50	60	70	80	90	100	110	120	130
FCFS	0	1	17	67	115	153	189	218	235
EOS	0	1	13	45	77	100	122	141	158
MCAW	0	1	4	6	8	9	10	10	11

Parameter values: $\mu=0.25$, $k=10$, $\omega=0.001$ and (i) $a=4.57$, $b=0.01$ (ii) $a=3.68$, $b=0.005$

Tables 4 and 5 show the sensitivity of the solutions to the model to variations in capacity and demand. Table 4 shows the effect on the equilibrium value of $\bar{t}$ of changes in the capacity of the queuing system to between 70% and 150% of the level assumed in Table 3; the results are generated by varying the parameter μ. As one would expect, increases in capacity cause queuing times to fall under all three regimes; reductions have the opposite effect. The lower the sensitivity of demand to waiting time, the greater is the effect of any given change in capacity on the average wait. Table 5 shows a similar analysis of the effects of fluctuations in the level of demand on average waiting times; in this case the results are generated by scaling the entry function (a-bt) up or down by the percentages shown along the top of Table 5. In this case, reductions in demand reduce waiting times (and *vice versa*); again, the effects are greater if demand is less sensitive to duration of wait. For each entry function and queue management regime, Tables 4 and 5 provide an indication of the magnitude of the shift in capacity or demand which would be required to cause the average wait to rise or fall to any particular level.

CHANGES OF POLICY REGIME

The framework we have developed can also be used to examine the theoretical implications for the queuing model of changes in the level of demand or in practices concerning referrals, changes in resourcing or funding, or changes arising from other types of policy directive. In this section, we provide two illustrations as follows: (i) a policy directive specifying a maximum waiting time within which all complainants who join the queue must be treated (as is currently specified in the Patients' Charter); and (ii) a change in funding arrangements which explicitly rations the number of complainants permitted to join the queue. In each case, we assume that before the relevant change takes place, the *'Equality of Suffering' (EOS)* queue management regime is in operation, so the 'initial' equilibrium (for comparative statics purposes) is as shown in Figure 2.

Imposition of a guaranteed maximum wait

In Figure 4, $\bar{d}$=OK and $\bar{t}$=OF represents the equilibrium position when the *EOS* queue management regime is in force, as in Figure 2. As we have seen, this equilibrium implies an expected wait of OE for the most marginal complainant who seeks and obtains treatment. Suppose that it is now decreed by politicians that it is unacceptable for any complainant to be kept waiting for as long as OE, and that hospital managers should achieve a maximum waiting time of OU<OE for all complainants who are eventually treated. The first implication is that more complainants than before seek treatment, attracted by the prospect of the shorter wait. In Figure 4, the equilibrium discharge rate increases from OK to OZ.

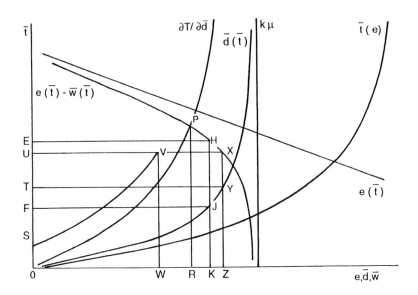

Figure 4

A second implication is that it is no longer possible for hospital managers to operate the *EOS* queue management regime, since the increase in demand dictates that waiting times (and therefore total discounted utility cost) for the more seriously ill must *rise*, while the discounted utility cost of the marginal complainant who joins with $\bar{t}$=OU must be lower than that of the marginal complainant who joins with $\bar{t}$=OE. The closest which hospital managers can now come to *EOS* is to offer the OW most seriously ill complainants shorter waiting times along the curve SV, which ensure equality of suffering within this group only; and the remaining WZ complainants a fixed waiting time of OU, which implies that suffering is less for the least ill within this group. The equilibrium position of $\bar{d}$=OZ, $\bar{t}$=OT is determined (in the same way as before) as the position at which the total wait measured by summing the individual waits (OSVXZ) is consistent with the total measured by multiplying the average wait by the discharge rate (OTYZ).

On efficiency grounds, the new equilibrium is unambiguously less favourable than the old one, because there is now *more* over-consumption of treatment than before (OR<OK<OZ) (although again, the difference between OK and OZ may be negligible if the system is operating close to capacity along the near- vertical section of $\bar{d}(\bar{t})$). The additional complainants who are encouraged to join by the guarantee of a maximum wait of OU create queuing congestion which imposes costs on the

complainants already seeking treatment which exceed the benefits the additional complainants themselves obtain. It is also interesting to note that the average wait *increases* as a result of imposing a maximum wait (OT>OF), because if the latter encourages more complainants than before to seek treatment, there is more queuing congestion in total, implying not only that the more seriously ill cases must wait longer (as was widely pointed out in the public debate at the time of publication of the Patients' Charter), but also that the average wait for the entire group increases (which was perhaps less widely recognised). If the average wait is itself a politically sensitive 'headline' statistic, this result should cause pause for thought before commitments of this kind are issued, notwithstanding the theoretical welfare analysis which, as we have seen, also argues against this type of guarantee.

Rationing at point of entry to the queue

In this section we consider the implications of the imposition of a quantitative limit on the number of complainants permitted to join the queue in any period. The idea that the creation of the NHS internal market represents a significant step along the path towards explicit rationing of access to treatment has been aired extensively elsewhere (see, for example Harrison *et al*, 1991; Harrison and Wistow, 1992). During the present (still transitional) phase of the reforms, the onus for determining access in individual cases appears to rest largely with hospital consultants (often operating within constraints imposed from above through District Health Authority decisions or recommendations); in future, one can imagine that their purchasing power will tend to give fundholding GPs greater influence over these kinds of decisions than may have been the case in the past. The potential within the internal market for the emergence of explicit rationing is a feature which proponents of the NHS reforms have been reluctant to emphasise in the public and political discussion; however, in our framework, explicit rationing can deliver benefits if the effect is to ease queuing congestion by reducing the numbers permitted to seek treatment, thereby allowing a more efficient use of resources without large queues starting to build.

The theoretical argument is illustrated in Figure 5, which compares the *EOS* equilibrium of Figure 2 with the position attained if the amount of treatment per period is explicitly rationed to OR. It is assumed that treatment is allocated to the most seriously ill complainants. A discharge rate of OR implies an average duration of wait of ON, and if hospital managers continue to manage the queue on the *EOS* principle, the waiting times for the OR treated complainants are determined along the curve $\alpha\beta$, which must satisfy the condition $O\alpha\beta R=ONQR$. Assuming that budgets are set at the appropriate level, it is possible *both* to attain the efficient, welfare maximising treatment level (the costs of the reduction in treatment are outweighed by the benefits of the reduction in queuing congestion), *and* to operate the most equitable of the three queue management regimes (which was not possible when attaining a discharge rate of OR under *MCAW* as in Figure 3).

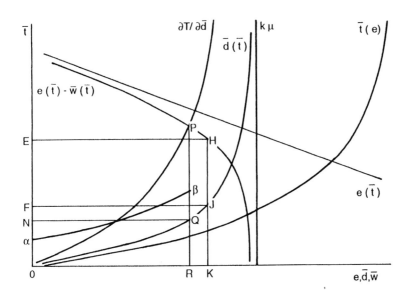

Figure 5

In common with some previous academic analyses (see Barzel, 1974; Cheung, 1974; Gravelle, 1990) our model is therefore in principle supportive of explicit rationing of access to treatment along the lines suggested above. However, it should also be emphasised that in the model, the benefits of such rationing arise solely from the reduction in queuing congestion; furthermore, the numerical simulations suggest that the system needs to be operating only marginally below capacity for congestion to be considerably eased. The disadvantage with explicit rationing of this type is that if waiting times do fall substantially, an increase in the numbers wishing to join the queue can be expected (i.e. more marginal complainants are attracted to seek treatment by the shorter expected wait). In order to remain at the welfare maximising equilibrium, these additional complainants must be denied access to the queue. As in any market in which the 'price' (in this case the waiting time) is artificially held below its 'market clearing' level, a situation of excess demand is certain to exist.

CONCLUSION

Starting from a theoretical interpretation of the NHS waiting list as a rationing device which restricts access to treatment for certain non-urgent conditions, this paper has used a queuing model to investigate the efficiency and equity implications of three theoretical regimes of waiting list management: firstly, treating complainants strictly in the order that they join the queue; secondly, affording higher priority to the more ill and lower priority to the less ill in an attempt to achieve equality between the total level of 'suffering' experienced by all treated complainants; and thirdly, offering rapid treatment to as many seriously ill complainants as the system can cope with comfortably without significant queues starting to build, and offering the remaining (less seriously ill) complainants a prospect of treatment which is so distant or uncertain that they are dissuaded from even joining the queue. We have shown that in the theoretical model, the numbers seeking treatment and the average duration of wait are highest under the first of these regimes and lowest under the third.

A welfare analysis provides strong efficiency arguments in favour of the third of these queue management regimes. The mathematical properties of the queuing model are such that it takes only a relatively small reduction in the numbers treated per period to achieve a large reduction in the size of the queue and the average duration of wait. The model suggests that the benefits to the large majority of more seriously ill complainants who would obtain treatment more rapidly if such a reduction were achieved would outweigh the costs to the small minority of less ill complainants who would thereby be excluded from treatment. In practical terms, it is more efficient for the pool of beds to be utilised at slightly less than full capacity with a negligible queue than it is for utilisation at full capacity with a very large queue. On the other hand, this approach would give cause for concern on grounds of equity, since it discriminates against complainants who are insufficiently ill to receive rapid attention but who are sufficiently ill that they would seek and obtain treatment under either of the other two regimes.

We have also used the model to investigate the theoretical consequences of two shifts of policy regime. On welfare criteria, the analysis tends to argue against the imposition of a guaranteed maximum wait, since the latter would be expected to increase the demand for treatment and therefore raise the level of queuing congestion experienced by all complainants. On the other hand, the model does tend to favour explicit (rather than implicit) rationing of entry to the queue, again due to the potential for efficiency gains through shorter waits for complainants whose need for treatment is most acute.

We have taken a deliberately mechanistic view of the NHS queuing process in order to permit an economic analysis of the type which has been attempted. Of course in practice, there are many ways in which decisions taken by clinical and managerial staff within the NHS can and do influence those characteristics of the service which correspond to the (supposedly fixed) parameters of our queuing model: e.g. GPs and consultants can give complainants greater or lesser encouragement to opt for in-patient treatment; patients can be discharged more or less rapidly after treatment; resources can be switched between different specialisms as priorities change or needs dictate; and so on. Naturally, the inherent flexibility and unpredictability of the NHS in these and many other respects makes quantification of the effects of any change of policy regime an infinitely more speculative and hazardous exercise than anything we have attempted in this paper. Nevertheless, we suggest that none of this fundamentally detracts from the relevance of the theoretical issues of efficiency and equity which we have discussed. In any case, these seem likely to continue to engage the attentions of both theoreticians and practitioners as the debate concerning the future shape and direction of the NHS proceeds.

REFERENCES

Barzel, Y. (1974), A theory of Rationing by Waiting, *Journal of Law and Economics*, 17, 73-95.

Cheung, S.C. (1974), A Theory of Price Control, *Journal of Law and Economics*, 17, 53-71.

Cullis, J. (1993), Waiting Lists and Health Policy, Frankel, S. and West, R. (eds.), Rationing and *Rationality in the National Health Service: the Persistence of Waiting Lists*, Macmillan, Basingstoke, 15-41.

Cullis, J.G., and Jones, P.R. (1985), National Health Service Waiting Lists: a Discussion of Competing Explanations and a Policy Proposal, *Journal of Health Economics*, 4, 119-135.

Cullis, J.G., and Jones, P.R. (1986), Rationing by Waiting List: an Implication, *American Economic Review*, 76, 250-256.

Donaldson, L.J., Maratos, J.I. and Richardson, R.A. (1984), Review of an Orthopaedic In-Patient Waiting List, *Health Trends*, 16, 14-15.

Frankel, S. (1993), The Origins of Waiting Lists, Frankel, S. and West, R. (eds.), *Rationing and Rationality in the National Health Service: the Persistence of Waiting Lists*, Macmillan, Basingstoke, 1-14.

Freemantle, N., Watt, I. and Mason, J. (1993), Developments in the Purchasing Process in the NHS: Towards an Explicit Politics of Rationing? *Public Administration*, vol. 72, 535-548

Frost, C.E.B. (1980), How Permanent are NHS Waiting Lists?, *Social Science and Medicine*, 14C, 1-11.

Gravelle, H.S.E. (1990), *The Efficiency of Rationing by Waiting for Health Care*, Discussion Paper no. 216, Department of Economics, Queen Mary and Westfield College, University of London.

Harrison, S., Hunter, D.J. and Pollitt, C. (1990), *The Dynamics of British Health Policy*, Unwin Hyman, London.

Harrison, S., Hunter, D.J., Johnston, I.H., Nicholson, N., Thunhurst, C. and Wistow, G. (1991), *Health before Health Care*, Social Policy Paper no.4, Institute for Public Policy Research, London.

Harrison, S. and Wistow, G. (1992), The Purchaser/Provider Split in English Health Care: Towards Explicit Rationing?, *Policy and Politics*, 20, 123-130.

Kleinrock, L. (1975), *Queuing Systems vol. 1: Theory*, Wiley-Interscience, New York.

Lindsay, C.M., and Feigenbaum, B. (1984), Rationing by Waiting List, *American Economic Review*, 74, 404-417.

Livny, M., Melamed, B. and Tsiolis, A.K. (1993), The Impact of Autocorrelation on Queuing Systems, *Management Science*, 39, 322-339.

Propper, C. (1990), Contingent Valuation of Time Spent on NHS Waiting Lists, *Economic Journal*, 100, 193-199.

Walters, A.A. (1961), The Theory and Measurement of the Private and Social Cost of Highway Congestion, *Econometrica*, 29, 676-699.

West, R. (1993), Joining the Queue: Demand and Decision-making, Frankel, S. and West, R. (eds.), *Rationing and Rationality in the National Health Service: the Persistence of Waiting Lists*, Macmillan, Basingstoke, 42-62.

Williams, A.H. (1985), Economics of Coronary Artery Bypass Grafting, *British Medical Journal*, 291, 326-329.

Williams, A.H. (1988), Applications in Management, in Teeling Smith, G.F. (ed.)., *Measuring Health: a Practical Approach*, pp. 225-243, Wiley, London.

Worthington, D. (1987), Queuing models for hospital waiting lists, *Journal of the Operational Research Society*, 38, 413-422.

APPENDIX

The queuing model in section 2 is solved and the expressions for p_0 and p_j (for j=1 to ∞) are derived by defining the queuing system to be 'in state j' whenever there are exactly j complainants in the system. Clearly, the system leaves one state and enters an adjacent state every time a complainant joins the queue, withdraws from the queue or is discharged from hospital. Over time, the number of times the system enters each state must approximate (to within one) to the number of times the system leaves the same state. Using the parameters we have already defined, we can therefore set up a series of equations which express these equalities between the rates of entry and exit to and from each state, as follows:

State	Rate at which system enters state		Rate at which system exits state
0	$(d_1 + w_1)p_1$	$=$	ep_0
$j\ (j \geq 1)$	$(d_{j+1} + w_{j+1})p_{j+1} + ep_{j-1} =$		$(d_j + w_j)p_j + ep_j$

These equations, together with the condition that the probabilities that the system

is in state j must sum to one over all values of j $\left(\sum_{j=0}^{\infty} p_j = 1\right)$, allows us to solve for

all values of p_j, as follows:

$$p_0 = \frac{1}{1 + \sum_{j=1}^{\infty} \prod_{h=1}^{j} \left(\dfrac{e}{d_h + w_h}\right)}$$

$$p_j = \prod_{h=1}^{j} \left(\frac{e}{d_h + w_h}\right) p_0 \quad \text{for } j = 1, \ldots \infty$$

Kleinrock (1975) provides a comprehensive exposition of the queuing theory which underlies these results.

The expression for t_j, the expected duration of wait for an 'average' complainant who enters the queue when there are j complainants already in the system (for j≥k) is obtained as follows. The new complainant will be called for treatment as soon as the (j-k) complainants already in the queue have either withdrawn or been called for treatment *and* a bed subsequently becomes available (which requires one further discharge to take place). The expected time for the (j-k) complainants to be cleared from the queue is obtained by defining y_t as the number of these remaining at time t (so y_0=j-k), and finding t such that y_t=0. y_t must satisfy the differential equation

$\dfrac{dy_t}{dt} = -\omega y_t - k\mu$, the solution to which is $y_t = -k\mu/\omega + [((j-k)\omega + k\mu)/\omega]\exp(-\omega t)$.

y_t=0 then requires $t = (1/\omega)\{\ln[(j-k)\omega + k\mu] - \ln(k\mu)\}$. The next bed then becomes available after a further expected wait of $(1/k\mu)$, so the final expression is

$t_j = (1/\omega)\{\ln[(j-k)\omega + k\mu] - \ln(k\mu)\} + (1/k\mu)$.

7 Health Care Planning and Priority Setting - A Modelling Approach

DEREK CRAMP & EWART CARSON

City University

INTRODUCTION

This chapter addresses the role that systems modelling can play in supporting decision making in an area that often presents policy makers and planners with considerable difficulties. This is the efficient allocation of resources, especially where demand exceeds supplies and thus involves the creation of some order of priorities. It requires the choosing of appropriate issues for attention, setting objectives, considering feasible courses of action and making choices from these alternatives. Fixing agenda, setting objectives and determining possible actions is usually called problem solving, while evaluating and making choices is called decision making.

Over the last 50 years or so there has been much research in the domains of operational research, economics, psychology, political science, and more recently artificial intelligence directed at gaining a better understanding of problem solving and decision making and formalising these activities. Particularly, much effort has been directed towards the development of subjective expected utility theory; a sophisticated mathematical model of choice that is the basis of much current econometric and operational research theory.

Complementing this prescriptive approach has been the more empirical study of how decisions are made. A noteworthy result of this research is a greater understanding of the limits that are imposed on rationality due to the complexity of the problems being considered.

Real world economic planning and policy making involves so many factors and activities that it is virtually impossible for the decision maker to give all of them adequate and balanced consideration. Inevitably, there is a tendency to "muddle through" (Lindblom, 1959) with subjective judgements rather than objective evaluation all too often determining choice.

Setting Priorities in Health Care. Edited by M. Malek
© 1994 John Wiley & Sons Ltd

THE SYSTEMS APPROACH

A new approach is required. However, there is some controversy as to the best way to address this problem. It certainly needs a method which is systemic as well as systematic, one that allows feedback and which includes all relevant data in a dynamic fashion. A more rigorous approach that could help in this task is that based on systems theory and modelling methodology. Introducing such models into management practice would be beneficial in the allocation of resources ensuring cost-effective, efficient and appropriate level of care delivery. For many years engineers have recognised the value of developing and making use of models that can assist in the design of systems and increase knowledge about the underlying processes which those systems support. In recent years these approaches have been usefully applied to clinical medicine and physiology (Carson and Cramp, 1985) and to a more limited extent to other clinical processes and activities.

Such systems-based ideas were also extant in management theory, which recognised two basic types of systems: the closed and the open. The closed system is not influenced by and does not interact with its environment while in contrast the open system recognises the dynamic interaction of the system with its environment. The archaic view of Taylor (1911), with its mechanical perception of people and organisations, was essentially a closed system, in contrast to the approach developed by Barnard (1938) who promoted the view, generally accepted today, of the organisation as an open system in constant interaction with its environment .

How can the systems approach be used to manage complexity in the planning and policy making process? (Flood and Carson, 1993). The systems approach envisages a problem, like an organisation, to be made up of, and needing, consideration of the connectivity between numerous interdependent factors, including individuals, groups, attitudes, motives, formal structure, interactions, goals, status and authority.

Thus the basic philosophy underpinning systems thinking is that consideration of isolated portions of complex situations is inadequate, and should involve a dialectic involving the interrelation and interdependence of events. This means that each individual event should not only be considered on its own but also as a part of a larger complexity in a manner that produces a unified whole. As long ago as 1977, Venedictov and Shagan noted that "the health care system is considered to be a complex dynamic system consisting of a set of interrelated subsystems, very closely related to external systems and joined by the common aim: the health of the population. This system also comprises several hierarchical levels -individual, district, national, regional and global" (Venedictov and Shagan, 1977).

MODELLING

A model is an image of reality or an abstraction from reality. It is a way to simulate reality and to represent a system (or problem) which incorporates the variables, constraints and relationships between variables, thought to be critical as a result of an in-depth analysis of the system (or problem). Salient elements are incorporated and minor factors ignored. Unnecessary complexity is minimised so that the system can be described in a form suitable for computer simulation. Provision is made for uncertainty and all the assumptions in making the model are considered explicitly.

MODEL DEVELOPMENT

The development of the model goes through three stages:

- the verbal model, at which stage the objectives for developing the model are identified and the conceptual framework is formulated;
- the symbolic model, the stage at which algorithms and computer models are developed as realisations of the structures and processes of the conceptual framework;
- the dialogue model, at this stage there is simulation of the model whereby various experiments are performed and the model is further adapted according to the needs of the user.

The main objective of the sequence is to allow the decision maker to experiment with different versions under altered external circumstances and to analyse the predictions in order to come up with an optimal strategy for achieving predetermined, although dynamic, goals. It is important that the policy maker or planner is involved in this step. This allows flexibility to be introduced, with the real life limitations recognised by the decision maker being incorporated. It also allows the selection of various resource allocation alternatives as well as needs and demand variations to be taken into account. Thus, if the initial model is not acceptable and often depends on the assumptions in the representation, then further options can be studies until the desired result is approximated and a valid model obtained.

THE CONCEPTUAL MODELS

The first conceptual model developed, shown in Figure 1, is a model which from a systems perspective provided considerable insight into the nature of decision support issues. It emphasised how, from a model-based view of the decision making, the relative importance of the health care process, the wider health outcome loop and resource considerations are all dependent on the clinical context. This could be expressed, from a systems standpoint, in terms of the nature of the system (clinical) problem and the time-scale of the decision process, and whether the decision involved emphasised either the diagnostic or the on-going care dimension.

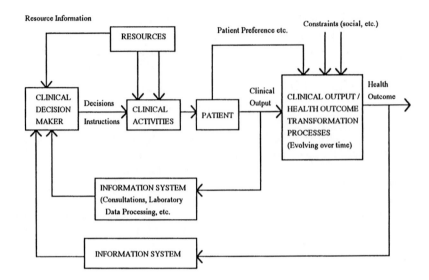

Figure 1. A conceptual model depicting a clinical perspective of health care delivery

This model is being used in the high dependency situation to study cost-benefit and cost-effectiveness issues relating to coronary care and intensive care units. It has also been used as the basis for a study of asthma clinic management at a London teaching hospital trust. The insight gained in these ongoing studies has encouraged the authors to develop the model further into a flexible "total health care" model.

Hitherto, in models of clinical process the patient output dimension (patient state) has been characteristically defined in terms of clinical variables. The concept of health outcome, which in part derives from transformation of such clinical variables, modulated by a wider range of features for a particular patient, is neglected. Similarly, such models do not recognise that a decision for clinical action is an irrevocable commitment to allocate and utilise resources and assumes the availability of such resources. However, it is in these very features that the planner has an interest.

The most recent version of our model is shown in Figure 2. This has been developed to enable greater emphasis to be placed on the resource utilisation element. The principal components are as follows.

Paralleling the previous figure, the lower half of Figure 2 comprises two feedback loops, an inner one with a specific clinical focus and a wider are focusing on health outcome. The decision makers in the context of this figure are the managers involved in health care planning and policy setting. The effecting agent "clinical activities" now includes the clinicians directly managing clinical activity, where the target of this clinical activity in Figure 2 is the patient population. A critical component of the feedback on clinical output provided to decision makers is the information gained via clinical audit.

The other principal feedback loops provide information relating to resources and the patient population. First looking at the patient population, a local feedback on to clinical activity is included reflecting patient choice and the voicing of concerns directly in relation to the health care delivered by the clinical professionals. The information system monitoring the wider and more general patient concerns and their political expression provides feedback to the managers as decision makers. For effective decision making in the context of resource allocation, information is requested on resource availability and cost, together with measures of the efficiency and effectiveness of their use. The first three of these are provided via the direct feedback loop from resources, whilst the issue of effectiveness is informed via outcome measures.

Figure 2 also depicts the means by which a model-based approach can assist management decision making. Through the provision of the relevant models of clinical epidemiology and health status, assistance can be provided in the tasks of needs assessment and advice generation. Simulation models offer a predictive capability, both for examining possible future trends, say on the basis of existing provision, and for examining the likely temporal impact of policy changes. The effectiveness of such model-based decision support provision is, of course, critically dependent upon the availability of necessary data and information relating to resource, clinical output and health outcome as indicated in Figure 2.

DISCUSSION

Prescriptive econometric models are prone to the criticisms that Ackoff (1979a) levied against operational research (OR) models for being concerned with "imagined realities" due to the lack of contact with "real world" situations. He condemned OR for being restricted to "the use of mathematical models and algorithms rather than the ability to formulate management problems, solve them, implement and maintain their solution in a turbulent environment". Ackoff sees the obsession with techniques as a handicap as it dictates the way a problem is envisaged and tackled. He states:

> in the first two decades of OR, its nature was dictated by three techniques it had at its command. The nature of the problems facing managers has changed significantly over the decades, but OR has not. It has not been responsive to the changing needs of management brought about, to a large extent, by radical changes taking place in the environment in which it is practised. While managers were turning outwards, OR was turning inward, inbreeding and inverting. It now appears to have attained the limit of introversion: a catatonic state.

This statement is worth quoting at length because it encapsulates and expresses the problem faced as decision makers try to grapple with the dilemma of trying to meet need, if not demand, with in real terms, diminishing resources. Systems models however, make clear the causal factors responsible for change from one point in time to the next, and thus enable behaviour to be predicted over time. A key emphasis in systems modelling is also placed on the presence of feedback loops. Their value is in helping the decision maker to better understand the relative

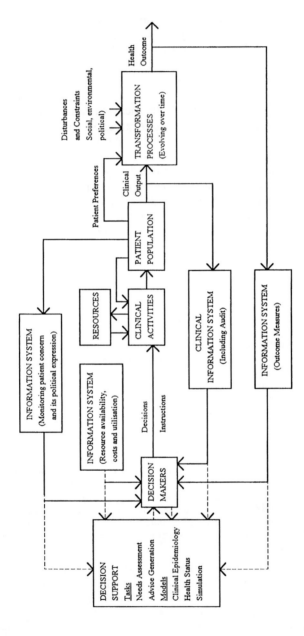

Figure 2. Conceptual model showing the role of decision support in relation to the local health care system

importance of alternative interventions being considered and also anticipate unintended outcomes of proposed plans and policies. This is somewhat different from other formalisms, as it allows the decision maker to be involved in choosing alternatives, which while not minimising costs might provide a better environment.

A further advantage of the systems approach is in the model building itself. This begins with the recognition of the factors responsible for a particular problem, or that might affect performance in a new situation. These factors are then represented in diagrammatic form so as to make their relationships quite clear. These steps when performed with the active participation of the decision maker not only ensure a true modelling of the real world situation, but also help the decision maker to gain a more incisive view of the problem. At the lowest level, involving the decision maker improves the likelihood of the model being used.

Following the development of the initial model structure, it is then expressed in the form of equations, or other appropriate symbolism, for computer simulation. This process of starting with structure rather than data enables decision makers to seek data prospectively and thus gain a better feel for the underlying influences impinging on the system. If actual data are not available estimates can be made. This contrasts with methodologies that are data driven rather than situational, and in which the decision maker can only be a passive participant.

Systems models are based on the holistic notion that all the relevant factors of a problem or situation should be taken into account, and that a problem or situation cannot be fully understood, and therefore modelled, unless these elements and the relationships between them are clarified. More prescriptive formal models tend to ignore the social and political (subjective?) aspects of a problem. Admittedly they do tend to impose constraints on potentially soluble problems!

"The optimal solution of a model is not an optimal solution of a problem unless the model is a perfect representation of the problem" as the writer, Ackoff (1979b), accepts this cannot be achieved but the aim of the system modeller should be to go as far down this path as possible and not to ignore important elements. It is for this reason that system modelling may well provide a valuable adjunct to the decision maker formulating policies and assessing priorities. There is just one caveat. As stated earlier it must be remembered that a model is an abstraction, an interpretation of reality; model behaviour must not be seen as true situational behaviour. It is rather a valuable aid to decision making in highly complex situations.

REFERENCES

Ackoff, R.L. (1979a), The Future of Operational Research is Past!, *Journal of Operational Research Society*, 30 (2), 93-104.

Ackoff, R.L. (1979b), Resurrecting the Future of Operational Research, *Journal of Operational Research Society*, 30 (3), 189-199.

Barnard, C. (1938), *The Functions of the Executive*, Harvard University Press, Cambridge, Mass.

Carson, E.R. and Cramp, D.G. (eds.) (1985), *Computers and Control in Clinical Medicine*, Plenum Press, New York.

Flood, R.L. and Carson, E.R. (1993), *Dealing with Complexity*, Plenum Press, New York.

Lindblom, C.E. (1959), The Science of Muddling Through, *Public Administrative Review*, 19 (3), 79-88.

Taylor, F.W. (1911), *Principles of Scientific Management*, Harper and Brothers, New York.

Venedictov, D.D. and Shigan, E.N. (1977) The IIASA Health Care System Model, Shigan, E.N. and Gibbs, R.J. (eds.), *Modelling Health Care Systems*, IIASA, Laxenburg, 11-19.

8 Health Care Requirements - A Framework for Progress in Priority Setting?

STEPHEN FRANKEL, JOANNA COAST &
JENNY DONOVAN

University of Bristol

INTRODUCTION - MODELS FOR PRIORITY SETTING

There are a number of practical options for priority setting which are advocated. In following any specific model, the priorities which are set will differ considerably from the priorities which would be set using an alternative model. No model is a perfect solution to the problem of priority setting. In fact there is no perfect solution. Each model can, however, be used to try to attain particular objectives, which must be decided upon by the purchasers of health care. In deciding on any specific option to follow, health authorities need to consider the principle behind the model, the resources required to pursue the option, and the likely results.

It would be impossible to assess every priority setting option here. However, the options which purchasing authorities might, perhaps, be considering at the current time are likely to include the following. The simplest option available is to maintain a system of implicit rationing, during which many of the difficult issues considered in this paper need not be confronted. This is unlikely to achieve any particular objectives with any consistency - except to maintain the status quo. A further option may be to set priorities on an arbitrary basis - again this is unlikely to achieve the objectives of health care provision with any consistency.

More structured methods for priority setting include methods based essentially on equity or efficiency principles. Methods based on efficiency principles include versions of cost utility analysis - either similar to the original Oregon formula (Oregon Health Services Commission., 1991) or using a "league table" approach (May, 1992) - or the system of programme budgeting and marginal analysis advocated by Donaldson and Mooney (Donaldson and Mooney, 1991; Mooney *et al.*, 1992). All these methods are based on the objective of maximising the benefit available from health care. Cost utility analysis conducted for particular localities is

Setting Priorities in Health Care. Edited by M. Malek
© 1994 John Wiley & Sons Ltd

likely to be relatively resource intensive, but there are problems with using the "league table" approach: both in the quality of available studies (Coast, 1993; Gerard, 1992) and in combining data from different locations, obtained at different times and based on different utility indices into league tables (Mason *et al.*, 1993; Drummond *et al.*, 1993; Gerard and Mooney, 1993) The programme budgeting method has a number of advantages, in particular that the data requirements are relatively modest, although there is some potential for bias resulting from powerful factions within the decision making group.

There are also methods based essentially on an equity principle: these include setting priorities on the basis of effectiveness (equality according to need defined as ability to benefit), on the basis of need (as assessed by burden of disease) and on the basis of age. Rationing by effectiveness has been advocated as a means of avoiding the problem of priority setting: by using only effective treatments, the health service would be able to cope with all potential requirements (Etzioni, 1991). As with cost utility analysis, either rationing by effectiveness or by "need" is likely to be relatively resource intensive. Rationing by age involves the particular equity principle that the young should be treated in preference to the elderly. Whilst the possibility of rationing by age has received some discussion in the USA (Callahan, 1987; Callahan, 1990; Relman, 1990) it is almost certain that it would be considered unacceptable as an *explicit* policy in the UK where the NHS aims to provide care for all.

Disadvantages of the models

Each of the options discussed above suffers various disadvantages. In particular, the majority of models are based on only one main principle: usually one of equity, efficiency or public participation, and it is this which may be their downfall. It may be inappropriate for the purchasing authority to base its priorities on only one principle, but combining models produces a new difficulty in that there is no mechanism for the trading off of one principle against another.

Further problems which arise with the majority of models are the massive data requirements which exist, particularly given the all-encompassing nature of many models (for example, the Oregon-type model). For most theoretical models the data requirements are large, so that their pursuit likely to be relatively costly: in many cases too costly.

HEALTH CARE REQUIREMENTS - A WAY FORWARD?

A framework for priority setting in health care which might overcome the problems detailed above is that of "health care requirements". This will be discussed in detail, in conjunction with an example of its application in practice. This framework aims to combine principles of equity with those of efficiency and public participation.

Within the framework of health care requirements, it is not expected that detailed analysis should be applied to all aspects of health care; indeed this is unrealistic given the complexities and costs of research in health care, and the practical difficulties of obtaining valid and reliable results.   Instead, priority setting in health care is developed at two levels. The first takes into account the climate surrounding priority setting within health care: the debate which informs attitudes to the different decisions which must be made. General preferences and priorities, therefore, will be informed by such debates as the treatment of the young versus the old, the treatment of so-called self-inflicted conditions versus the treatment of "victims" of disease, as well as general considerations of effectiveness and cost-effectiveness.

At the second, more detailed level, and to be applied selectively to specific areas, is the framework of health care requirements. Each of the principles of equity, efficiency and public participation is taken into account. The equity principle is considered in two ways: firstly by the examination of the distribution of the disease in the population (equity of access according to the general burden of disease within the population) and secondly by the examination of information on effectiveness (equity of access according to ability to benefit). Efficiency is taken into account by combining information on costs with information on effectiveness (in the form of utility). Public preferences are taken into account as the final part of the model and relate to the principle of public participation.

Because each of the different principles is considered explicitly, the resulting priorities are less likely to suffer from omissions of important data than many other models. A particular problem that occurs with all models that aim to take account of more than one principle is that the data must be traded-off in some way - so that all aspects can be taken into consideration. This is a notoriously difficult area (for example, consider the controversy which surrounds the trading-off of quality and quantity of life which is attempted in the quality-adjusted life-year), basically involving a value judgement about the relative importance of each of the relevant areas. It is important to stress that these decisions are concerned with making value judgements rather than applying some form of scientific methodology.

There are two main methods by which data may be traded-off. The first is analogous to the method used in the QALYs (Quality Adjusted Life Years): attempting to develop a formula which takes into account each of the different principles. In practice this is likely to be impossible with such different areas as the population distribution of a condition, the effectiveness and cost-effectiveness of interventions and public opinion about treatment: each of these is likely to be expressed in different and non-comparable ways, thus making any sort of formula unusable.

The second alternative is to consider each aspect of the model in terms of the levels of support reached. This is somewhat analogous to the method of "sieving" advocated by the document *Choices in Health Care*, which sets out the method to be used in the Netherlands for priority setting (Government Committee on Choices in Health Care, 1992). In *Choices for Health Care* it is recommended that care is passed through each of four "sieves" in turn, with each sieve representing one important aspect of health care. Using this alternative for the health care requirements framework would imply that any intervention would have to reach a particular level of effectiveness, cost-effectiveness and public support to be provided by the purchasing authority. Again value judgements, which may vary by condition or circumstances, need to be made by the purchasing authority to determine these specific levels. In addition, the model of health care requirements would attempt to assess the distribution of a disease in the community, in part to assess the relevant margins for health care, and in part to ensure that access to treatment for different conditions with similar effectiveness, cost-effectiveness and public support is equitable.

Grand plans and statements of intent are associated with most models which are advocated for the purposes of priority setting, and generally these models are unsuccessful in achieving their objectives. It is important here, therefore, to stress two particular aspects of the framework of health care requirements. Firstly, it does not aim to investigate all the possible areas of health care intervention at one time, and secondly, three practical steps for action are contained within the framework. Each of these aspects will be discussed in turn.

Areas for investigation

In practice it will take much time and hard work before the health service is able to set priorities in any realistic sense. This is recognised explicitly here and therefore detailed examination of specific areas with particular difficulties, within a general framework of debate and rational choice, is advocated. Fitting particular areas into the general framework will be difficult and is likely to take place on a relatively crude basis. It is impracticable, however, to attempt to change the whole pattern of services at one time. The process is comparable to doing a jigsaw in which certain parts of the picture are concentrated on at any one time.

Particular areas of health care may be chosen for more detailed study for a number of reasons. Areas of concern may include interventions aimed at treating particular common and expensive conditions, for example stroke; interventions which aim to service particular client groups, for example the mental health services; interventions which have something particular in common, for example the large volume elective surgery conditions; interventions from one particular specialty; etc.. It is important, however, that the not inconsiderable resources involved in applying the model of health care requirements, should be allocated, at least in the first instance, to areas of particular uncertainty or confusion or of particularly high cost. Prioritising areas for prioritisation is, inevitably, a priority!

Three steps for action

Having chosen a specific aspect of health care intervention for study, three steps are advocated, as shown below. Each step should consider carefully and methodically the evidence for the essential aspects of priority setting: population distribution of disease, effectiveness, cost-effectiveness and public preference which, as outlined above, enable the process of priority setting to take into account the principles of equity, efficiency and public participation.

Examination of existing literature and routinely available data

The first step which should always be pursued with regard to the area of interest is to consider the existing literature and routinely available data. It is important that these analyses include the evidence regarding the population distribution of indications for an intervention, the effectiveness of treatment, the cost-effectiveness of treatment, and any information on the public desire for the intervention to be provided. Such forms of analysis are becoming more common and are supported, for example, by the Department of Health funding the production of both the Effective Health Care Bulletins (Long and Sheldon, 1992) and the Epidemiologically Based Needs Assessments (Donovan *et al.*, 1992; Williams *et al.*, 1992b; Williams *et al.*, 1992c; Williams *et al.*, 1992a; Williams *et al.*, 1992d) and are also a major output of health services research units. These analyses are useful for considering particular conditions, although they are generally insufficient for the purposes of priority setting in that they do not usually involve comparisons between different conditions, and do not always set the particular intervention in the context even of its own specialty.

Research without data collection - utilisation of consensus

The second step is to consider the conduct of research without dedicated data collection. Such research is concerned with obtaining consensus about the priorities which should be set, and in particular, the formulation of guidelines to assist in decision making. Such consensus is generally obtained from experts in the field, but it is not inconceivable that those making decisions should include other interested parties such as members of the public or particular pressure groups. Of other available methods for priority setting, this second step is perhaps closest, in form at least, to the method of programme budgeting and marginal analysis as advocated by Mooney *et al.*,. (Mooney *et al.*, 1992). For the purposes of the health care requirements model, however, the analysis should consider each of the essential aspects of priority setting, and should not be limited exclusively to the consideration of efficiency, as in the programme budgeting and marginal analysis model.

Dedicated research

The third step is to perform dedicated research in each of the essential areas, using a methodology to enable the maximisation of the research potential from limited resources. The population distribution of disease will be assessed by studies of the prevalence and incidence of the chosen conditions in specific areas. Assessment of the effectiveness (or outcome) of an intervention and of the costs of treatment will be performed using observational studies, or where possible, experimental studies such as randomised controlled trials, with untreated patients being identified from the population study. The public desire for the treatment of particular conditions will need to be elicited by qualitative and quantitative research with patients and members of the public.

Priority setting in Health Care Requirements

It is important to consider how each of these steps can contribute to the overall priority setting process. The first step, of literature review and routine data analysis, can provide information about each of the areas of interest (population distribution, effectiveness, efficiency, public opinion). It is likely, however, that in many cases the research will be either inadequate or non-existent (Donovan *et al.*, 1992; Williams *et al.*, 1992b; Williams *et al.*, 1992c; Williams *et al.*, 1992a; Williams *et al.*, 1992d; Robbins *et al.*, 1992) In the short term, however, such reviews will provide purchasing authorities with at least some systematic basis for the decisions that they must take. Where there is already adequate information for the setting of priorities, even if not previously identified, this information can be used and steps two and three need not be pursued. The second step is intended to provide a medium term solution for those interventions for which there is insufficient evidence contained in the existing literature and routine data sources. Whilst such consensus research is unlikely to be adequate in the longer term, it can give purchasers further basis for priority setting where the existing information is inadequate for such important decisions. It is when the evidence which experts draw on to reach decisions is inadequate that step three is required. The conduct of rigorous research in step three will provide detailed information for the setting of priorities in the long term and must then be combined with empirically obtained data about public preferences.

Earlier in this paper brief consideration was given to the problems associated with trading-off the different principles which inform the priority setting process. Two methods of trading-off one principle against another were mentioned: neither of these seem practical at the present time, given the current state of knowledge in this area. To develop formulae of the type:

$$\text{priority} = 0.5 \text{ effectiveness} + 0.3 \text{ efficiency} + 0.1 \text{ public preferences} + 0.1 \text{ population distribution}$$

is patently ridiculous, given the numerous ways in which each of these variables can be measured. It is similarly impossible, at the present time, to set levels of each of the variables which must be reached, as there is no basis upon which to identify such levels for most conditions. There is also little information about the costs of different forms of health care, without which it is impossible to know what quantity of different items could be provided and therefore the relative levels which should be set.

One solution may lie in the use of a "balance sheet" approach to inform particular areas of decision making. These "balance sheets" could contain all the available information regarding the principles outlined above for each of the interventions being considered. Ideally the information should be collated for differing severities of each condition. Purchasing authorities may then use their own value judgements to decide, on the basis of this information, which specific treatments for which specific severities of illness should be considered priorities. In a country such as the UK, where health authorities are being encouraged to think about priorities on a local basis, each purchasing authority could be encouraged to make its own value judgements about the relative importance of these principles.

It may be argued that many purchasing authorities already combine this sort of information implicitly. It is important, however, that each of the different forms of data is explicitly considered and compared across the interventions for which the decision is being made. Detailed and methodical scrutiny of each of the component areas is required in the schema of health care requirements.

It is important to stress here that this model does not require that any principle be subordinate to any other. Each purchasing authority will wish to make its own value judgements about the relative importance of each principle in line with its policy objectives, and will therefore wish to be relatively consistent in the weight it gives to each item across decisions.   The quality of evidence in particular cases may additionally affect the relative weight given to each item in the balance sheet. In general, therefore, a purchasing authority might give greater weight to public preferences rather than effectiveness, but where evidence about effectiveness is good and that concerning preferences is weak, it might prefer to put more weight on the evidence concerning effectiveness.

"HEALTH CARE REQUIREMENTS" IN PRACTICE - THE EXAMPLE OF ELECTIVE SURGERY

The area of elective surgery is one which has been covered in confusion since the initiation of the National Health Service: there is much uncertainty about the appropriate levels of provision (Coast, 1993), and thus it is an appropriate area in which to apply the model of health care requirements. Within the general area of elective surgery there are many interventions for many conditions - too many for the detailed consideration discussed above. For this example it was, therefore, necessary to further reduce the interventions of interest to a manageable number. This was done by using the criteria that the chosen interventions should be important in terms of the volume of activity, and the cost to society, that they represent. A further criterion in this case was that study of the conditions and interventions should be feasible in the general population.

For the first step of the analysis, reviews incorporating existing literature and routine data were conducted.(Donovan *et al.*, 1992; Williams *et al.*, 1992b; Williams *et al.*, 1992c; Williams *et al.*, 1992a; Williams *et al.*, 1992d)   These reviews highlighted the great level of uncertainty regarding all aspects of these interventions: for none of the interventions was it possible to provide detailed unequivocal information about the population distribution of disease, the effectiveness or the cost-effectiveness of treatment, or the level of public desire for the intervention to be provided.

The second and third steps of the analysis are presently being undertaken.   The second step aims to set criteria for treatment of each of the conditions based on the consensus of clinicians.   Researchers are experimenting with a number of methods of obtaining consensus about the indications for treatment.   During this early use of the health care requirements model, concern has focused mainly on the effectiveness of treatment, with less consideration being given to cost-effectiveness, public preferences and the prevalence and incidence of the condition in the population.

The Somerset and Avon Survey of Health (SASH), being conducted by the Health Care Evaluation Unit, is presently accumulating data to establish the prevalence and incidence of these conditions in the local population.   The SASH study also incorporates a qualitative assessment of public preference for treatment of the various conditions and provides non-concurrent controls for the investigation of effectiveness and cost-effectiveness of interventions.   These latter two assessments will be conducted observationally using cohorts of individuals being treated by surgery in hospital, with specific questions of effectiveness and cost-effectiveness being answered using randomised controlled trials.

An example of the type of data produced by the Health Care Requirements framework is given below, based on the balance sheet approach, and utilising data on hip and knee replacement obtained from the Epidemiologically Based Needs Assessments. Because of the poor quality of the data obtained during these literature reviews, it is not possible to classify the data for the varying degrees of severity of conditions requiring hip or knee replacement.   Clearly attempts to form such balance sheets at the present time suffer from the poor quality of the majority of the data, and it is essential that the quality of the data should be classified as part of the process of forming the balance sheet.   Methods for the assessment of the quality of evidence thus need to be devised which can be applied to each of the four areas.   These could be similar to the scheme developed to assess quality of effectiveness evidence by the US Preventive Services Task Force (Report of the US Preventive Services Task Force, 1989) and adapted by Williams *et al.,*. (Williams *et al.*, 1992a) This is shown in table 1, and is used to assess the quality of the evidence concerning effectiveness in table 2. It is vital that, where evidence is relatively poor (for example regarding the comparative cost-effectiveness of the different procedures), this is acknowledged.

Table 1. Quality of evidence according to US Preventive Services Task Force, 1989 (Report of the US Preventive Services Task Force, 1989) adapted by Williams *et al.*, (Williams *et al.*, 1992a)

I	Evidence obtained from at least one properly designed, randomised controlled trial.
II-1	Evidence obtained from well-designed controlled trials without randomisation.
II-2	Evidence obtained from well-designed cohort or case-control analytic studies, preferably from more than one centre or research group.
II-3	Evidence obtained from multiple time series with or without intervention. Dramatic results in uncontrolled experiments (such as the results of the introduction of penicillin treatment in the 1940s) could also be regarded as this type of evidence.
III	Opinions of respected authorities, based on clinical experience, descriptive studies or reports of expert committees.
IV	Evidence inadequate owing to problems of methodology (e.g. sample size, length or comprehensiveness of follow-up) or conflicts in evidence.

Table 2. Balance sheet comparing hip replacement with knee replacement for each of the four elements of health care requirements

	Population Distribution of need for surgery	Q	Effectiveness	Q	Cost-Effectiveness	Q	Public preferences	Q
KNEES - treatment by total knee replacement	Various estimates of prevalence and incidence based on small clinical samples. No clear estimates available for indications for surgery.		Pain relief & satisfactory function in 90% cases, but deep wound infection occurs in 0.5-2% cases, and for all cases there is a 2-3% probability of revision after 6 years [various studies - see Williams *et al.* - knee]	III	Poor estimates of cost per QALY - not sufficiently robust for decision making.		No evidence yet	
HIPS - treatment by total hip replacement	No clear estimates available for indications for surgery.		72-100% obtain pain relief and improved mobility, but 5-10% of patients experience complications. There is a 1-2% failure rate per annum [various studies - see Williams *et al.*, - hip]	III	Poor estimates of cost per QALY - not sufficiently robust for decision making.		No evidence yet	

Q = Quality of evidence (based on table 1 for effectiveness column)
Williams M - hip (Williams *et al.*, 1992c), Williams M - knee (Williams *et al.*, 1992b)

Given the poor evidence in table 2, it is likely that any immediate decisions made on the basis of health care requirements would be related mainly to the effectiveness of treatment and the distribution of illness at this stage. Decisions will therefore relate to the value judgements made by the purchasing authority about the relative importance of equity, as assessed by equality of treatment according to ability to benefit, and equity as assessed by equality of treatment according to the numbers of individuals suffering from a condition. The balance sheet helps to indicate areas where resources should be most urgently directed. Research currently underway at the HCEU seeks to inform each of the elements. When these data are available it will be possible to use the scheme to its full potential to illuminate this one small area. There is also the intention to put other elective surgery conditions alongside, but the work is still very much in progress.

Although this table is of use in illustrating the possible methodology of the framework of health care requirements, it is just that: an illustration. It indicates the kind of decisions and information which are required, as well as the poverty of information which exists. In this example only two particular interventions are compared, but in the future the model could be used to compare a number of different interventions concurrently.

CONCLUSION

Whilst there are no easy answers to the choices which purchasing authorities must make if they are to set priorities, and there are no perfect options which will produce a simple formula for priority setting, a series of steps which could be followed by a purchasing authority is outlined above. "Health Care Requirements" is not a solution to all the difficulties associated with setting priorities explicitly, but sets out a framework within which the available empirical evidence can be assessed. The framework is particularly useful for identifying areas which would benefit from further research. Where such data are not available it suggests both medium and long term solutions.

With the Health Care Requirements framework each of the principles of equity, efficiency and public participation is considered, but the value judgements about the relative importance of each of these remains to be decided by those setting priorities for particular localities. While this framework does not intend to be the final solution to the setting of priorities, it marks an attempt, currently in progress, to illuminate and elaborate the factors involved in an important and confused area of provision: elective surgery.

REFERENCES

Callahan, D. (1987), *Setting limits. Medical goals in an ageing society*, Simon and Schuster, New York.

Callahan, D. (1990), *What kind of life. The limits of medical progress*, Simon and Schuster, New York.

Coast, J. (1993), The role of economic evaluation in setting priorities for elective surgery, *Health Policy*, 24, 243-257.

Donaldson, C. and Mooney, G. (1991), Needs assessment, priority setting, and contracts for health care: an economic view, *Br Med J*, 303, 1529-1530.

Donovan, J., Frankel, S., Nanchahal, K., Coast, J. and Williams, M. (1992), *Epidemiologically based needs assessment: Prostatectomy for benign prostatic hyperplasia*, Health Care Evaluation Unit, Bristol.

Drummond, M., Torrance, G. and Mason, J. (1993), Cost-effectiveness league tables: more harm than good? *Soc Sci Med*, 37(1), 33-40.

Etzioni, A. (1991), Health care rationing: a critical evaluation, *Health Affairs*, 10(2), 88-95.

Gerard, K. (1992), Cost-utility in practice: a policy maker's guide to the state of the art, *Health Policy*, 21, 249-279.

Gerard, K. and Mooney, G. (1993), QALY League tables: handle with care, *Health Economics*, 2, 29-64.

Government Committee on Choices in Health Care, (1992), *Choices in Health Care*, Ministry of Welfare, Health and Cultural Affairs, Rijswijk.

Long, A.F. and Sheldon, T.A. (1992), Enhancing effective and acceptable purchaser and provider decisions: overview and methods, *Quality in Health Care*, 1, 74-76.

Mason, J., Drummond, M. and Torrance, G. (1993), Some guidelines on the use of cost effectiveness league tables, *Br Med J*, 306, 570-572.

May, A. (1992), Perfect purchasing, *Health Service Journal*, 16 July, 23-24.

Mooney, G., Gerard, K., Donaldson, C. and Farrar, S. (1992), *Priority setting in purchasing. Some practical guidelines*, NAHAT, Birmingham.

Oregon Health Services Commission, (1991), *Prioritization of Health Services. A report to the Governor and Legislature*, Oregon Health Services Commission,

Relman, A.S. (1990), Is rationing inevitable? *New Eng J Med*, 322(25), 1809-1810.

Report of the US Preventive Services Task Force, (1989), *Guide to the clinical preventive services*, W and W, Baltimore.

Robbins, M., Frankel, S., Nanchahal, K., Coast, J. and Williams, M. (1992), *Epidemiologically based needs assessment: Varicose vein treatments*, Health Care Evaluation Unit, Bristol.

Williams, M., Frankel, S., Coast, J., Nanchahal, K. and Donovan, J. (1992a), *Epidemiologically based needs assessment: Cataract surgery*, Health Care Evaluation Unit, Bristol.

Williams, M., Frankel, S., Nanchahal, K., Coast, J. and Donovan, J. (1992b), *Epidemiologically based needs assessment: Total knee replacement*, Health Care Evaluation Unit, Bristol.

Williams, M., Frankel, S., Nanchahal, K., Coast, J. and Donovan, J. (1992c), *Epidemiologically based needs assessment: Total hip replacement*, Health Care Evaluation Unit, Bristol.

Williams, M., Frankel, S., Nanchahal, K., Coast, J. and Donovan, J. (1992d), *Epidemiologically based needs assessment: Hernia repair*, Health Care Evaluation Unit, Bristol.

9 Marketing in the National Health Service

SHARON SCAGGS[1], LOUISE BELL[2], REVA BERMAN BROWN[3] & SEAN MCCARTNEY[3]

[1]*Thameside Community Health Care NHS Trust*
[2]*Southend Health Care NHS Trust*
[3]*University of Essex*

INTRODUCTION

The activities of service industries worldwide are increasingly dominated by large private and public sector organisations (Howells and Green, 1988). The NHS is a large public sector industry and is said to be the largest single employer in the UK. It is a multistage organisation providing health care services to the vast majority of the UK's population. Changes in the NHS, such as those outlined in *Working for Patients* (1989) and the Patient's Charter (1992), have created a service that is beginning to introduce certain marketing techniques to help achieve business success.

The White Paper, *Working for Patients*, proposed the development of an internal market within the NHS. It suggested that certain General Practitioners (GPs) would be given their own budgets with which to purchase certain treatments for their patients. Some hospitals would become autonomous, self-governing trusts. Individual responsibilities of clinicians would increase, with these professionals gaining greater responsibility for treatments and care given to patients.

This paper begins with a discussion of current marketing theories, discussing their relevance for the NHS. We describe what is emerging in the Service and what theorists suggest may be appropriate in order to consider whether or not there is a need for marketeers in the NHS.

THE MARKET PHILOSOPHY

In the NHS, the creation of the internal market and autonomous, self-governing trusts in both the community and acute sectors have meant that there is increasing pressure on health service institutions to sell their services. Selling services has

Setting Priorities in Health Care. Edited by M. Malek
© 1994 John Wiley & Sons Ltd

required the development of strategies to market them in such a way that the institutions succeed financially, to ensure their existence in the future.

Marketing is a matter of overall strategy, rather than a series of uncoordinated initiatives. It can be of value, even in the absence of competition, as it offers an effective means of deploying resources and transfers some power to consumers.

There is increasing evidence throughout the NHS relating to the way the Service has begun to incorporate strategies and activities which have previously been the domain of commercial and industrial enterprises. There are now quality departments, communications and public relations departments, information departments etc.

Previously, these kinds of departments were seen solely in the commercial sector, and NHS activity focused on providing health care services. Advances in technology, changes in treatments, and demographic, political and social changes have created the need for commercial activities within the service. The essence of the Griffiths Report (1983) was that the NHS needed to become more business-like in its approach.

One of the ideas currently in vogue in the NHS is the notion of corporate, or strategic planning, which looks at the long-term of the organization. In commerce and industry, the corporate planning process aims to produce a statement which includes corporate financial objectives for the long-term planning period of the company. These are often shown as turnover, profit, or return on investment. The long-term horizon for corporate planning is usually five years, but fluctuates depending on the nature of the markets in which the company operates.

The NHS is beginning to initiate various long-term planning type activities, which can be seen in various guises. The consolidation of property in community trusts, selling of land, creation of private wards in trusts are all measures designed to improve the long-term future success of the organization. This kind of corporate planning will, it is hoped, create additional revenue which may be used to support the organization, reduce expenditure, consolidate services, and lead to a more efficient and effective use of staff.

Since *Working for Patients* (1989), the NHS has begun to strengthen its skills in the field of marketing, taking examples of techniques from those already in use in industry and commerce. Competitive strategies, outcome measurements, and the establishment of data relating to costs have begun to play a far larger part of the NHS's activities because of the need to be effective in the selling of services to purchasing consortia and GPs.

Competitive strategies may not yet be of the same importance or significance in the NHS as in the world of business and commerce. Health Service managers, however, are coming to terms with working in a more competitive environment. Regardless of the organization and the nature of its business, knowledge of the environment in which it operates and the competitive forces that play on it are crucial to survival (Coad and Kennedy, 1992: 11).

The introduction of a managed market in health services has necessitated the emergence of the need to gather information about market share and market penetration, because the NHS trusts and provider units need to sell services to ensure their survival as separate entities.

Certain Trusts have the geographical monopoly on market share while others are surrounded by competitors who challenge NHS provision and have entered the market, providing cheaper, better quality, or outcome-focused treatments that sell to GPs. This is leading some Trusts to become isolationist, guarding information relating to their services, rather than sharing and disseminating information which they consider might give local competitors a business advantage.

As a consequence, it can be said that, to some extent, the NHS has become more dynamic, and hospitals are beginning to establish viability in the business sense. The increasing number of GP fundholders, and the need to maintain a competitive edge within a market, has allowed various outside agencies (such as MIND or housing associations) to establish contracts to provide services that were previously in the domain of the NHS (Coad and Kennedy, 1992).

Business plans and marketing strategies have been seen as ways of improving quality, monitoring activity, reducing costs, and increasing revenue and productivity. The need to develop commercial-type skills is highlighted when one considers the possibility that certain units may cease to be viable if they lose revenue because their purchasers prefer competitors' services.

THE MARKETING PROCESS IN THE NHS

While selling is part of marketing, marketing itself is far more than simply selling. Once a Trust decides that it needs to market its services, it needs, initially, to define its market, and then to decide upon and implement its marketing mix. The commercial marketing process is described below, with emphasis placed on how one might go about marketing in the NHS, using a hypothetical NHS Trust as the example.

DEFINING THE MARKET

The decision of a Trust to market its services requires it to define the constituency in which its marketing will operate. Kotler and Clarke (1987) define the 'market' as the set of all people who have an actual or potential interest in a product or service. In the case of a Community Trust, for example, the market may be those people living or working within its catchment area.

While, many people living within the defined market area will need to use the health services which the organization is providing, some doubtless will not. The Trust's Board will have to decide whether to serve all sectors of the community, that is to provide for a mass market, or whether to focus efforts on selecting more appealing markets, thus restricting business to a smaller, but potentially more needy target market. A health market may be sectorized in a number of ways, for example by age, gender, a   of domicile, employment status or even medical condition.

THE MARK   ING MIX

After defining the intended market, the Trust will need to develop a marketing mix to maintain its ability to compete within the market. A marketing mix is defined by

Kotler and Clarke (1987) as the particular blend of controllable marketing variables which an organization uses to achieve its objectives within the target market.

McCarthy (1978) categorised the marketing mix as consisting of the four "Ps": product, price, promotion, place. These are discussed more fully below from the point of view of the provision of health care.

PRODUCT

In the language of marketing, 'product' is not necessarily a material object. It can be a service, and for the NHS, 'products' are all health care services provided to 'consumers', as patients would be termed.

In the community setting, the products cover such services as Mental Health, Primary Care, or Learning Disabilities. There are also professions allied to medicine in community settings such as Dentistry, Chiropody, Occupational and Speech Therapy.

In the acute setting, hospitals provide both in- and out-patient services such as medical, surgical, and rehabilitative care, as well as offering facilities for out-patients in areas such as diabetic or renal care. Separate individual product lines (as marketeers would term health care treatments and interventions) exist within the services provided by the NHS. These are specialist treatments provided by separate professions such as Psychiatrists, Psychologists, Psychotherapists, Radiologists, or Surgeons, or specialist nursing staff working in the Mental Health Services, or Health Visitors in the Primary Care setting, or Paediatric Nurses in the Acute setting. Consumers (in their guise as patients of the NHS) receive 'packages of care', which comprise all elements of treatments given by the gamut of different professionals.

If our hypothetical trust is an Acute Trust, it needs to bear in mind when implementing its marketing strategy, that there are certain products (services) which it must offer because they are statutorily required core services, for example Accident and Emergency. There are, however, other products which it can regard as optional extras, and it can choose to provide these because they are lucrative, effective, reduce waiting times or increase consumer choice. Services like Podiatry (minor foot surgery) are included in the list of optional extras. Survival of the Trust within the internal market will depend upon its making successful choices of product mix by selecting the most appropriate optional extras, while meeting statutory requirements.

The Trust must also take into account that their products will be at different stages in their life cycle; some will be in the developmental stage, others will be functioning well and creating revenue, and for some, there will be a drop in demand.

Marketeers use the term 'product life cycle' describe four different stages of a product: introduction, growth, maturity, and decline. The life cycle of the Trust's mix of product lines is considered in more detail below.

Introduction

In the introduction phase, new products are developed, refined and introduced into the market place - in the case of the NHS, this is likely to be the local community.

This initial stage is the most resource-intensive for any Trust wishing to enlarge its product range by means of the establishment of new products (in non-marketing-speak, to develop their services). Costs will be high in the introductory stage because of slow take-up, initial capital expenditure and promotional expenses.

For the hypothetical Trust, an example of this process could be the development and introduction of a Podiatric service for patients who would otherwise have to wait for referral to orthopaedic surgeons with long waiting lists. The advantages of the introduction of such a service are that it reduces waiting times, increases consumer choice, and is more cost-effective than orthopaedic surgery. The Trust will need to consider the initial expenditure for any new service, which in the case of Podiatry, includes the need for an operating theatre, a sterile environment, equipment, and qualified assistants.

The Trust may establish new products at the request of its purchasers (GP fundholders or purchasing consortia), or may use the information it has derived from market research to persuade purchasers of the need for the new product. Market research is a useful exercise where resources are constrained because the results could be used to establish both the need for, and the requirements of, new and already-established services.

The need for the Podiatry service in the Trust may for example, have been highlighted subsequent to the receipt of high numbers of complaints about long waiting times for minor surgery, long-term pain, increased use of other services due to disability etc. Minor surgery carried out by orthopaedic surgeons is resource-intensive and often waiting lists are long; Podiatry where appropriate, however, provides an alternative that is quick, cheap and offers patients greater choice.

Kotler and Clarke (1987: 339) point out that

> Unfortunately, it is the norm in the health care environment to provide inadequate support to new products and services. As a result, insufficient demand is generated, leading managers to conclude the new product or service was not a good idea.

We will assume, however, that the hypothetical Trust will support the introduction of new products, leading to the next stage in their life cycle, that of growth.

Growth

The growth stage for new NHS products begins when the expectations of those consumers who comprise the health market grow, and demand begins to increase. Consumers using the product early on in its life (the guinea pigs, or in marketing language, the 'early adopters'), and satisfied with it, will carry on using it. This sets a reassuring pattern for other future consumers who may then follow their example and utilise the service.

GP fundholder consortia, for instance, regularly discuss 'product offers' and new products in order to make purchasing decisions. These purchasing consortia may become increasingly instrumental in influencing service developments because what they wish to purchase for their patients will become that which will sell. If the consortia hear of products that are more cost-effective, of better quality, or which create additional consumer choice, the availability of services will grow.

The growth of the health market generally (outside the growth of new products provided within the NHS) is attracting new groups of competitors such as chiropractors and osteopaths into what was previously a closed service which did not include such alternative professional groups. GPs now employ such professionals on contracts to work on their behalf with patients who had not responded to medical interventions.

The failure of the medical model to treat specific disorders such as eczema has led to Chinese medicine and acupuncture being used within the health service. The adoption of these new product lines can be viewed as the beginnings of an inclusive service within the NHS.

Where both potential and actual treatments are concerned, marketing may be useful in selling their benefits and in increasing consumer choice. The current philosophy of the NHS is basically about using available resources to treat patients effectively and efficiently. Using alternatives to the existing medical paradigms does increase consumer choice, and marketing has its place to play in this process. Such 'fringe' professions (previously marginalised by the NHS) as osteopathy have been encouraged by the creation of the new health market and they are in the process of taking up the possibilities that this has created for them.

It is here that the technique of market research will benefit the NHS, as it is an effective means through which to establish the market relevance of these newly emerging professional groups, and will provide information about the efficacy of harnessing their services for inclusion within mainstream services. Such inclusion may well result in the reduction of market competition and the introduction of further sources of revenue into the NHS.

Private practitioners present competition to the NHS, and many agencies have been set up which are able to provide a range of health services and products. These agencies may be able to offer competitively priced products because of reduced overheads or variations in product delivery, enabling them to provide products which cost less than the same product provided by local Trusts. These are issues which would benefit from the existence of marketing specialists who can examine such challenges and suggest strategies which would enable trusts to maintain their market share.

While the introduction of new products and the ensuring of their growth are never problem-free, the next stage in the product life cycle involves a different set of difficulties.

Maturity

The attainment of the maturity stage of a product can be recognised as the time when the rate of sales growth slows down but sales continue at a satisfactory level. It is suggested that once this stage has been reached, marketing can fall back to the level necessary to maintain brand loyalty (Sheaff, 1991). A product can be seen to have reached maturity in marketing terms is the baby clinic offered by GPs. From a marketing perspective, such a clinic is no longer a new product, and it has passed its introduction and growth phases. It has reached maturity in that it is consistently utilised by the market - parents who have a new child - and take-up of the product has reached a satisfactory level.

In commerce and industry, the achievement of the maturity stage of a product is likely to result in efforts to step up promotional activities to maintain market share. Improvements in the product line are another technique used to hold onto market share, and this may lead to expense which requires cost cutting. Maintenance of market share can result in higher costs, and weaker competitors who are unable to maintain the processes will leave the arena for well-established competitors who aim to gain greater competitive advantage.

The hypothetical Trust, now that it has developed its marketing process, may well find itself involved in these kinds of difficulties in its attempts to maintain the market share of its products which have reached maturity. If it is unsuccessful, its products will enter the last phase of the product life cycle, that of decline.

Decline

A number of reasons may result in the decline of a product. In the health care setting, these may include technical innovation, advances in medicine and increased knowledge, which results in the reduction of the need for what were previously essential services.

A clear example of the decline of a product is the tonsillectomy. Whether the explanation given for the drastic reduction in the number of those treated with this surgical intervention is attributed to increased knowledge about the non-necessity for this operation as a treatment for tonsillitis, or explained as a change in fashion in the practice of medicine, the tonsillectomy is a product clearly in decline.

The hypothetical Trust will eventually have to face the implications of carrying weak products for which there is a declining market. Although it is difficult to estimate the full cost of continuing to provide weak products, the price of would have to include management time, staffing, promotional activities, and resources which conceivably would be better focused on more efficient products. The continuance of a weak product may also have cost implications relating to damage to the corporate image of the organization because of maintaining a treatment or service which is seen as ineffective or unnecessary.

PRICE

Cost leadership may be a strategy that the Trust chooses to pursue, although cash limiting may impede this process in the future. The rising numbers of GP fundholders results in diminishing resources available to purchasing authorities. Direct competition for resources between both these groups is designed to gradually introduce the GP purchasers into the health market. This does, however, effectively reduce income for purchasing consortia.

Unlike the commercial sector, the NHS is discouraged from making 'profits' on the products it supplies. It is here that the NHS is between a rock and a hard place. It is actively encouraged to seek value for money initiatives but the purpose of these is not to accumulate surplus revenue or profit but rather to improve effectiveness and efficiency.

The general idea appears to be one of reducing costs by increasing efficiency whilst not making any profits. This goal is achievable through actions like an examination of the staff skill mix, changing the qualification status of health care professionals, introducing National Vocational Qualification (NVQ) trainees, or developing day-stay surgery.

Recent years have seen the increased introduction of unqualified staff who perform certain specific tasks previously carried out by qualified staff who belong to one of many professional registration bodies. Speech Therapy Assistants, Foot Care Assistants and National Vocational Trainees are in evidence throughout the NHS, performing various tasks from nail clipping to assessing patients' needs. On occasion, this process has led to the reduction in costs for providing certain services, which has resulted in more competitive pricing rather than accumulation of profit.

PROMOTION

Sheaff (1991) states that in a commercial setting, the heart of promotion is selling techniques, among which branding, merchandising and packaging are basic components. Active advertising and promotion of health care services is not (yet?) a feature in the United Kingdom, although the radio station Classic FM carries advertising for a private hernia treatment centre.

The hypothetical Trust will encounter difficulties with promotion because it is prevented from using many of the commercial promotion activities. There are advertising guidelines which exist for health care professionals from the various associations, and doctors are forbidden from advertising themselves as better or more qualified than their colleagues. An acceptable promotion activity which the Trust could initiate would be to provide leaflets and service directories that are given to potential purchasers, describing services on offer, explaining how they can be accessed, and discussing referral criteria. Already pricing tariffs are a feature in such literature and in the future, as the Trust refine its approach to pricing policy, this will doubtless increase.

PLACE

In marketing terminology, the 'place' is the location where the product is available. In the NHS, the term 'place' can be applied to locations such as hospitals or clinics where product lines are delivered. The NHS and Community Care Act (1990) required purchasers to buy health care for the local population. Data collected by Public Health Departments are used to assess areas of service deficiency, and enable purchasers to make informed purchasing plans.

MARKETING EXPERTISE IN THE NHS

Because use of marketing is relatively new to the NHS, there are, as yet, few studies of its efficacy or of the extent of marketing expertise currently in place. The study by Bournes and Miles (1993) therefore is of value in supplying much-needed data about the current situation. Bournes and Miles surveyed four hospital regions and showed that there was wide variety in interpretation of the role and place of marketing in health services. This variety caused differences in the way that the various Trusts in the study dealt with the responsibility for marketing. The survey revealed that there were vast differences in the level of skill, experience and knowledge of those personnel employed in marketing positions.

The responsibilities of the Marketing Departments in these four regions varied from, at one end, having complete control of contractual negotiations, marketing, planning and quality, to having no responsibility, apart from the production of brochures (public relations) at the other. There was also diversity of the marketing activities and responsibilities of clinical directorates, some having total control of marketing and others having none.

Currently, the skills, knowledge and expertise of NHS marketing personnel varies considerably. Some individuals have marketing experience gained outside the NHS, others have marketing qualifications and degrees, and others have neither.

CONCLUSIONS

If there were no benefits, potential or actual, to the use of marketing in the NHS, it would be unnecessary to use a marketing approach. The identified benefits, however, are as yet small because the use of marketing is comparatively new.

One of the more intangible benefits is that marketing provides a viewpoint that is relatively fresh. For instance, Gronroos (1991: 147) suggests that health care can be seen as a consumer service along with insurance, financial and transport services. In health care, there has been an increase in looking at consumer issues and a marketing approach can provide a new focus for this.

The internal market philosophy has already resulted in the establishment of inter-departmental service level agreements for support services such as personnel, information and finance. Competitive tendering has been a common strategy for Trusts in the pursuit of value for money in areas such as hotel services (catering, domestic and laundry etc.). Market testing is an exercise whereby a Trust will actively seek an alternative source of supply for an existing service. Areas such as transport and supplies have become the latest focus for this approach.

Of more benefit in the long-term, however, is the fact that the existence of marketing highlights issues of quality. There have been national attempts to improve quality in the NHS. One of the purposes behind the issuing of the Patient's Charter has been to bring the issue of quality to the fore. Quality is about customers, and using a marketing approach aimed at users has implications for improvements to services.

Various standards relating to individual service areas have become well-defined over the past two years and are included as separate schedules in most contracts. Knowing the service standards facilitates the marketing of services, and conversely, the need to market services accentuates the need for quality in the service being marketed.

Companies in the commercial sector consistently analyse the full range of benefits that they can offer their customers by listing major product features and what these mean for the customer. Differential benefits (those features that make one service better than another) emerge from this kind of analysis. A company which fails to identify its own differential benefits will be unable to assess whether what it is offering is of the same standard as, or better or worse than, what their competitors are providing.

Approaching the marketing of NHS services by means of the application of differential benefits is somewhat problematic, however, because many professionals are not allowed to present data about the differential benefits that exist between themselves and other service providers. For example, both dentists and doctors are forbidden from advertising themselves as better qualified than other colleagues, thus preventing them from stating they are, or that the service they provide is, better than their competitors. As the situation now exists, data relating, for example, to rates of success in treatment that could be used to draw comparisons between groups, would have to be informally collected..

In any organization, marketing faces outward and inward. 'Out there' are existing and potential customers who need to be provided with the service; and 'in here' are the personnel who need to be aware of, and brought into, the process of providing for the customers 'out there'. Gronroos (1990: 13) highlights the need for the marketing role to be shared at every level of the service industry, rather than in specific departments. The establishment of Marketing Departments in NHS institutions is not sufficient; all the personnel be involved in the marketing approach. Restricting marketing to the Marketing Department's 'experts' prevents the putting forward of valuable or helpful ideas from other staff who are personally involved (and expert) in the products (services) which the Marketing Departments are concerned to market. As Parasuraman *et al.*, (1988: 88) suggest:

> Marketing has an outside focus of understanding, communicating with, and providing for, existing and potential customers, while at the same time having an internal role in influencing the management of services so that they can reach and exceed customer expectations. The two cannot be separate, particularly in service organizations.

Commercial marketeers insist that selling is seen an activity which is separate from marketing. In the NHS, selling takes the form of the sale of services within the context of promoting them to users, or those placing contracts. Yet, selling in the commercial sense, resembles what is happening within the internal market in two main ways: the first involves Trusts selling their services directly to purchasers and

GPs, and the second highlights the need to examine data about the local health needs of the local market.

Common sense will confirm that it is only by selling something to someone that financial goals can be achieved, and that advertising, pricing, service levels, and so on, are the means (or strategies) to that achievement. But promotion objectives and advertising objectives should not be confused with marketing objectives.

Everything in the garden is not lovely, however. Despite the obvious benefits that a marketing approach can offer, there is resistance to the incorporation of the approach into the NHS. An objection made by health care staff to the marketing of their services is that marketing is incompatible with professional decisions, and has no place in a health care setting. Health care professionals believe that a patient's trust is a pre-requisite to the relationship between professional and patient, and it is believed that any form of salesmanship (as marketing efforts are perceived) being inherently manipulative, would harm this basic relationship.

A counter-argument here is that the Community Care Act (1990) explicitly states that services should be tailored to meet the needs of consumers, and marketing is a way of ensuring that these needs are met because, as Sheaff (1991) suggests, marketing plays an important role in revealing consumer views. Thus, it can be considered that marketing in the NHS is can result in the introduction of new services and an increase in consumer choice.

The underlying ethos in the health care setting is the need to demonstrate value for money in the services provided. Even though commercial marketing is concerned with increasing market share or profit, marketing in the NHS can contribute to the provision of value for money by highlighting deficiencies in services, or indicating where services could be more appropriately targeted, delivered or improved.

It is possible that the NHS will limit its marketing activity to its Marketing Departments despite the fact that marketing is an organization-wide activity. Even if an institution does encourage all personnel to contribute to its marketing approach, there is as yet no guarantee that they will be willing to do so. There are grounds for supposing that negative attitudes by personnel resistant to the idea of marketing may limit the benefits which the marketing approach makes possible. Outright rejection of the marketing approach may well lead to the situation where the baby is thrown out with the bathwater, while resistance, resulting from a misunderstanding of the nature and purpose of marketing in the NHS, may well lead to mistakes such as the misapplication, or the inappropriate adaptation, of commercial marketing techniques. This would be a great pity, because, all things considered, it seems likely that both market research and marketing techniques have the potential to be of great use and benefit to the NHS.

REFERENCES

Bourne, H. and Miles,. C. (1993), Marketing: Its Place in Organizational Structure. *Health Services Management*, 89 (6), June, 18-19.

Coad, H. and Kennedy, B. (1992) Competitive Strategies in the NHS. *Health Services Management*, 88 (2), April, 11-13.

Gronroos, C. (1990), *Service Management and Marketing*, Lexington Books, Toronto.

Howells, J. and Green, L. (1988) The location of research and development: Some observations and evidence from Britain. *Regional Studies*, 18, 13-29.

Kotler, P. and Clarke, K. (1987), *Marketing for Health Care Organizations*, Prentice-Hall Inc. New Jersey.

McCarthy, E.J. (1978), *Basic Marketing: A Managerial Approach*, Homewood, Irwin.

Parasuraman, A., Zeithaml, B., and Berry, L. (1988), Servqual: A Multiple Item Scale for Measuring Consumer Perceptions of Service Quality. *Journal of Retailing*, 64 (1), 12-40.

Patients Charter. (1992), HMSO, London

Sheaff, R. (1991), *Marketing for Health Services*, Open University Press, Buckingham.

Secretaries of State for Health, Wales, Northern Ireland and Scotland, *Working for Patients*, Cmnd 555, (1989), HMSO, London.

10 De-marketing - A Strategy of Rationing for Equity?

ANNABELLE MARK

Middlesex University Business School

INTRODUCTION AND BACKGROUND

The development of the marketing discipline within the NHS has been seen as something new and innovative (Health Services Management 1993) within the context of the reforms to the system brought about by the introduction of the internal market. The question for many managers now however, is not so much how can marketing help to raise the income of the part of the NHS for which they are responsible, but how can marketing help in the management of the market to contain and control demand. The focus on demand and supply and the move away from need (Mark 1992) which was a feature of the reforms when first implemented (Roberts 1989) is now increasingly open to question. The demand/supply dynamic alone does not provide an adequate solution to the problems of disentangling excess demand from need in health care.

The reforms have also had a second but significant impact in the transfer of responsibility, implied by the internal market, from individual clinicians to purchaser organisations, including GP fundholders, for the allocation of health provision. In return the doctors have been encouraged to transfer their decision making skills from the individual patient to the organisation, where their involvement in management has been encouraged, with some success (Health Service Journal 1993) particularly through the introduction of clinical directorates, and GP fundholding. This refocusing of perspectives has confused the issue of whose definition of need is now being applied, is it any one of Bradshaws (1972) felt, expressed or comparative needs which rest for their interpretation on the consumer, or is it, as seems more likely, still a normative definition of need which has moved from one set of professionals, that is the patients own clinician, to another set namely public health specialists and managers, neither of whom necessarily have the consumers trust or any real legitimacy (Hunter 1993) to make decisions on behalf in the community in this way. This attempt to transfer responsibility from individual clinicians to population managers has led to an increasing concern with the ethics and values implicit in this

Setting Priorities in Health Care. Edited by M. Malek
© 1994 John Wiley & Sons Ltd

rationing activity (Weale 1988, Wall 1989), especially when paraded under the rationing banner of health gain (Hotchkiss *et al.* 1993). Such explorations indicate that the application of yet a further set of principles, this time those associated with marketing, within this context, will need to become   more sophisticated   and sensitive, if, as a discipline, it is to develop and retain credibility as an activity appropriate to the health sector in the UK, where the debate on health rationing is currently seen as "lacklustre and naive" (NAHAT 1993). The search is on therefore to find appropriate marketing tools for the health sector which could help in the management of health care needs as well as demands.   However, the problem may well prove to be that such tools will require marketing managers, together with their purchaser rather than their provider colleagues, to embark on a less attractive set of activities and decisions than they have associated with the discipline so far.   As a consequence such activity may further put at risk the future reputation of the marketing disciplines role in health care.   The emphasis on the provider side involvement in marketing, and the absence of such developments to anything like the same degree within the purchasing organisations, is a powerful demonstration of this point (East Anglia RHA 1990), which is now being addressed at ministerial level by the introduction of the seven stepping stones to effective purchasing (NHSME 1993)

SEVEN STEPPING STONES TO EFFECTIVE PURCHASING

- a strategic view
- robust contracts
- knowledge based decisions
- responsiveness to local people
- mature relations with providers
- local alliances
- organisational fitness

Purchasers not only need to understand the activity of marketing as it has been initially interpreted in the UK (Baker 1985) but could also reflect on the contribution that one of the purchasers key resources, epidemiology, has made to the early developments of marketing in identifying how patients or clients can become "infected" respectively with a disease or a desire for a given product for example Pessemiers (1982) discussion of the Bass (Epidemiological) Model of 1st purchaser behaviour. A further reason why marketing needs to develop as a purchaser activity is that it would hopefully balance any disproportionate advantages that providers may already have in their familiarity with what it has to offer, this is a form of information asymmetry associated with internal markets themselves (Coase 1960), and could reveal, through the purchasing rather than the providing activity, those aspects of marketing which are underdeveloped because of the general absence until now, of markets in public services in the UK and the unique problems which they generate. Without attempting a survey of all the tools available to marketing, this paper does explores the implications of the application of one of marketings less well used instruments, namely demarketing, to see what it has to offer for the future, and also what light it can shed on past work within the NHS, to allocate according to patient and population needs to provide improved health care and health outcome (DoH 1993).

MARKETS IN HEALTH CARE - THE CONTEXT.

If the aim of marketing is to make selling unnecessary (Drucker 1990), the NHS has always been involved in marketing when as Kotler (Drucker 1990) suggests it is understood as finding needs and filling them to provide positive values for both parties. The mistake of many of the new NHS marketing managers is to see their main function in the context of selling as the promotion of a set of products you have, and want to push into any market you can find (Drucker 1990). More recent UK definitions of the activity of marketing place at least equal emphasis on providers capabilities as on clients needs and wants, "The marketing concept is the process of matching a providers capabilities and the needs and wants of the clients to achieve the objectives of both parties" (MacDonald 1989). As such this definition should send alarm bells to policy makers and managers alike as it implies for health care that historically entrenched groups, institutions and services should dictate what needs can be met, presumably to the exclusion of those needs for which their is a market but currently no appropriate resource.

These definitions of the role of marketing still fall short of the key issues for public services, which is why the relatively obscure alternative marketing tool of demarketing is now being considered here. Demarketing, has so far been largely dismissed as too difficult or restricted in its use (Sheaff 1991) to be of value to the NHS as an organisation, yet it can be argued that such difficulties have already been addressed explicitly by others, using non marketing techniques, who have wished to solve the same problems addressed by the demarketing process. Examples of this are:

- RAWP (DHSS 1976), a rationing device originally based on an assessment of needs using morbidity as a measure of need rather than normative (provider) or demand (purchaser) assessments, and latterly amended and discredited for its insensitivity (Hacking 1993);
- or QALYS (Williams 1983) which places explicit values on needs, which are determined by the notion of the quality adjusted life years, calculated from user judgements about the value of various states of health, which consequently determines who may or may not receive treatment, these also have had their critics (Smith 1987).

The implications behind what so far have been the rather negative view of the potential of demarketing (Sheaff 1991) implies that solutions which present problems in seeking to address "chronic over popularity" (Kotler & Levy 1971) can be dismissed from the marketing arena. This attitude implies that either there must be elsewhere, outside of marketing, solutions to the problems if only we can find the right discipline, construct or methodology; or more worryingly that as a discipline marketing is severely restricted in its scope or unwilling to become associated with the negative aspects of controlling demand for humanitarian needs other than via the price mechanism. Pricing however is value laden and when brought into play (Birch 1986, Judge 1988), in normally free services, is likely to have some deterrent effects on the transaction and this can be potentially devastating for those affected by the transaction, be it a woman seeking infertility treatment or an elderly person requiring nursing or psychiatric care. Furthermore, transaction costs themselves are likely to act as a deterrent (Harrison *et al.* 1989), especially if they fall in to line with the US experience where at the start of the UK reforms they represented 20% of total expenditure on health compared to 6% in the UK.(Prowse 1990).

Marketing and the use of the price mechanism is the latest method which is being applied in the evolution of the health service as an organisation. The NHS is, as we have already seen, littered with examples of explicit methods such as RAWP and QALYS which have been applied to address the problems of priority setting or rationing. However what is also well recognised (Klein 1989, Harrison *et al.* 1993) are the more implicit devices which have rested predominantly with the medical profession and the myth of clinical freedom (Hoffenberg 1986). What has also remained constant since 1948, until the introduction of the internal market, is the context in which such attempts have been undertaken, that is of a hierarchically based organisation (Thompson *et al.* 1991). This context is important, if as Williamson suggested in 1975, the decision as to whether an organisation chooses to follow, markets or hierarchies, is dependent on which is perceived as providing the cheapest and thus most efficient transaction costs. Demonstrably the UK has provided one of the most efficient health care system in the world both in terms of input and outcomes (Schieber & Poullier 1991) and transaction costs (Prowse 1990), and it is somewhat surprising therefore that in attempting to contain costs further markets, which have demonstrably failed the organisation of health care in the USA, should have been introduced to the UK. Indeed, recent evidence suggests (OECD 1992, 1992a) that of all the developed nations the USA is, in fact, the only one which has failed to contain health care costs. Meanwhile, the rest of the world looks on with interest at the rush towards market mechanisms in the UK, to see what the outcomes might be for their own tentative steps in that direction, even though the macro issues which separate Europe and the USA may make comparisons inappropriate (Abel Smith 1992).

Making this clear distinction between markets and hierarchies however has been contested (Ouchi 1981) on the basis that elements of both can coexist and lead to a third form of organisation based on trust and co-operation. The complexity and conflict (Mark & Scott 1992, Harrison, Hunter, Marnoch & Pollitt 1992) inherent in the NHS as an organisation suggests that this view may be somewhat naive, and such conflict, even in commercial terms, is increasingly seen to be essential to successful organisations (Pascale 1991). Other distinctions which may be made between purchasers, representing a form of demand side socialism, and by implication providers, representing a form of supply side capitalism, may prove to be more appropriate to understanding what happens to the UK health sector. Based on this analysis, the NHS now *organisationally* incorporates the notion of the mixed economy of welfare and the conflicting value systems inherent in these two differing approaches. Understanding why the transition from hierarchies to markets has occurred involves both the more obvious political agendas of the Thatcher years (Kingdom J 1992,) but also changes in the cultural (Storey 1992) and social policy (Ginsburg 1992) agendas within UK society and foreseen in respect of marketing as a move "away from the Christian ethic of deferred gratification to a more hedonistic and short term view of life which emphasizes immediate gratification" (Baker 1985). More significant perhaps than either of these issues was the need to find a mechanism which contests the worst aspects of the very hierarchical organisation of healthcare and the power which it confers on the tribes who inhabit it, rather than those who use it. It was inevitable therefore that, given the declared preference for the market which has been a feature of all aspects of the Conservative administration which came to power in 1979 (Massey 1993), a change to the structure of the health care organisation in the UK away from hierarchy towards markets with the introduction of the internal market, would be seen as the appropriate fix for health systems which needed to be contained.

It is in this organisational context that the NHS and government is seeking solutions to the demand/supply/need conundrum. The demand/supply problems have been to a large extent the prerogative of the economists (Culyer 1976, Mooney 1986). Needology has been the major concern of the sociologists (Bradshaw 1972 Townsend 1979) and the epidemiologists (Hannay 1979) who more particularly share a concern with identifying and providing for need which the consumer has not presented to the health system. These may be the comparative and felt needs for the sociologists and the iceberg of the epidemiologists but looked at with the new marketing perspective both fall within the definition of marketing as the *finding* and filling of needs to provide positive values for both parties, attempts to bring together these two perspectives for purchasers are now in evidence through such devices as the Lifecycle Framework for assessing health need (Pickin & St Leger 1993). Such morally justifiable activity does not however address the problems of expressed need (Bradshaw 1972) or demand as defined by the economists (Mooney 1986) which represent the main problem of rationing for health care providers. The central question is thus, given limited resources, what proactive rather than reactive responses are available to manage the demands of the health care market. Furthermore, what mechanism is available to enable unmet needs, especially those for which no normative solutions currently exist, to be allocated a proportion of the health care provision.

DEMARKETING

One possibility is demarketing which is defined as "that aspect of marketing that deals with discouraging customers in general or a certain class of customers in particular on either a temporary or permanent basis" (Kotler & Levy 1971). It can be divided into four areas all of which have relevance for the UK health service. They are:

General demarketing

General demarketing is required when an organisation wants to shrink the level of total demand. In the NHS this has been a major policy activity of the last ten years which has resulted in for example a reduction of 30% in the number of public hospitals (Abel Smith 1992). Another example of this shrinkage is the Tomlinson Report (Tomlinson 1992)on the future of health care in London where provision or supply (but not necessarily demand) is said to exceed the norm for elsewhere in the country. Evidence from twelve European countries has also confirmed that health care costs can be contained by regulating supply rather than demand (Abel Smith 1992), but it may also be because until now at least supply is the only thing which managers and governments have thought can be manipulated, either by reducing facilities or manpower, certainly the evidence from this European study supports this in noting the absence of demand side strategies.

Selective demarketing

Selective demarketing occurs when a company wants to discourage the demand coming from certain customer classes. This occurs both directly and indirectly, in the first case there are those services for which contracts from purchasers are not going to be placed with providers, or for which partial payment is required (e.g. tattoo removal or infertility treatment respectively). In the second more indirect approach the whole Health Education and Promotion activity implies not just the encouragement to maintain a healthy lifestyle, but also as a on sequence the reduction in requirements for health care provision, best exemplified by the warning on cigarette packets.

Purchasers who now need to incorporate the Health of the Nation (DoH 1991a) targets, for reductions in for example cardiovascular disease or suicides, in their placing of contracts are also thus now involved in this activity.   However, contradictory objectives may prevent such targets being met, for example the introduction of limited list prescribing for GPs and tighter monitoring and control of drugs budgets has in some cases prevented GPs from using the very latest non toxic psychiatric drugs with which it is not possible to take an overdose, in favour of the cheaper but still potentially lethal older forms of drugs. The patient is thus given the potential by the health service itself to increase rather than decrease demand through the para suicide rate, such a situation pushes the example into the ostensible demarketing category described below.

Commercial awareness of the selective demarketing approach in health care is confirmed by the advertising industry which has in the past acknowledged the innovative nature of health care marketing and its contribution to new areas, for example the indirect approach applied in Health Promotion in Scotland in the 1980s, which was highly thought of by advertising professionals, winning several awards. This work not only involved promoting the benefits of non smoking in reducing death and disease in the adult population, but in addition showed increased sensitivity to the needs of the other groups in the target population by refocusing the approach for adolescents, for whom threats of death were too distant or too uncertain; instead they used asocial (smokers are not nice to be near) rather than a health message although the outcomes in preventing ill health would be the same (Leathar & Hastings 1983).

Further selective demarketing examples which are becoming more specific in terms of the classes or groups targeted are:

- the use of information on the risks to patients of putting themselves forward for specific treatments or surgery, for example the "Prostectomy or Watchful Waiting Video" being piloted under guidance from the Kings Fund at Central Middlesex Hospital which results in self rationing by those who after watching the information provided in the video, decide that they do not feel ready to encounter the risk normally associated with a surgical procedure of this kind.
- proposals to introduce a system which would select the patients who would benefit most from treatment (Williams 1990), which already occurs in relation to ITU through the use of the APACHE scoring system (IEZZONI 1992) and has been made more explicit in the American Oregon experiment (Honigsbaum 1991) with all its attendant problems (Davies 1991).

Ostensible demarketing

Ostensible demarketing involves the appearance of trying to discourage demand as a device for actually increasing it. This seems now less likely to occur within the internal market as doctors do not necessarily have a direct say over who gets what any more although a study of extra contractual referral utilisation (DoH 1992a) may reveal otherwise. The initiatives to reduce waiting lists both centrally and locally, together with the Patients Charter which came into force in April 1992 (DoH 1991b and 1992b), have attempted to stop long waits, even though there is evidence that many waiting lists seem to stabilize at a particular length (Mullen 1993). However, a strategy well known to hospital managers in the past and adopted by many hospital clinicians was one of maintaining long waiting lists, this "ostensible demarketing" gave out the message that "by having long lists you (the patient) will know I am the best around and will therefore be prepared to wait in the queue that much longer to get the best" or "even be prepared to seek my attentions more quickly by paying for it through the private sector" as Yates (1987) had found, and which led the Parliamentary Health Committee to request a special study of the issue (House of Commons 1991). Further examples which will make the public and private health sectors interactive are now occurring, for example the refusal by some hospitals to undertake certain procedures (e.g. varicose veins surgery), may well result in increases in demand within other public and more particularly private sector facilities for this non provision.

Unintentional demarketing

Unintentional demarketing is when attempts to increase demand actually results in driving customers away. In the NHS this can be the inappropriate or insensitive provision of treatment or care, for example family planning or cytology screening services, which fail to reach certain ethnic groups because of the unreliability of ensuring an all female environment which makes it unacceptable for cultural, ethnic or religious reasons (Ahmad 1993). It also occurs in relation to waiting lists when long waits lead to recovery from a condition without intervention (Wightman 1980).

This set of definitions of the activities associated with demarketing must be seen in the context of the main activities associated with the marketing discipline and the way such mainstream activities now exist within the health sector. The general perception of marketing rests on the five ideas of:

- *studying the market,* for which the NHS equivalent is epidemiological and planning activities relating to the population to be served, as well as utilisation rates and outcome information when available.
- *segmenting the market,* in NHS terms this may be the division into either care groups for example the elderly, children; or activities, for example surgical or medical services or even the new largely speciality based clinical directorates;
- *targeting the groups you want to serve,* in the reformed NHS this should be consumers but is more likely to be purchasers and providers for the NHS jointly or separately who will identify those groups for whom treatment will be provided and thus by default rather than design those who will be excluded;
- *positioning yourself in the market,* in the health sector this is particular to the provider organisations both public and private, but also increasingly applies to GP fundholders and purchasers who may offer alternative non NHS contracts for NHS providers to compete against;
- and lastly *creating a service which meets needs,* within health care; the current emphasis on the economists definition of need must be set in the historical context of the sociological and epidemiological definitions and the fact that interest groups will identify any form of provision as meeting a need which exists somewhere in what Kotler and Levy(1971) described as the real but rare situations where an organisation is faced with chronic over popularity, this exists for the NHS even with those who choose to use alternatives in the private health sector(Calnan *et al.* 1993).

These five ideas and their consequent activities add up to what have been described as the "fair weather activities" (Kotler & Levy 1971) of marketing and the challenge of them for the NHS has been complicated by the diversification of customers who are now not just clients/patients, their GPs or their families but also the professionals representing the purchasing arm of the internal market. There is also a political imperative implicit in the activity of marketing in the public sector as a proactive and positive set of public relations related activities endorsing New Right ideologies (Massey 1993) which can mask real concerns about what is in fact the down sizing of the public sector. However, the competitive behaviour implicit in the reforms of the 1980s (Common Flynn and Mellon 1992) indicate that in general there are limited views of what competitive actions are open to the public sector as organisations now using marketing methods, be they

- the pursuit of new markets and customers for example European trade or former private sector purchasers;
- developing new products and services and dropping less valuable ones, without necessarily asking all the relevant interested parties be they professionals, providers, purchasers or consumers;
- changing the way in which goods and services are produced, for example by changing or re profiling staff, developing day surgery;
- adjusting prices to take advantage of market conditions now seen as the negotiations between providers and purchasers, or
- investment and access to capital markets which could be the eventual outcome required by the Tomlinson (1992) proposals to change the structure of health care provision in London, or what Common Flynn and Mellon (1992) describe as the differences between choice in the public and private sectors "If public sector markets are not to generate privileged groups of service recipients, either everybody has to have access to the same amount of purchasing power according to their need for the service, or mechanisms other than the markets should be used for the distribution of services."

Demarketing as an alternative set of activities could meet these objectives in a different way which still relates to marketing, but also provides the tools to ration for equity, if used explicitly, and could thus provide some answers to such dilemmas.

So how would demarketing help? A number of issues are apparent and are briefly summarised as:

Intervention

It implies intervention, this needs to be an explicit activity for purchasers and not just an implicit activity for purchasers or providers as at present, examples of this implicit activity are found in the use of technological rationing devices such as APACHE (Iezzoni 1992) which seeks to assess patient viability, as a way of determining access to treatment, such systems may not have the flexibility, sensitivity and ultimately trust which until now has been invested in the doctor by patients and their relatives. Unless, when made explicit to consumers, they are demonstrably seen as a guide over which the doctor has a veto. Otherwise such rationing methods will damage the consumers relationship with the health care system, unless of course that is the intention in which case it may be seen as a implicit, but somewhat unethical, selective demarketing activity.

Collaboration

Greater collaboration between purchasers for health gain would mean the use of selective demarketing techniques to ensure that an equitable distribution of health provision was targeted at the most vulnerable as Williams (1990) suggests rather than those who are most effective at gaining access to the system, also implied within this is a requirement for a degree of trust and collaboration from providers with purchasers (Stockford 1993), which may be in keeping with Ouchis' (1981) more positive assessment of the possible combination of hierarchies and markets. Providers might otherwise wish to discriminate in favour of the most treatable in order to establish a good outcome record, and may already be discriminating in various ways to attain this via various implicit demarketing activities.

Decentralisation

Decentralising power and responsibility if, as has been established (Abel Smith 1992) most methods of cost containment are on the supply side and generated centrally to a greater extent in most countries, demarketing offers the opportunity to become proactive on the demand side of the equation especially where this is a purchaser led activity, thus moving further away from Kleins (1989) assessment that most rationing decisions "have always been made in a highly dispersed and *only partly visible* way"

Explicitness

Explicitness where rationing decisions are taken using this particular mechanism of determining explicitly in the context of "chronic over popularity" (Kotler & Levy 1971) it will make the actions of those now so empowered, particularly the managers, more understandable and the acceptability can thus be established perhaps in the context of Walls (1993) notion of managerial utilitarianism, and confirms Harrison *et al.* (1993) assumption that under the "provider market the visibility of rationing may also increase".

Ethics

In taking the ethical issues, which seem to have bedevilled the discussion of demarketing as a reasonable strategy for health care, on board, and discussing them in the context of current and more particularly past practices, both implicit and explicit, a general question arises about the degree to which demarketing might have always been the major activity indulged in by public services, which is probably why marketing has kept away from all but the "fair weather" (Kotler & Levy 1971) activities so far; this explanation does also confirm the assumption that "The NHS market will be a most unusual and distinctive one, to which lessons drawn from a business background may not apply in any straight forward way" (Harrison *et al.* 1993).

Finally perhaps this exploration of demarketing as an appropriate device has revealed that if the notion is not applied and utilised in any overt way, the continued application of what are clearly demarketing strategies implicitly, may mean that we end up just revisiting under another name the notions of professional and provider preference at the expense of alternative strategies for health improvement or gain by the consumer, for as Reisman suggests (1993) in a market for health there must also be a market for ideas. As a new device, in the search to maintain rationing for equity in health, demarketing could be a useful mechanism for driving forward both central and local agendas in the context of health care for the 1990s after all as Shakespeare said,

"What's in a name? that which we call a rose
By any other name would smell as sweet"
(Shakespeare: Romeo and Juliet)

REFERENCES

Abel Smith B (1992) Cost Containment and New Priorities in the European Community *The Millbank Quarterly* Vol. 70 No 3

Ahmad Waquar Ihsan-Ullah (ed.) (1993) *Race and health in contemporary Britain* Open University Press Buckingham England

Baker Michael J.(1985) *Marketing Strategy & Management,* Macmillan Basingstoke England.

Birch S (1986) Increasing Patient Charges in the National Health Service: a method of privatizing primary care *Journal of Social Policy* 15(2):178

Bradshaw J S (1972) *A taxonomy of social need* in McLachlan G(ed.) Problems and progress in medical care: essays on current research. 7th Series Oxford University Press

Calnan M , Cant S Gabe J (1993) *Going Private why people pay for their health care* Open University Press Buckingham England

Coase R. H. *The problem of social cost,* Journal of Economic Literature October 1960.

Common R Flynn N & Mellon E (1992) *Managing Public Services* Butterworth Heinemann ISBN 0 7506 0452 2

Culyer A (1976) *Need and the National Health Service* Martin Robertson London.

Davies P *Thumbs down for Oregon rations* Health Services Journal Vol. 101 No 5278 p10-11.

DHSS(1976) *Sharing Resources for health in England.* Report of the Resource Allocation Working Party

DoH (1991a) Department of Health *The Health of the Nation : A consultative document for health in England.* HMSO London.

DoH (1991b) *The Patients Charter Department of Health*

DoH (1992a) *Department of Health Guidance on Extra Contractual referrals,* Issued under EL(92)60 Department of Health.

DoH (1992b) *Implementing the patients Charter* Circular HSG(92)4, Department of Health.

DoH(1993) Department of Health *Managing the new NHS: a background document.* Department of Health London.

Drucker P (1990) *Managing the non profit organisation* Butterworth Heinemann London

East Anglia Regional Health Authority, Office for Public management. *Contracting for Health Outcomes* East Anglia RHA Cambridge.

Ginsburg N (1992) *Divisions of Welfare - a critical introduction to comparative social policy* Sage London.

Hannay D R (1979) *The symptom iceberg: a study of community health* Routledge London.

Harrison S Hunter D J Johnston & Wistow G (1989) *Competing for Health* Nuffield Institute for Health Service Studies Leeds.

Harrison S Hunter D Marnoch G Pollitt C.(1992) *Just managing: power & culture in the National Health Service.* Macmillan London.

Health Services Management (1993) News Vol. 89 No 7 p 5.

Health Services Journal (1993) *The power to change* News Focus Vol. 103 No 5374 p14-15.

Honigsbaum F (1991) *Who shall live ? Who shall die? - Oregons Health Financing Proposals.* Kings Fund College papers. Kings Fund College.

Hotchkiss J Watson P Boydell L (1993) *Health Gain: from Rhetoric to reality.* Journal of Management in Medicine Vol. 7 No 4 34-41.

House of Commons (1991) *Public Expenditure in Health Services*: Waiting Lists Parliament House of Commons Health Committee 1st Report Vol. 1 429-1 8th May.

Hunter D (1993) *Something rotten in the state* Health Services Journal Vol. 103 No. 5360 p21 8 July.

Iezzoni L (1992) *Predicting in-hospital mortality a comparison of severity measurement approaches.* Medical Care 30 (4) April.

Judge K(1988)(ed.) *Pricing the social services* London Macmillan

Kingdom J *No such thing as society- individualism & community* Open University Press.

Klein R (1989) *The Politics of the NHS* (2nd Ed) London Longman.

Kotler P & Levy S J (1971) *De marketing yes demarketing* Harvard Business Review Nov/Dec Vol. 49 no 6 p74-80.

Leathar D S & Hastings G.B. (1983) *Basic Research into Women & Smoking.* University of Strathclyde, Glasgow, Advertising Research Unit.

Loveridge R & Starkey K (1992) *Continuity and Crisis in the NHS* Open University Press

MacDonald M (1989) *Marketing Plans how to prepare them: how to use them* Heinemann

Mark A (1992) *How has the symbol changed - a community care consumers dilemma* Health Services Management March.

Mark A & Scott H (1992) *Management in the National Health Service* in Willcocks L & Harrow J (eds.) Rediscovering Public Services Management McGraw Hill. Maidenhead England

Massey A (1993) *Managing the Public Sector* Edward Elgar.

Mooney G H (1986) *Economics Medicine & Health Care* Harvest Press Brighton.

Mullen P (1993) *The future of waiting lists* Journal of Management in Medicine 7 (4) pp 60-70

NAHAT (1993) *Rationing Dilemmas in Healthcare* NAHAT Birmingham.

NHSME(1993) *Purchasing for Health: a framework for action.* Speeches by Brian Mawhinney and Sir Duncan Nichol. NHS Management Executive Publications Unit. Leeds.

OECD (1992) *US Health Care at the Crossroads* Organisation for Economic Co operation and Development Health Policy Studies Series 1.

OECD (1992a) *The reform of health care - a comparative analysis of 7 OECD countries* Organisation for Economic Co operation and Development Health Policy Studies Series 2.

Ouchi W G (1981) *Theory Z* Addison Wesley Reading Mass.

Pessemier Edgar A (1982) *Product Management strategy and organisation* 2nd ED J Wiley & Sons Chichester. p 156.

MacDonald M H B (1989) *Marketing Plans how to prepare them: how to use them* Heineman

Pascale R.(1991) *Managing on the Edge* Harmondsworth Penguin.

Picken C & St Leger S (1993) *Assessing Health Need using the Life Cycle Framework* Open University Press Milton Keynes

Prowse M (1990) *Buying on behalf of patients* Financial Times Wednesday Feb. 28th

Reisman D (1993) *Market & Health* Macmillan Basingstoke

Roberts J A (1989) *The National Health Service: from myths to markets* Health Policy & Planning Vol. 4 No 1 62-71

Hoffenberg R (1986) *Clinical freedom - the Rock Carling Fellowship* Nuffield Provincial Hospital Trust London

Sheaf R (1991) *Marketing for Health Services* Open University Press

Shieber G J & Poillier JP (1991) *International Health Spending* Health Affairs vol. 10 no 1 106-16

Smith A (1987) *Qualms about QALYS* Lancet N0 1. pp. 1134-6

Storey J.(1992) *Cultural theory & popular culture - an introductory guide* Harvester Wheatsheaf.

Stockford D (1993) *Perspectives on Purchasing* The Health Service Journal Vol. 103 No 5382 9 Dec.

Thompson G , Frances J Levacic R Mitchell J. (1991) *Markets, Hierarchies and Networks - the co-ordination of social life.* Sage/Open University London.

Townsend P (1979) *Poverty - in the United Kingdom* Pelican Penguin Harmondsworth England.

Wall A (1989) *Ethics and the Health Services Manager.* King Edwards Hospital Fund for London

Weale (1988) *Cost & choice in Health Care - the ethical dimension.* King Edwards Hospital Fund for London

Wightman J.A.K. *The Management Problems of a Rising Waiting List, Waiting for Hospital Treatment* DHSS 1980 pp. 40-43

Williams A (1983) *The economic role of health indicators* in G Teeling Smith (ed.) *Measuring the social benefits of medicine* Office of Health Economics London.

Williams A (1990) *Escape the trap* The Health Services Journal Vol. 100 No 5188 pp. 242-3

Williamson O E (1975) *Market & Hierarchies: analysis and antitrust implications.* New York Free Press

Yates J (1987) *Why are we waiting - An analysis of Hospital Waiting Lists* Oxford University Press Oxford.

11 Funding the National Health Service - Policy Maintenance or Policy Change?

ALLAN BRUCE & STEPHEN BAILEY

Glasgow Caledonian University

INTRODUCTION

In financial year 1991-92 expenditure by the National Health Service (NHS) amounted to £31.3 billion (Central Statistical Office, 1992), almost all of which was financed by central government from its general tax revenues. NHS expenditure represents some 12% of total public expenditure, or to put it another way, some 5.2% of Gross Domestic Product (GDP). In 1990-91 taxation financed 78%, National Insurance Contributions 15.5%, charges 5%, land sales 1% and charitable donations 0.5% (Ensor, 1993).

Income available to the NHS in the UK had shown a modest increase during the 1980s, but the infinity of demand, demographic change and increased unit costs had all conspired to make health authorities run harder in an effort to stand still. For example, it was estimated that real expenditure on health and personal social services would have to rise by 1% per annum 1983/84-1993/94 simply to take account of demographic change (Cmnd 9189). Failure to achieve this led to allegations that the NHS had experienced a shortfall in funding of some £1.8 billion between 1981-82 and 1987-88 (House of Commons, Social Services Committee, 1988).

With the 1990 reform of the NHS, inspired as it was by the White Paper - *Working for Patients* (Cm 555) - the Government was clearly intent upon intensifying its pursuit of efficiency, effectiveness and economy and of leading a more direct challenge to the prevailing culture of the NHS. Notably, however, the Government had elected not to pursue more radical options that had been floated prior to the publication of *Working for Patients* relating to alternative sources of funding (Butler, 1992). Adherence to the status quo is not without precedent, previous review bodies - Ministry of Health 1956 (Cmnd 9663) and The Royal Commission 1979 (Cmnd 7615) - had been given potentially radical remits to explore alternative courses of action, though at the end of the day had been reluctant to recommend radical

Setting Priorities in Health Care. Edited by M. Malek
© 1994 John Wiley & Sons Ltd.

changes. For example, the Royal Commission that reported in 1979 had, amongst other things, examined the funding of the NHS but had also been keen to promote some degree of continuity. Given the highly politicised and emotive nature of health care provision, fundamental reviews of the NHS must always run the risk of reopening old wounds, so that there might well be a strong rationale for preferring policy maintenance to policy change.

With this caveat in mind, this chapter examines the funding of the NHS within the context of a general acceptance of the status quo. It recognises that, whilst political and economic ideology will suggest particularly radical 'solutions' to 'problems' perceived in this light of partisan stances, in practice both 'problems' and 'solutions' will be re-evaluated for their pragmatism and ability to maintain broad political consensus. The inheritance of past programmes upon the change of political persuasion of governments and the incremental nature of change serve to moderate radical principles.

ISSUES AND PROSPECTS

In addition to restricted general financing, there are additional reasons for examining alternative and/or supplementary sources of funding. These sources are not necessarily mutually incompatible and may be used in varying combinations. Their objectives are not simply to bridge a financing gap. They can:

- Promote equity: those who can afford to pay more should do so.
- Encourage cost-effective management: establish a clearer link between income and expenditure by, for example, giving management some discretion and responsibility for income generation.
- Improve accountability: failure to separate NHS finance from general taxation means that it is not entirely clear to the electorate what proportion of tax revenue is spent on the NHS. Moreover, identifying a separate NHS component could facilitate patient opting-out with private insurance.
- Shift the tax burden: to more palatable sources of finance for example, voluntary participation in a lottery.
- Reduce demand: general taxation may actually serve to increase demand for health care - the 'we've paid for it so let's consume it' syndrome and moral hazard (failing to adopt healthy lifestyles if the NHS is perceived as providing a 'fall-back' facility).
- Fend off cries of wolf: claims that the NHS is 'under siege', that 'patients are dying on waiting lists', or that the NHS may eventually 'go down the tubes' have been common throughout the history of the NHS because funding is not guaranteed.
- Secure additional revenue: assuming there are no offsetting reductions in revenue from general taxation.
- Depoliticise the NHS: if alternative sources of finance could be found that required less support from tax revenue.

Most of these objectives are discussed in detail below. Not all are clearly separable and not all relate to each alternative source of funding. However, they illustrate that a plurality of financing options have much more subtle objectives than simply increasing available finance. Indeed, this may not be an objective at all. Whatever the financial arrangements, they must fulfil the basic purpose and criteria of the NHS.

LOCAL TAXATION

Introducing an element of locally-raised funding into health services is hardly innovative, it would have been a corollary of an option floated during wartime negotiations about the future of health care, to allocate responsibility for acute hospital provision to local government. Local government was regarded as something of a logical choice for administering the hospital service since it had inherited the poor law hospitals and had in any case been responsible for a 'rag bag' of health and health-related functions. Principally, however, opposition to this possibility had come from the medical profession and in particular, General Practitioners (GPs) who were always wary (indeed fearful) of municipalisation and of becoming salaried employees of the state (Eckstein, 1958).

The local government issue appeared again in the late 1960s with proposals for reorganising the NHS (Klein, 1989), but a fundamental problem remains in that local government is also extremely heavily dependent on revenues from central government general taxation. Sole reliance upon local taxation would require Council Tax levels to nearly double, almost certainly unacceptable to the Government and householders. One of the painful lessons of the local government property tax was that, too great a financial demand was being placed on too narrow a tax base. The end result was an increasing dependence by local government on central government's intergovernmental grants (themselves financed out of general taxation) at the cost of increasing central control over local affairs and increased fiscal stress (Bailey and Paddison, 1988; Bailey, 1991).

Local taxation may also exacerbate problems relating to equality of access and level of service since income would vary from authority to authority. Hence, there would be a continuing need for redistribution of financial resources via central government. Moreover, local government's own local taxing powers have been both severely constrained and reduced over recent years. Health would still be in a position of competing for resources with other public services such as education, roads and refuse. It may seem disadvantageous to be placed within the constrained resource envelope of local government services as a whole rather than occupying a more salient public position on its own.

Clearly the local government experience of local taxation is not an obvious way out of financial constraint and health is unlikely to be given its own local tax. The only real result may be increased local political accountability, not a sudden lifting of resource constraints. Even the former is questionable, since local government is not unanimously regarded as successful in that respect. General taxation, therefore, may have to remain the main source of NHS funding as recognised in 'Working for Patients'.

EARMARKED TAXES

An alternative to a local tax with local control over tax rates (if not tax base) is an earmarked tax. Here, the rates and base of the tax are determined by central government, but the revenues are dedicated to the NHS. Revenues can be assigned in whole or in the form of a predetermined and fixed percentage.

It has recently been argued that the general public has lost track of the uses to which general taxes are put (Mulgan and Murray, 1993). It is argued that the separation of the tax bill from the benefits it finances ('disconnection') has led to an opaque and excessively centralised governmental structure. People have become unwilling to sign 'blank cheques' to the State, accepting its decisions on spending totals and distributions. Indeed, past surveys have shown that the electorate would be prepared to pay additional taxes in order to secure a higher level of funding for the NHS (Game, 1984). While the electorate is prepared to see an increase in taxation for the NHS, it may not wish to see additional taxation used for other purposes, a danger that is ever present with the use of general taxation for all public services. It is here, therefore, that the justification for an earmarked tax for the NHS is derived. It is argued that such an arrangement would 'reconnect' taxes and services, sharing sovereignty between elected representatives and citizens. Voters would be given an effective choice over the real level of the NHS budget, rather than decisions being made downwards from the top.

If the tax were a buoyant tax (its yield increasing in line with a growth in the economy) then the NHS would enjoy a rising income. A property tax (concomitant with the local government option) has long been criticised for its inelasticity (e.g. Cmnd 6453). Whilst a health tax on earnings is much more buoyant, aggregate real earnings tend to rise and fall with the national economic cycle. Hence, the NHS may face periodic funding crises. It is, therefore, not self-evident that an earmarked tax would depoliticise health care or provide greater stability. The only real advantage is that the Government may not be so cavalier as to attempt to reduce or divert it for other purposes.

The most popular contender for the earmarked tax would appear to be National Insurance Contributions (NICs) whose total revenue is greater than total spending on the NHS. However, NICs are already notionally used to finance a wide range of benefits (including health) so they would have to be increased if specifically earmarked to health. The problem here is that NICs tend to be regressive in that rates do not vary substantially across the range of incomes. In particular, the narrow exempted range of low earnings and the open-ended Upper Earnings Limit mean that workers on low earned incomes pay proportionately more than those with high earned incomes. Suggested reforms of NICs (including merger with income tax) have been refused during the 1980s (Cmnd 9756) with the result that, if earmarked to health, those on low incomes would disproportionately finance health.

In fact as Klein (1988) points out, the problems run deeper than this. Health care may not merely be about redistributing income over time - like pensions. It is also about redistributing expenditure between groups with high and low medical risks. If NICs were used to fully finance health, would it be fair to expect that responsibility for funding the NHS to come only from the wage packets of the working population rather than also from business through corporation tax and from the general population through expenditure taxes etc.? Who would pay the contributions of the non-working population - for example, the chronically sick? The answer to this is undoubtedly the Treasury, using general taxation.

NICs would effectively be an income tax and could have an impact upon the incentive to work. In this case, the very process of earmarking may itself cause the tax base to shrink. Furthermore, governments often dislike earmarked taxes precisely because they reduce their freedom to allocate resources. Here again there is a sense in which policy maintenance may be preferred to policy change.

Another option from within the earmarked taxation fold is what are described as 'sin taxes' which include taxes on tobacco and alcohol. These taxes can be levied upon individuals with a view to deterring 'self-abuse' and if used to finance the NHS, could also be regarded as an indirect form of user charge (Wagner, 1991), but crucial questions can be asked about what this type of tax is likely to achieve.

An important issue that must be considered when examining the potential for a tobacco tax to contribute to the funding of the NHS is the extent to which its potential yield is influenced by the market for tobacco, The UK's consumption of cigarettes has fallen markedly from over 120 billion in 1980 to less than 90 billion in 1992, a trend which seems likely to continue. Consequently, success in deterring smoking by highlighting health risks, in conjunction with possible increases in the level of tax levied upon tobacco products could very easily deprive the NHS of future income raised from this source. Not only might a shrinking tax base create its own funding crisis for the NHS, but a tobacco tax may also bring ethical and moral dilemmas for surgeons who refuse to operate upon heavy smokers because of their poor prognosis. If a tobacco tax was specifically earmarked to provide for health care, it would arguably be immoral to deny treatment to those who were financing a disproportionate share of NHS costs. In addition, however, smokers are not exclusive consumers of health services and the fact is that many smokers die at an earlier age than their non-smoking counterparts, so that the latter may make more use of services that have been disproportionately financed by the former.

PATIENT CHARGES

The debate about user-charges for GP and hospital services pre-date the NHS, so many of the arguments are familiar. The case for charges is that they generate more revenue, they make patients more cost-conscious, they ration services and deter frivolous demands, they relieve pressure on general taxation and they improve efficiency if based on costs. On the down side, asymmetry of information may afford the medical practitioner the opportunity to persuade individual patients to demand the same amount of health care (or even more) when chargeable compared with when free. Patients may also be encouraged to stay in hospital longer than medically necessary, especially if (say) the daily charge is constant while daily in-patient costs fall during post-operative recuperation.

Charges will also tend hit the poor the hardest and so contradict both equity of contribution and the principle of access on the basis of need, irrespective of income and wealth. Indeed, charges might have the perverse effect of discouraging people from seeking early treatment, so perhaps increasing costs. This would be neither efficient nor humanitarian, nor effective. But can we dismiss the charging option on this basis, particularly if the Government is seeking to limit the amount of tax revenue being devoted to the NHS. To counter these criticisms of charges, increasing revenue from charges would have to be considered in conjunction with exclusions. The main options for charging are identified as follows:

Hotel Charges

Unlike charges for GP services, hotel charges may not have the effect of discouraging the consumption of health care, decisions about referral and admission to hospital are primarily the preserve of doctors. A hotel charge would be more akin to a tax that is incurred involuntarily by the patient. Yet there remains a problem here about the rather narrow base of such a tax when one considers exclusions from such a tax. Some 80% of all prescriptions issued in the UK are exempt from charges (Le Grand, Winter and Woolley, 1990) and if this level of exemption was replicated for hotel charges, then charges would have to be relatively high for those who do not qualify for exemption in order to generate a reasonable income. Recent estimates suggest £10 per day could raise an annual total of some £200 million. Billing patients, recovering outstanding charges and sorting out exemptions would also lead to increased administrative costs.

However, given that patients are in hospital often less than a week, and further, that people could take out insurance to cover hotel charges, can hotel charges be dismissed? Insurance premia are likely to be regressive given both their lack of means-testing and the general association between ill-health and low income. Poverty traps would be evident where some people would be better-off receiving social security and categoric exemptions could result in the affluent elderly being exempt while the young poor have to pay. Insurance may also result in cost-push inflation in that they (unlike direct taxes) are included in the cost-of-living index. Whilst hotel charges could raise substantial amounts of revenue, it may not be additional money for the NHS but merely used to cut the amount of tax finance devoted to it. Hence, it might be politically unpopular if the additional revenue were not spent directly on patient care (i.e. earmarking may be necessary).

Prescription Charges

Between 1979 and 1993 there was about a 21-fold increase in prescription charges, based on the assumption of a one-item prescription. In 1979 the cost of a prescription was 20 pence regardless of the number of items, whereas April 1993 saw prescription charges increase to £4.25 per item. Prescription charges would have to be increased substantially in order to make a significant impact in terms of additional revenue and given the percentage of the population who regularly receive prescriptions but are exempt from paying, this increase would be borne by a minority of the population.

However, the usefulness of charges extends beyond the need to raise additional revenue. Charges also reduce costs by deterring frivolous consumption. They also have the added advantage over charges for GP services in that they do not directly deter people who have a potentially serious illness from seeing their GP. Indirect deterrence may occur if someone expects that a visit to their GP may be expensive as a result of, say, a four-item prescription. Even here, though, patients have the option of not taking prescriptions to retail chemists (indeed, a proportion do not). Selective self-prescribing may also occur where an individual may ask the pharmacist to supply the most important items on the prescription or ask for a cheaper less effective alternative over the counter. There may also be a perverse effect of more expensive prescriptions' reducing revenue, especially where it is cheaper to buy medicines over the counter.

INCOME GENERATION

The 1988 Health & Medicines Act allows the NHS to generate income by selling support services where there is excess capacity as long as additional costs are fully recovered and there is no significant disadvantage to the NHS or its patients. The intention is to raise additional finance for improved health care, to encourage managers to be more innovative, cost conscious and consumer orientated and to enhance the professional image of the NHS. A wide range of income generation schemes is in operation, directed at patients, staff, visitors and the private sector. These initiatives range from charging patients for private facilities, renting hospital floor space to florists, newsagents and banks to offering specialist laboratory services to the private sector, fitness testing, catering for functions and property leasing. In total, 57% of income is derived (almost equally) from the lease of buildings and land, laundry services and car park charges. Retail shops raise 14% with no other single category raising more than 8% (NAO, 1993).

Within the reformed NHS there is clearly more emphasis upon income generation than before. Competition between providers of health care gives rise to a more pronounced entrepreneurial culture with fewer inhibitions to income generation, though there are important questions to be asked about such initiatives. Some schemes do not in fact resolve the long-term problems of funding the NHS. Selling capital assets such as land, for example, will at best only postpone the inability of the NHS to reconcile infinite demand with finite resources. Indeed, some initiatives might even exacerbate the problem in the longer term. For example, recent deals with property developers to build new hospital wings in exchange for land will ultimately create additional financial demands for staffing and associated running costs. Experience in the past has demonstrated that a critical factor is the revenue consequences of capital projects where investment may generate additional expenditure in years to come.

There are also questions of integrity, accountability and ultimately of how such additional resources are to be spent. What are the prospects that additional resources will find their way directly into patient care? Is there good reason to suspect that additional resources of this nature are being used to build empires or to invest in projects that do not have a direct bearing upon patient care? For example, car parking charges may be used to improve security for parked vehicles rather than to provide services for patients. Moreover, is it appropriate for management to invest considerable time and effort into income generation (the cost of which will probably be ignored for charging purposes) particularly if the potential sums are so low relative to total income.

In practice, income generation will remain of extremely modest proportions with limited benefits shared by patients, staff and visitors alike. Its importance lies in the attitudinal changes which it generates (particularly for management), the benefits of which will be potentially more substantial and longer-lasting though intangible. It is certainly not a major potential source of net income and comes a very long way behind the other options already discussed.

A LOTTERY

A lottery could provide additional income for the NHS based upon willingness rather than ability and/or obligation to pay. However, the yield could be low and unpredictable and the costs of collection high relative to yield. Income may be disproportionately sensitive to fluctuations in the economy and, if substantial funds were to be generated in this way, there may be considerable opposition from the gaming industry. Some people may find it morally objectionable that the NHS be funded in part by the proceeds of gambling and there is also no guarantee that the additional income raised by a lottery will actually be a real gain for the NHS. It may instead be used by the Government as a means of reducing its financial commitment to the NHS by way of general taxation.

CHARITABLE DONATIONS

Given the highly visible and often emotive nature of health care provision - particularly acute hospital services that are actively engaged in saving lives - the NHS has consistently been able to attract charitable donations over the years. Indeed, one might expect that, if anything, charitable donations may have a tendency to increase as the nature of the funding crisis becomes increasingly politicised and as concern over the future of the NHS spreads amongst the electorate. For those on the right of politics, there may be an opportunity to articulate this in terms of 'the active citizen', where individuals and organisations have increasingly been encouraged to play a more active part in society, donating their time and/or money to a variety of worthy causes (Ignatieff, 1991).

However, while often well-meaning, charitable donations can be regarded as little more than a windfall for minor programmes. Furthermore, they may seek to promote the cause of sectional interests to the exclusion of more needy or deserving cases. In other words, there is a sense in which the responsibility for the allocation of scarce resources would be displaced, especially where general revenues are levered by donations for particular treatments (e.g. kidney dialysis) and/or are for capital projects and items which incur future spending commitments.

In addition, charitable donations are neither formalised nor regularised. They rely upon the rather loose idea of the 'active citizen' and may ignore the legitimate role of the state in ensuring that society has a more structured approach to equity and of specifying the obligation that individuals and organisations might have. Thus, while taxation is inherently unpopular, its yield is much more predictable. Charitable organisations may insist upon a capital project to see a return that is both tangible and enduring and to avoid the possibility of money being sucked into services that had little or nothing to do with the donor. Hence, existing priorities may be distorted by the need to service a new capital asset, the provision of which may not be able to be thwarted as a result of potentially unwelcoming publicity - of 'looking a gift horse in the mouth'.

CONCLUSIONS

Of the possible additional sources of finance discussed above, perhaps the greatest potential lies in some form of earmarking. Earmarked taxes are likely to be more acceptable than local taxation for two reasons. First, it is unlikely that the NHS will be incorporated into local government as it stands at present. There is currently a trend towards less reliance being placed upon local government as a natural vehicle for providing strategically important services locally, in favour of arrangements where services and levels of spending are being controlled centrally. Second, it is unlikely that local government's tax base can be significantly increased. In addition to central government not wishing to increase devolved responsibility for raising revenue to the locality, crucial questions must be asked about whether local taxation has access to a sufficiently broad tax base to support a significant increase in its responsibilities. With reference to the latter, this position is likely to be exacerbated here in Scotland with the impending reorganisation of local government and the creation of smaller administrative units.

In terms of other sources of finance that have been discussed, a lottery is effectively a voluntarily incurred, earmarked payment. Patient charges and income generation appear to be limited by political and administrative issues and charitable donations would seem to be of limited potential. Consequently, without exception, all of these sources can do little more than offer income to the NHS at the margins. They are not alternatives in the sense that they can claim to reduce significantly the burden of general taxation, they are at best supplementary sources that may be able to bolster NHS resources. There is also the danger that their existence could be used to justify a reduction in central government's general taxation commitment to the NHS at the margins.

There are dilemmas here too in that the NHS operates within an economic environment in which it is unlikely to receive additional and substantial financial resources from general taxation or for that matter, at the cost of other publicly funded programmes. Therefore, perhaps one of the few alternatives available to policy makers at a local level would be to seek refuge in the development of supplementary sources of funding as a means of ameliorating the funding crisis. Crucially, however, some alternatives may generate additional expenditures as well as income, namely charitable donations and income generation. However, these expenditures may not be directly related to patient care and as such may constitute specific examples of budgetary rigidities which may accrue within the health service.

Budgetary rigidities are also an inescapable feature of earmarked taxes, so that while they may have a potentially higher yield than other options identified herein, problems remain. For example, accepting the principle of earmarking for one service will only lead to claims for similar treatment by others which are arguably of equal social importance (e.g. education). If all services were to become financed by earmarked taxes then severe budgetary rigidities may negate any early benefits for individual services. It also serves unnecessarily to limit public accountability and democratic decision-making by side-stepping decisions on incremental change. There may be a tendency for pressure groups to exploit earmarked taxes for their own purposes and to redefine them as fees or charges, even though incurred on a compulsory basis. Indeed, buoyant earmarked taxes may lead to over-expansion of service, something which would not have occurred as a result of specific democratic decisions. On the other hand, inelastic earmarked taxes will lead to unintended fiscal restraint for particular services.

The likely response, that such outcomes could be avoided by compensatory adjustments in general tax revenue (i.e. if earmarked taxes do not fully finance the service) begs the question, why bother with partial earmarking at all? Such outcomes could also be avoided if a service were financed by several earmarked taxes and by other incomes sources as well. A mix of income sources would probably lead to less income instability. But the greater the number of income sources the more the financing arrangements approach the current situation of financing health out of general taxation. The inescapable fact is that decisions about the levels and quality of public service provision and their financing are ultimately matters of democratic accountability, decisions which cannot and should not be side-stepped by dedication of income sources.

Finishing on an unexciting, but realistic note, it is clear that there are no easy solutions to the perceived financial problems of the NHS. The nature of those problems will change both with ongoing reforms (such as internal markets) and with any diversification of income sources. It is unrealistic and naive to search for a panacea. Nonetheless, a diversity of income sources may allow greater flexibility and responsiveness to current financial problems. The real question is the extent to which the various income sources discussed above can supplement general tax revenues, not substantially to increase revenue but rather to change the public's, management's, medic's and patient's perception and appreciation of the health service.

Unless the finance and delivery of health care is subjected to radical change, then central government will necessarily continue to be concerned with the availability of health care and continue to finance the vast bulk of it from general taxation. Nevertheless, there is scope for selective use of partial earmarking, for example increases in NICs or of voluntary participation in lotteries, both specifically devoted to health. There is also scope for increased use of patient charges to deter frivolous consumption, for example of prescribed medicines, provided exemptions safeguard the needy poor and for various forms of income generation. Private hospitals and health insurance will continue to have a role peripheral to the NHS.

The objective of these initiatives is less to raise revenue than to improve operational procedures within the NHS. They are a partial solution to a different question: how to improve service delivery rather than simply to increase its financing. These principles and potential practices are not unique to the NHS. They are already a concomitant and increasing part of most local government and other public sector services and there is no reason why they cannot be used for health care. However, it is unrealistic to see them as an escape from the fiscal restraint which affects the rest of the public sector. The NHS is not in a unique category of its own.

REFERENCES

Bailey, S, J. (1991), Fiscal Stress: The New System of Local Government Finance in England, *Urban Studies*, 28 (6), 889-907.

Bailey, S, J. and Paddison, R. (1988), *The Reform of Local Government Finance in Britain*, Routledge, London.

Butler, J. (1992), *Patients Policies and Politics: Before and After Working for Patients*, Open University Press, Milton Keynes.

Central Statistical Office, (1992), *Annual Abstract of Statistics*, HMSO: London.

Cm 555, *Working for Patients*, HMSO, London.

Cmnd 6453, (1976), *Local Government Finance: Report of the Committee of Enquiry*, (The Layfield Report), HMSO, London.

Cmnd 9189, (1984), *The Next Ten Years: Public Expenditure and Taxation into the 1990s*, HMSO, London.

Cmnd 9756, (1986), *The Reform of Personal Taxation*, HMSO, London.

Eckstien, H. (1958), *The English Health Service*, Harvard University Press, Cambridge Mass.

Ensor, T. (1993), *Future Health Care Options: Funding Health Care* IHSM Policy Unit, The Institute of Health Services Management: London.

Game, C. (1984), Axeman or Taxman - Who is Now the More Unpopular?, *Local Government Studies*, 10, 9-14.

House of Commons, Social Services Committee, (1988), *First Report 1987-88 Resourcing the National Health Service: Short Term Issues*, HMSO, London.

Ignatief, M. (1991), Citizenship and Moral Narcissism in Andrews, G. (ed.) *Citizenship*, Lawrence Wishart, London, 26-36.

Klein, R. (1988), Financing Health Care: The Three Options, *British Medical Journal*, 296, 735-736.

Klein, R. (1989), *The Politics of the NHS*, Longman, London.

Le Grand, J. Winter, D. and Woolley, F. The National Health Service: Safe in Whose Hands, in Hills, J. (ed.), *The State of Welfare: The Welfare State in Britain since 1974*, Clarendon Press, Oxford, 1990, 88-134.

Ministry of Health, (1956), *Report of the Committee of Enquiry into The Cost of The National Health Service*, (Chairman: C. W. Guillebaud), HMSO, London, Cmnd 9663.

Mulgan, G. and Murray, R. (1993), *Reconnecting Taxation*, DEMOS, London.

National Audit Office, (1993), *Income Generation in the NHS*, Report by the Comptroller and Auditor General, HMSO, London.

Royal Commission on The National Health Service, (1979), *Report*, HMSO, London, Cmnd 7615.

The Economist, (1993), Full Charge, 29th May, 30.

Wagner, R, E. (1991), *Charging for Government: User Charges and Earmarked Taxes in Principle and Practice*, Routledge, London.

12 NHS Corporate Governance - Myth or Reality ?

JAMES HARRISON

Aston Business School

INTRODUCTION

Public Sector Context

Reform in the public sector has been endemic for more than a decade. Gunn (1989) describes a process of transition from public administration through business management to public management. Hood (1991) characterises this "new public management" as having seven key elements:

- hands on professional management
- explicit standards and measures of performance
- greater emphasis on output controls
- shift to disaggregation of units
- shift to greater competition
- stress on private sector styles of management practice, and
- stress on greater discipline and parsimony in resource use.

Pollitt (1990) conveniently coined the term "managerialism" as a descriptor for this doctrine, which he depicts as a "a set of beliefs and practices, at the core of which burns the seldom-tested assumption that better management will prove an effective solvent for a wide range of economic and social ills" (p1).

These themes are easily discerned in the series of initiatives to which the NHS was subject throughout the 1980s and early 1990s. Initial measures were directed to making the then system more efficient such as Rayner Scrutinies in 1982 and the introduction of performance indicators in 1983. These eventually gave way to a qualitatively quite different set of strategies which sought much more profound change:

Setting Priorities in Health Care. Edited by M. Malek
© John Wiley & Sons Ltd

- the introduction of general management (DHSS 1983) as the means of changing the *organisation and management* of the service
- the community care initiatives (DHSS 1986; DHSS 1989a) designed to change fundamentally the *pattern of service* delivery
- the nation wide health targets (DHSS 1991a) which promulgated *explicit outcomes*, and
- quality (DHSS 1989b) and charter (DHSS 1991b) initiatives which reinforced a customer-centred *orientation*.

Arguably, however, of these substantive strategies, the most important and the most radical was the *Working for Patients* (WfP) (DHSS 1989b) reforms. These were published first as a White Paper and subsequently brought to law as the NHS & Community Care Act 1990.

The WfP reforms introduced a revised financial framework based on capitation funding, separate roles for "purchasers" and "providers" within a newly established internal market, and, allowed for the creation of NHS Trusts and GP Fund Holding (GPFH) practices. Of particular interest, however, are those aspects of the reforms which sought 'better' management, which included the following specific proposals:

- the creation of a Policy Board and a Management Executive nationally
- new roles for NHS Authorities
- new membership of NHS Authorities, and,
- devolution of decision making. (DHSS 1989b)

HEALTH AUTHORITIES AND MEMBER PERFORMANCE

Farnham & Horton (1993, p46) assert that the public sector "is predicated on the view that private sector economistic, rationalist and generic management is the ideal model..." It is no coincidence, therefore, that reformed Health Authorities display a remarkable similarity to the private sector board. Indeed, as Fitzgerald & Pettigrew (1991 p1) observe:

> The ideas draw on the experience of commercial, free market competition... [in which] the boards of companies act as the market managers

Thus the size and structure of the reformed Health Authorities together with the characteristics of the 'new' non executives are consistent with a more "business-like" approach. This is embodied in the modelling of these important public authorities upon the private sector institution of the company board.

It is important to note, however, that the performance of Health Authority members themselves has had a significant influence upon the changes to and within Health Authorities. Although the term Health Authorities did not come into existence until 1974, there has been an enduring interest in their activities and performance and that of their predecessor bodies (Farquharson-Lang, 1966; Kogan *et al.*, 1978; Haywood & Alaszewski 1980; Haywood & Ranade 1985; Ham, 1986a 1986b; Ham *et al.*, 1990). In terms of the members of such bodies Kogan *et al.*,

(1978 p75) felt "their impact upon the service was slight", a view supported by Haywood & Alaszewski (1980 p 89) who concluded that they "had little impact on the conduct of health authority affairs." This latter view was subsequently qualified further:

> Members must either adapt to the new emphasis on expectations and performance or accept that they are simply the 'dignified' element of the NHS constitution, the public facade of the private machine."
>
> (Haywood & Ranade, 1985 p112)

This then gives a flavour of the circumstances which pre dated and, in part, prompted some of the WfP reforms. The post reform functions of DHAs now include:

- assessing the population's need for health care
- purchasing services for residents
- public health
- statutory responsibilities, and,
- managing Units which remain under their control.

(DHSS, 1989c p1)

The greatest change, however, is in the reduction from 16-19 members to 6 non executive (including a Chair) and 5 executive directors (which must include the Chief Executive and Director of Finance). This on the basis that,

> If health authorities are to discharge their new responsibilities in a business-like way, they need to be smaller and to bring together executive and non-executive members to provide a single focus for effective decision making
>
> (DHSS 1989b, p65)

FOCUS OF THE RESEARCH

Corporate Governance is the term used to describe "the purpose and methods of how we structure and control companies large and small" (Midgley 1992, pvii) or "the system by which companies are directed and controlled" (Cadbury 1992, p15). A more comprehensive view, however, holds that:

> "the governance role is not concerned with running the business of the company, per se, but with giving overall direction to the enterprise, with overseeing and controlling the executive actions of management and with satisfying legitimate expectations, for accountability and regulation by interests beyond the corporate boundaries. If management is about running business; governance is about seeing it is run properly. All companies need governing as well as managing"
>
> (Tricker 1984, p6).

Tricker also provides a model in which he defines the four dimensions of governance (see Fig 1). This model offered a helpful insight in shaping the investigation and a convenient framework for the reporting of its findings.

Emphasis on external issues	Direction	Accountability
Emphasis on internal issues	Executive Management	Supervision

Focus on the needs of the business	**Focus on the needs of the shareholders and other stakeholder interests**

Figure 1. A Conceptual Model of the Activities of Corporate Governance

Source: Tricker, 1984 p. 174

Although much interest revolves around the evaluation of the reforms, for example, the effectiveness of the new purchasing organisations etc. This interest can obscure a more fundamental and growing unease with the 'fitness' of such organisations and thus, their ability to undertake effective assessment, sensitive purchasing etc. The much publicised and embarrassing debacles in the Wessex and West Midlands RHAs -particularly when coupled with the growing number, if less prominent, difficulties in some DHAs - reinforce these concerns. Such events have attracted scrutiny by the Committee of Public Accounts (Committee of Public Accounts 1993a and 1993b) and led directly to the establishment of the Corporate Governance Task Force, in June 1993 (Bottomley, 1993 p13). As Tricker observed,

> accountability is not an ex gratia activity on the part of those governing a company, but a precisely bounded duty based on the reality of power, and with appropriate and effective sanctions, if it is not properly performed.

(Tricker, 1984 p131)

The research reported here is concerned with exploring the expression and efficacy of corporate governance. It will focus upon *how* Authorities conduct themselves and their business rather than with the success or failure of a particular functional component of that business. If one doubts the value of such an investigation it is worth recalling that, at 1989 prices, the NHS accounted for 6% of GDP, some £29b in 1990. A typical DHA has an annual budget of between £13m-183m with which to purchase health care for between 89,000-860,000 inhabitants. It is also important to demonstrate whenever possible the validity of policy reform, to both illuminate current practice and future policy making. The findings of such research will therefore have organisational, economic and social implications for the management of the NHS and indeed beyond in the wider public sector.

APPROACH & METHODS.

The research concentrates upon the changes within English District Health Authorities (DHA). English, because the statutory framework and cultural diversity prevent meaningful national comparison, and DHAs, because of their functional and political centrality to local communities. Although similar changes have taken place in Regional Health Authorities (RHA), NHS Trusts and Family Health Service Authorities (FHSA) these have been excluded from consideration on the basis that RHAs currently exercise a 'strategic' role and NHS Trusts are providers. FHSAs are purchasers, but are different historically, culturally and organisationally. DHAs are, therefore, (currently) quite distinct as purchasers and in terms of their relationship with their local community as a natural 'constituency'.

The approach to the overall study is to collect data via a postal survey of Non Executive and Executive directors in a representative number of DHAs. This will be augmented by further and detailed investigation in a number of case study sites over time. This paper reports the findings from an initial proving study. Accordingly, the sample - of all the DHAs within a single RHA - may not be representative and have only limited *statistical* significance. They do, however, provide a snap shot at a particularly critical time and may indicate a level of perception and practice during the period of the Corporate Governance Task Force's deliberations.

THE FINDINGS

The Respondents

All Non Executive and Executive members of the constituent DHAs from within a single RHA were invited to complete a postal questionnaire during the course of July 1993. Of the 63 Directors then in post, 49 returned a completed questionnaire which was equal to a response rate of 77.8%. Of those who replied, 53% were Chairs/Non Executives and 47% were CEOs/Executives.

Of the Executive members, CEOs and Directors of Finance were the most likely to respond and together they represented 43.4% of all Executive respondents. In terms of the executive's antecedent discipline, a small proportion were clinical, the highest proportion, however, came from an Admin. & Clerical background. The latter have clearly been more successful in terms of an occupational strategy in the ratio of 2:1.

Two thirds of non executive directors had occupied their present role for 2 years or more, one third for less than two years. This tends to support the contention of 'continuity' rather than 'change' in the membership of DHAs (Ashburner *et al.,* 1991). 73.5% of respondents were male and 26.5% female. The majority of women respondents were Chairs/Non Executives; women Executives remain under represented. The proportion of women recently appointed is, however, now on a par with their male colleagues - see Table 1.

Table 1. Cross tabulation of Gender by Tenure

	Base	Male	Female
	49	36 73.5%	13 26.5%
Less than 2 years	15 30.6%	7 14.3%	8 16.3%
2-5 years	22 44.9%	19 38.8%	3 6.1%
More than 5 years	12 24.5%	10 20.4%	2 4.1%

All age ranges between 20 and 79 years were represented, with the majority falling in late middle life.

Of those respondents who were Chairs/Non Executives, (effectively) the smallest proportion was drawn from the private sector and the largest from the public sector. This again implies continuity rather than change. Free text comments would suggest that respondents from a private sector background were, perhaps, less satisfied with issues of corporate governance than those from other backgrounds.

Strategic Direction

In reply to questions asking respondents if their Authority had discussed its purpose and established a mission statement, strongly affirmative responses were received to both i.e. 95.9% and 98% respectively. However, when asked if the mission stated to whom and for what the Authority was to be held accountable the response, while still positive, fell to 77.6%. Equally, when asked if the mission statement outlined the values the Authority would use as the basis of its judgements, the response was again 77.6%. See Fig 2.

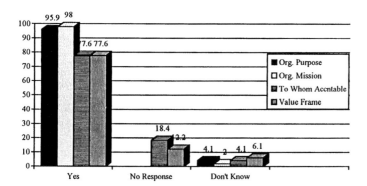

Figure 2. The Relationship of Purpose and Mission to Accountability and Values (percent)

These figures suggest that while purpose and mission have been discussed and documented this has not gone far enough. The rhetoric does not match reality. About 1:5 Directors are unclear about their wider obligations to stake holders and slightly less deny or are ignorant of any moral or ethical under pinning for the organisations decision making.

In terms of the single most important strategic issue facing respondents, the greatest number identified questions of the organisation's boundaries/merger (55.1%) followed by a combined group of those who specified contracting or commissioning (38.8%). No other single issue emerged to any significant degree, including finance, marketing etc.. This would suggest that these issues are either under control, not an identified priority, or are viewed as (relatively) insignificant. See Fig 3.

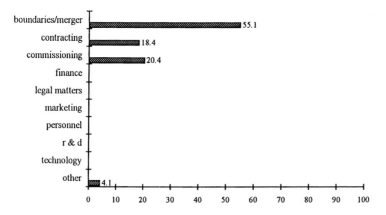

Figure 3. The Most Important Strategic Issue Facing District Health Authorities (percent)

When asked if priorities had been set for member involvement 61.2% stated this was the case, 34.7% that it was not. This would suggest that for 1:3 respondents there is no explicit or systematic involvement in the key strategic areas they had identified.

Executive Management

When asked if the atmosphere in the boardroom encouraged frank discussion and permitted both non executives and executives to challenge assumptions 98% of respondents agreed that this was so. A similar level of agreement was expressed when respondents were asked if non executives and executives could disagree with the chair and therefore influence his/her decision.

If the atmosphere and the nature of the debate is as open as such responses would seem to indicate, what of the substance of executive management ? When asked if non executives and executives have the opportunity to place items on the Authority agenda 81.4% replied that they did. Nearly 1:5 denied or did not know if this was the case. Of those respondents in the latter categories, non executives formed the highest proportion and women directors were twice as likely to hold such views as their male counter-parts.

When the substance for debate was clear, however, the overwhelming manner of decision making was by consensus (85.7%) and voting (14.3%). The majority of directors saw their contribution as being generalist (42.9%) or corporate (36.7%) in character. Only 20.4% saw themselves as specialists. Of the executives in this latter group, Directors of Finance and of Public Health were more likely to hold this view.

Whatever the perception of the nature of their contribution, when asked who made most decisions 91.8% of respondents identified executive directors.

Supervision

Those surveyed were asked to indicate the existence of audit, remuneration or management review committees. *No single respondent did so.*

When asked if timely and appropriate information was provided to the Board 69.4% of respondents agreed that this was so. 79.6% agreed that the information provided supported monitoring and strategic control.

Respondents were asked to indicate if the Authority reviewed its own working style on a regular basis; 63.3% agreed. When asked if the Chair reviewed the performance of non executive directors on a regular basis 36.7% agreed. Although, without exception, Chairs indicated that this was the case, a significant proportion of [their own] non executives did not support this view - see Table 2. However, when asked if the Chair and non executives regularly scheduled reviews of the executives only 16.3% agreed that these took place. See Fig 4.

Table 2. Cross tabulation of Chair's Review of NEDs by Non Executive Role

	Base	No Reply	Yes	No	Don't Know
		1	7	4	14
	26	3.8%	26.9%	15.4%	53.8%
Chairman	3		3		
	11.5%	0	11.5%	0	0
Non Executive Member	23	1	4	4	14
	88.5%	3.8%	15.4%	15.4%	53.8%

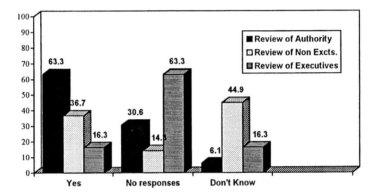

Figure 4. Review Practice within District health Authority (percent)

The nature of the relationship between non executives and executives was characterised as close (30.6%), cordial (67.3%), tense (2%) and distant (0%).

Accountability

When asked if there was a shared sense of corporate identity, 95.9% of respondents agreed that this was the case. 89.8% agreed that there was clarity about the boundary between the Chair and the CEO. We are able to conjecture, therefore, that there is a high level of agreement amongst respondents as to the nature of the shared organisational reality they inhabit, and, that the focus of leadership - and therefore accountability - is unambiguous.

When asked how frequently their Authority met in public, the majority (83.7%) indicated 4-6 times per annum. Given that many pre reform DHAs met publicly on a monthly basis, this represents a reduction in transparency by nearly half.

Respondents were asked if they thought it was important to act in an ethical manner, to which there was 100% agreement. However, when asked if their Authority had an explicit ethical code only 30.6% agreed that this was so. This was brought into sharp relief when respondents were asked if any non executive had declared a potential conflict of interest - 38.8% of respondents indicated that they had. See Fig 5. In short all agreed the importance of acting ethically, yet only 1:3 had any explicit ethical framework. Against this backdrop, there was an unexpectedly high level of reported conflict of interest, a perception Chairs did not appear to share - see Table 3.

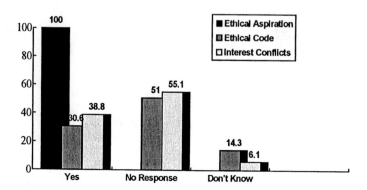

Figure 5. The Relationship of Ethical Aspiration to Practice and Experience in DHAs (percent)

Table 3. Cross tabulation of Conflict of Interest by Member Type

	Base	Yes	No	DK
		19	27	3
	49	38.8%	55.1%	6.1%
Chairman	3 6.1%	0	3 6.1%	0
Non Executives	23 46.9%	7 14.3%	13 26.5%	3 6.1%
Chief Executive	4 8.2%	3 6.1%	1 2.0%	0
Executives	19 38.8%	9 18.4%	10 20.4%	0

Key Influences upon Performance

Induction

A little more than two thirds (67.3%) of respondents reported receiving an induction or orientation into their role as a director. This was not the case for about half the non executives and about a quarter of executives. The number reporting this, however, reduces when one compares the experience of recent and past appointees - see Table 4.

Table 4. Cross tabulation of Induction by Tenure

	Base	Yes	No	DK
		33	14	2
	49	67.3%	28.6%	4.1%
	15	12	3	0
Less than 2 years	30.6%	24.5%	6.1%	
	22	13	7	2
2-5 years	44.9%	26.5%	14.3%	4.1%
	12	8	4	0
More than 2 years	24.5%	16.3%	8.2%	

Statutory Obligations and Legal Responsibilities

55.1% of respondents indicated that they had been provided with this information, 36.7% had not and 8.2% did not know. In short, nearly half of all respondents were unclear about their obligations and responsibilities. This was fairly evenly distributed amongst directors of all types, except for Chairs who do appear to be much clearer about such matters. Recently appointed directors are somewhat more informed than those of longer standing.

Personal Influence

When asked who had the most significant influence upon their role locally, a varied picture emerged. Two things are clear. Firstly Chairs are generally most influenced by their CEO and vice versa. A not unexpected finding (Stewart, 1986). Secondly, 4.8% of Chairs, 11.9% of non executives and 38.1% of executives - 54.8% in all - claim that the CEO is the most significant influence upon them. This compares with a total of 23.8% for DHA Chairs. The CEO is clearly a pivotal figure and therefore a significant focus for promoting and sustaining effective performance.

DISCUSSION

In common with much research, this study raises more questions than it answers. It is, of course, important to remember that the sample is small and therefore not necessarily representative, and so, the findings need to be interpreted with caution. That said, however, the study does provide a timely insight into the perceptions and practice of board members in the constituent DHAs within a single English RHA.
    Key themes to emerge are as follows.

Strategic Direction

It is clear that directors perceive the importance of their contribution in this area but these data suggest that there is some discrepancy between the apparent and the real e.g. the existence of a mission statement but some uncertainty about stake holders. Equally, a clear pattern of priorities is evident but little systematic involvement of some board members.

Executive Management

A litmus question in this area concerned the ability of directors to place items on the board's agenda. 20% of respondents were uncertain or doubted their ability to do so. Given that many of those who hold such a view were non executives/women this may imply a difference between the powerful and the powerless. The presence of outside directors / women may not in itself guarantee either acceptance or an acceptable performance. Also important is the perception of about a quarter of executives who saw themselves as specialists. Such a view may both narrow their own contribution and reduce the nature and quality of the wider debate. Whilst matters of health policy and management - at this level - are complex and must in part be 'technical', this may also be used as a device to subdue non executive involvement. Were non executives to be so influenced, they may be reluctant to raise agenda questions ? They may also be reluctant to shape or challenge the decisions which, by common consent, are made predominantly by executives?

Supervision

The evidence here is unequivocal. No respondent reported the existence of an audit, remuneration or management review committee. Equally, the level of agreement that the Authority, the non executive directors, and, the executives are explicitly reviewed falls progressively and sharply. This is not to suggest that supervision is absent. Clearly this is not the case, but subtle mechanisms may be both less obvious and less robust. Effective corporate governance demands that such processes be made manifest. Also important, is the near unanimous view that relations between the parties are close or cordial; this may suggest a degree of non executive capture.

Accountability

Here again the picture is one of inconsistency. As noted above, respondents had only a partially formed view of, and their responsibilities toward, stake holders. This may offer some explanation of the substantial reduction in the extent to which DHAs feel the need to conduct their business in public. The level of ethical aspiration expressed was commendably high but, not unlike strategic direction, actual performance was somewhat different. With 1:3 reporting a conflict of interest by a non executive director, evidence of a formal ethical code was slight.

Whilst the picture detailed above is far from unremitting gloom - particularly in terms of recent appointments - there is scope for improvement. To what extent therefore do the findings of the Report of the Corporate Governance Task Force encourage or facilitate this ? The principal means by which it seeks to effect change is by promulgating a Code of Accountability for the NHS and a Code of Conduct for NHS Boards. Helpfully the report clearly identifies the role of NHS boards:

- to set strategic direction, priorities and objectives
- to oversee the delivery of planned results

- to ensure effective financial stewardship
- to ensure high standards of corporate governance and personal behaviour
- to appoint, appraise and remunerate senior executives, and
- to ensure effective dialogue between the organisation and the local community.

(Shaw *et al.*, 1994 p22)

This is supplemented by specific additional responsibilities concerning mental health legislation, external relations, staff relations, personnel policy and employment practice. All of which are to be carried out with due regard to the public service values of "accountability", "probity" and "openness" (Shaw *et al.*, 1994 p15).

Using Tricker's taxonomy, a more detailed analysis of the report reveals an emphasis upon accountability, supervision, executive management and direction in that order of importance. In terms of the *accountability* domain:

- personal/organisational accountability to the Secretary of State (and thus Parliament) is made abundantly clear
- this duty is reflected in the Code of Accountability to which all board members are *required* to subscribe
- in the sense of 'accounting to' the community, NHS bodies will have to:

    - publish an annual report of their stewardship and performance
    - publish the remuneration of directors
    - provide/ensure reasonable access to information by the public, patients and staff

- directors will be required to declare private interests which are material and relevant to NHS business.

Whilst these measures go a considerable way towards addressing concerns about accountability, some encouragement to meet and conduct business more frequently in public would have been welcome. As Sir Adrian Cadbury (1993) has observed, "openness is the basis of public confidence in any corporate system"

The *supervision* dimension is addressed in the report in terms of:

- an obligation to establish both audit and remuneration committee(s)
- a requirement to co-operate with the NHS Management Executive and the Audit Commission/external auditors
- the adoption of, yet to be published, "good practice guides" on finance and performance.

Such proposals again go a considerable way to addressing concerns in this area. However, whilst recognising that the report does require boards to,

> ensure that management arrangements are in place to enable responsibility to be clearly delegated to senior executives for the main programmes of action and for

performance against programmes to be monitored and senior executives held to account

(Shaw *et al,*, 1994 p23)

more emphasis could have been given to the need for the Chair review the effectiveness of non executive directors. A statement upon how to deal with dysfunctional Chairs would also have been welcome and more even handed.

The *executive management* aspect of Corporate Governance is addressed in terms of:

- defining clearly the roles of the Chair and non executive directors
- emphasising the difference between the executives and the non executives who "are not on the board to manage the authority or trust and must not compromise their detachment" (Shaw *et al.*, 1994 p34).
- discouraging unreasonable constraints being placed upon the chief executive.

These particular proposals, together with a clear view of the role of the board, adequately distinguish between management and governance.

Finally, the element of corporate governance concerned with *direction*. The report has least to say about this component, other than:

- to identify the need to set strategic direction as a key board responsibility
- identifying the boards key stake holders
- encouraging dialogue with the local community.

Whilst separate and earlier guidance exists in this area, what appears to have been assumed is that the national agenda and priorities will have primacy and that strategic direction is little more than adapting macro policy to local circumstance.
This being framed in the context of 'business management', it becomes a rational rather political process. However, the notion that Health Authorities and Trusts will be prepared or able to subordinate their local and market interests in this way seems both unrealistic and unlikely. Ironically it is in defining and pursuing such interest that the public interest has been shown to be at its most vulnerable.

CONCLUSION

This paper sets out, against the backdrop of public sector reform and concerns about Health Authority member performance, the findings from an initial study of corporate governance in the NHS. The findings - which are compared with the recently published Report of the Corporate Governance Task Force - begins to explore the extent to which corporate governance in a post reform NHS exists and whether it is, or is not, an effective focus for organisational performance. Against the backdrop of some spectacular examples of organisational failure, and, the as yet unknown influence of recent guidance in this regard, this must remain an open question. What is clear is that such collapses and their underlying dysfunction, raise important moral questions, reduce public acceptability and participation and diminish and distort the effective setting of priorities in health care.

REFERENCES

Ashburner L, Ferlie E & Pettigrew A (1991) Organisational Restructuring and the New Health Authorities: Continuity or Change? *Paper presented at the BAM Conference*, University of Bath, September

Cadbury Report (1992) *A Report of the Committee on The Financial Aspects of Corporate Governance* Gee: London

Cadbury A (1993) Effective Boards *Paper presented at NAHAT Conference on Building Effective NHS Boards*, Queen Elizabeth Conference Centre, London, September.

Bottomley V (1993) *Conference Focus* Health Service Journal 24th June 11-16

Committee of Public Accounts (1993) Fifty-seventh Report *West Midlands Regional Health Authority: Regionally Managed Services Organisation*, HMSO: London

Committee of Public Accounts (1993) Sixty-third Report *Wessex Regional Health Authority Regional Information Systems Plan* HMSO: London

DHSS (1983) *NHS Management Inquiry* [Griffiths Report] HMSO: London

DHSS (1986) *Neighbourhood Nursing: A Focus for Care* [The Cumberlege Report], HMSO: London

DHSS (1989a) *Caring for People - Community Care in the Next Decade and Beyond*, HMSO: London

DHSS (1989b) *Working for Patients* White Paper HMSO: London

DHSS (1989c) *Role of District Health Authorities: Analysis of Issues*, HMSO: London

DHSS (1991a) *The Health of the Nation* HMSO: London

DHSS (1991b) *The Patients Charter* HMSO: London

Farquharson-Lang W M (1966) *Administrative Practice of Hospital Boards in Scotland*, SHHD: Edinburgh

Farnham D & Horton S (1993) *Managing the New Public Services* Macmillan: Basingstoke

Fitzgerald L & Pettigrew A (1991) *Boards in Action: Some Implications for Health Authorities*, NHSTD: Bristol

Gunn L (1989) A Public Management Approach to the NHS *Health Services Management Review* 2(1) 10-20; March

Ham C (1986a) *Strengthening the Role of Health Authority Members* Kings Fund: London

Ham C (1986b) *Managing Health Services: Health Authority Members in Search of a Role*, SAUS: Bristol

Ham C, Huntington J & Best G (1990) *Managing with Authority* NAHA/NHSTA/SFPC: London

Haywood S C & Alaszewski A (1980) *Crisis in the Health Service* Croom Helm: London:

Haywood S C & Ranade W (1985) *District Health Authorities in Action: Two Years On - A Progress Report* HSMC: Birmingham

Hood C (1991) A public management for all seasons? *Public Administration* 69(1): 3-19

Kogan M *et al.,* (1978) *The Working of the NHS,* Royal Commission Research Paper Number 1, HMSO: London:

Midgley K (Ed) (1982) *Management Accountability and Corporate Governance,* Macmillan: London

Pollitt C (1990) *Managerialism in the Public Service* Blackwell: Oxford

Shaw J, Askew B, Burgess S, Marchment M & Punt K (1994) *Public Enterprise: Governance in the NHS* Report of the Corporate Governance Task Force NHSME: Leeds

Stewart R (1987) *Templeton Series on General Management* Issue Study No.1 'DGMs and Chairmen: A Productive Relationship?' NHS Training Authority: Bristol

Tricker R I (1984) *Corporate Governance* Gower: Aldershot

13 Referrals from Primary Care - Priorities and Strategies for Change

ELAINE MCCOLL[1], JOHN NEWTON[1] &
ALLEN HUTCHINSON[2]
[1]*University of Newcastle*
[2]*University of Hull*

BACKGROUND AND INTRODUCTION

Wide variations in referral rates by general practitioners from primary care to secondary care have been noted by a number of authors and over a period of many years. For example, in a study of Manchester general practitioners, Wilkin and Smith (1987a) reported a four-fold difference in referral rates between the highest and lowest quintiles (11.8 and 2.9 per hundred consultations respectively). Examining practices in the National Morbidity Surveys, Crombie and Fleming (1988) found a similar difference, while Noone and colleagues (1989) identified a threefold difference in referral rates amongst 25 practices in the Oxford Region. These observed differences have been a matter of concern, particularly for policy-makers and managers. In 1985, the then Chief Medical Officer (Acheson, 1985) was concerned that 'a phenomenon so gross can continue to defy analysis'. A later report by the National Audit Office (1991) suggested that differences in referral rates placed a question mark over issues of quality of care and resource use. Marked variations suggest that some doctors may be over-referring and using scarce hospital resources inefficiently while others are failing to refer patients who might benefit from specialist opinion and care. However, there is no consensus as to the most 'appropriate' referral rate. The average is 8 per 100 consultations but there is no empirical evidence as to whether this is optimal in terms of patient well-being (Metcalfe, 1991). Clearly, further examination of the relationship between referral behaviour and patient outcome is required before guidelines can be given on appropriate referral patterns. Nonetheless, there is considerable pressure from managers and politicians to reduce existing variations in referral rates.

Structural factors such as levels of morbidity, age structure and relative deprivation of practice populations (Wilkin and Smith, 1987a; Wilkin and Smith, 1987b), as well as the experience of general practitioners (Reynolds *et al.*, 1991;

Setting Priorities in Health Care. Edited by M. Malek
© John Wiley & Sons Ltd

Newton *et al.*, 1991) and the availability of secondary care facilities (Noone *et al.*, 1989) have been shown to have some influence on referral behaviour, but are unable to explain much of the variation. Qualitative studies have shown that referral behaviour is also influenced by factors internal to the doctor (such as tolerance of risk) and general practice and by external pressures and structural constraints.

But a general understanding of the factors affecting referral behaviour may not be sufficient to trigger behavioural change amongst doctors. Metcalfe (1991) believes that "personal and educational factors are not amenable to administrative influence, and crude administrative measures used to shift the balance by intruding in the situational field are unlikely to achieve the desired result". He argues instead for an educational approach based on self- and peer-review. Stocking (1992) further suggests that the implementation of change is most likely to succeed if those who will be ultimately responsible for the process of change are also involved in setting the agenda. These concepts of identifying opportunity for change through peer-review are also central to the doctrine of medical audit.

It was in this spirit that Northumberland Family Health Services Authority (FHSA) embarked on a local initiative, focusing on an informed review of current referral practice. To this end, quantitative analysis of 1990-1991 referral rates was carried out by Cambridge Medical Information on behalf of the FHSA (Northumberland Family Health, 1992). Data supplied by individual practices in their annual reports were analysed according to the criteria outlined by Coulter *et al.* (1991). Each practice was supplied with individualised feedback, comparing its referral rates across a range of specialities with those for all practices in Northumberland. Guidelines on interpreting high and low referral rates were included, along with suggestions for auditing the referral process. It was explicitly recognised that this information was a stimulus to exploring the factors which affect referral and to understanding why they were as they were, rather than a judgement of what was an appropriate referral rate. To complement this quantitative approach, Northumberland Medical Audit Advisory Group (MAAG) commissioned a qualitative study to establish general practitioners' own agenda for change with respect to the referral process. This study was carried out at the Centre for Health Services, University of Newcastle upon Tyne.

THE DELPHI APPROACH

The Delphi approach was employed to derive general practitioners' views regarding priorities for change. This technique (the name derives from the Greek Oracle at Delphi) is a method for establishing a consensus view on a chosen topic. It was developed at the RAND Corporation in the late 1940s (Quade, 1967); early applications were in the area of forecasting technological events, but it has been increasingly applied in the fields of education, social planning and the health services (Bond and Bond, 1982; Burns *et al.*, 1990; Hutchinson and Fowler, 1992). In the Delphi approach, the knowledge or opinions of a group of "experts" are combined to quantify variables "which are either intangible or shrouded in uncertainty" (Pill, 1971); an "expert" may be any individual who is competent to make a relevant input. The technique involves a series of self-administered questionnaires, thereby guaranteeing anonymity for the individual respondents. The first questionnaire generally presents a series of statements and asks the chosen experts to make a judgement or express an opinion on each of these statements (Duffield, 1989). The results are then analysed and fed back to the experts; this second (and any subsequent rounds) provide the opportunity for respondents to refine their views until a consensus is reached.

The Delphi technique therefore represents a relatively quick and inexpensive means of achieving a representative consensus view. It also overcomes some of the main drawbacks associated with the consensus conference or committee approach to decision making, such as problems of adverse group dynamics and practical difficulties in convening a meeting. The technique, with its key characteristics of expert input, anonymity of response, controlled feedback and statistical group response was therefore considered to be highly appropriate in determining general practitioners' priorities for change with respect to the referral process.

In this study, two postal questionnaires were used to identify five areas of potential change in referral practice and to elicit suggestions of strategies for change. The ideas put forward in these questionnaires were then discussed in depth with a random selection of practices across the county; these discussions provided a list of topics or projects which, it was suggested, could form the basis for a referrals initiative to be further developed by Northumberland MAAG.

THE FIRST ROUND DELPHI QUESTIONNAIRE

Methods

The first round Delphi questionnaires contained a list of twenty seven factors known to or held to influence referral behaviour, based on the findings of previous research in the Northern Region and elsewhere (Newton *et al.*, 1991; Healey and Ryan, 1992). These included doctor characteristics (e.g. the doctor's need for reassurance), patient characteristics (e.g. social and economic circumstances) and structural factors (e.g. the range of open access services available). Doctors were asked to rate each factor, on five-point scales, in terms of both perceived amenability to change and of the doctor's own keenness to see change with respect to that factor. A score of 1 indicated "not at all amenable to change" or "not at all keen", while a score of 5 denoted "amenable to change without any difficulty" or "very keen".

Since all general practitioners were involved in the referral process, all were considered to be "experts" for the purpose of this work. Accordingly, in April 1992, the questionnaire was sent to all 178 general practitioners then on Northumberland FHSA's list. The questionnaire was accompanied by a letter from Northumberland MAAG, explaining the nature and purpose of the study. A reminder, enclosing a second copy of the questionnaire, was sent to all those who had not responded after three weeks.

Response rates

A total of 121 questionnaires were returned, a crude response rate of 68%. Of these, five were returned completely blank, yielding 116 usable responses. Unfortunately, the timing of this first questionnaire coincided with a major survey of general practitioners' views on health service commissioning by Northumberland District Health Authority; this undoubtedly had a detrimental effect on response rates. Some respondents also had some conceptual difficulties in completing the questionnaire, as evidenced by their comments both to the Centre for Health Services Research and to Northumberland MAAG. Nevertheless, the usable response rate of 65.2% was highly satisfactory for this type of approach. 88% of all practices in the county were represented. A higher response rate (72.3%) was obtained from doctors in practices which were in the upper tertile on overall referral rates than those in the middle and lower tertiles (60.7% and 56.5% respectively); however, this difference was not statistically significant. Response rates were not significantly associated with location (urban, mixed or rural), list size (< 4000 patients, 4000-8000 or > 8000 patients) or fund-holding status. However, doctors from vocational training practices were significantly over-represented; those from such practices were much more likely to respond (75.9%) than were their colleagues from non training practices (48.6%).

Findings

For each of the 27 statements presented in the questionnaire, and for each of the dimensions of amenability to change and keenness for change, a mean score was computed across all 116 valid responses. On the amenability dimension, a high mean score is indicative of greater amenability to change. On the keenness dimension, a high mean score indicates a greater desire for change. The findings are summarised in Table 1.

Amenability to change

Factors relating to practice structure and to attributes of individual doctors were seen as most amenable to change. For example, the mean score for "the degree to which I can call on the expertise of partners or colleagues within the practice" was 4.0, equivalent to "amenable to change without much difficulty". By contrast, factors relating to patient characteristics were seen as less amenable to change. The mean score for "patients' social and economic circumstances" was 2.0, indicating that doctors considered that these could be changed only with great difficulty. Practice referral rates, categorised as high, medium and low, did not significantly affect doctor's overall views on the amenability to change of the factors presented; when the 27 factors were ranked on the basis of their mean scores, a high degree of agreement was achieved across all three groups (Kendall's coefficient of concordance W = 0.93, p < .001). However, opinions on the amenability to change of "referral policy in this practice" did show a significant association with referral rates; doctors in practices with medium referral rates saw this as more amenable to change than their counterparts in high referring practices or low referring practices.

That doctors in practices with low referral rates rate this factor significantly lower on the amenability dimension may be an indication of a "floor effect" - a perception of little scope for further reductions. Consensus on the ranking of the factors was also achieved across rural, mixed and urban practices (W = 0.86, p < .001). However, the setting in which doctors practised did appear to influence their views on the amenability to change of patients' social and economic circumstances; doctors in rural practices were significantly more optimistic that these could be changed than were there colleagues in mixed and urban areas. This may reflect the relative levels of deprivation across these settings.

Table 1. Round I Delphi Questionnaire Results: Mean Scores for Amenability to Change and Keenness for Change

Factor	Amenability to change [a]	Keenness for change [b]
1. The range of specialist care available to me	3.4	4.0
2. The pressure my patients put on me	3.0	3.4
3. My tolerance of uncertainty	3.2	3.4
4. The length of hospital waiting lists	2.9	4.7
5. My sense of clinical autonomy	3.4	2.8
6. Referral policy in this practice	3.9	3.0
7. My perception of the benefits of what is available in secondary care	3.5	3.7
8. What my partners may think of my referral rate	3.8	3.2
9. My medical knowledge and training	3.5	4.0
10. The personal characteristics of patients I see in this practice	2.2	2.8
11. My need for reassurance	3.1	3.1
12. What consultants may think of my referral rate	3.2	3.3
13. The type of cases and conditions I see in this practice	2.2	2.9
14. Patients' expectations of referral	2.8	3.5
15. The pressure of work in this practice	2.7	3.9
16. What the FHSA may think of my referral rate	3.4	3.0
17. The cost of the referral to the NHS	2.9	3.4
18. My knowledge of and relationship with consultants	3.6	3.8
19. The degree to which I can call on the expertise of partners or colleagues within the practice	4.0	3.3
20. Patients' need for reassurance	2.8	3.5
21. My estimation of clinical probabilities	3.3	3.6
22. Patients' social and economic circumstances	2.0	3.8
23. Concern about possible legal action by a patient	2.8	3.6
24. The distance patients live from specialist care	2.3	3.4
25. The financial implications to patients of being referred	2.7	3.4
26. My freedom to refer to the hospital of my choice	3.2	3.6
27. The range of open access services available to me	3.4	3.8
Overall mean across all 27 factors	3.1	3.5

[a] A higher mean score indicates greater amenability to change
[b] A higher mean score indicates greater keenness for change

Keenness for change

In general, doctors were most keen to change factors relating to the provision of secondary care services and to their relationship with consultants. Almost all doctors expressed a desire to change the length of hospital waiting lists, with 72% declaring that they were "very keen" for change. External opinion appeared to be comparatively unimportant; the mean scores for "what my partners may think of my referral rate" and "what the FHSA may think of my referral rate" were 3.2 and 3.0 respectively. These scores are attributable mainly to a high endorsement of the "indifferent" category for these items (66.1% and 68.2% respectively); indeed some respondents commented that they had no idea what anyone thought of their referral rates. Doctors were also largely indifferent or even actively opposed to changing the mix of patients they cared for; the mean scores for "the type of cases and conditions I see in this practice" and for "the personal characteristics" of patients I see in this practice" were 2.9 and 2.8 respectively. They appeared to guard their sense of clinical autonomy; over 30% of respondents said that they were "not very keen" or "not at all keen" for change with respect to this factor. Overall, the ranking of the 27 factors on the basis of mean scores for keenness indicated close agreement between doctors from practices with high, medium and low referral rates (Kendall's coefficient of concordance $W = 0.91$, $p < .001$). A high degree of consensus was also achieved across all practice settings ($W = 0.92$, $p < .001$).

Priorities for change

Where the aim is to generate a local agenda for change by voluntary action, success in bringing about change is most likely for those factors perceived as relatively easy to alter and for which there is a strong desire for change. In setting the agenda for change, such factors should be accorded high priority. By contrast, those factors which were perceived as difficult to alter and about which doctors were indifferent or opposed to change should be regarded as lower priority. To determine overall priorities for change it was therefore necessary to synthesise respondents' views across the two dimensions. To do this, the overall mean scores for amenability to change and keenness for change were computed to be 3.1 and 3.5 respectively. The average scores across all respondents, shown in Table 1, for each of the 27 factors were then plotted in a matrix defined by these two values; for example, "my tolerance of uncertainty" (mean score for amenability 3.2, mean score for keenness 3.4) was categorised as "high amenability - low keenness". The results are summarised in Table 2 and are shown graphically in Figure 1. Seven factors were rated as highly amenable to change and highly desirable to change. Five of these related to the availability of secondary services and to the provision of information on such services. The remaining two were related to general practitioners' own skills, both in a general sense ("my medical knowledge and training") and more particularly as these related to clinical judgement ("my estimation of clinical probabilities"). Those factors which were accorded low ratings on both dimensions related in the main to patient characteristics and case-mix. Low priority was also given to economic factors, with both "the cost of the referral to the NHS" and "the financial implications to patients of being referred" falling into this quadrant of the matrix.

Table 2. Round I Delphi Questionnaire Results - Amenability to Change vs Keenness for Change

Low amenability High keenness (mean score for amenability < 3.1 mean score for keenness ≥ 3.5)	High amenability High keenness (mean score for amenability ≥ 3.1 mean score for keenness ≥ 3.5)
The length of hospital waiting lists* The pressure of work in this practice Patients' need for reassurance Patients' social and economic circumstances Concern about possible legal action by a patient	The range of specialist care available to me* My perceptions of the benefits of what is available in secondary care* My medical knowledge and training* My knowledge of and relationship with consultants * My estimation of clinical probabilities* My freedom to refer to the hospital of my choice* The range of open access services available to me*
Low amenability **Low keenness** (mean score for amenability < 3.1 mean score for keenness < 3.5)	**High amenability** **Low keenness** (mean score for amenability ≥ 3.1 mean score for keenness < 3.5)
The pressure my patients put on me * The personal characteristics of patients I see in this practice The type of cases and conditions I see in this practice Patients' expectations of referral The cost of the referral to the NHS The distance patients live from specialist care The financial implications to patients of being referred	My tolerance of uncertainty My sense of clinical autonomy Referral policy in this practice * What my partners may think of my referral rate My need for reassurance What consultants may think of my referral rate What the FHSA may think of my referral rate The degree to which I can call on the expertise of partners or colleagues within the practice

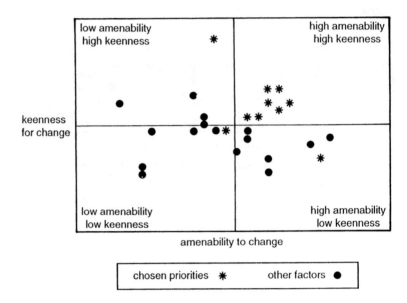

Figure 1. Priorities for Change

THE SECOND ROUND DELPHI QUESTIONNAIRE

Methods

From the responses to first round Delphi questionnaire ten priority areas for change were identified. These included the seven factors rated as highly amenable to change and highly desirable to change, as shown in Table 2. It was also decided to include the factor which doctors were keenest of all to change, but perceived as potentially difficult to alter - "the length of hospital waiting lists"- as well as "referral policy in this practice", which respondents perceived as reasonably amenable to change, but were relatively indifferent about altering. Finally, the factor "the pressure my patients put on me" had a mean score on both the amenability and keenness dimensions which fell close to the threshold values and this was also included. These ten target areas for action and change were fed back to the panel of 116 first round respondents in the second Delphi questionnaire, sent out at the beginning of July 1992. As before, a single reminder with a second copy of the questionnaire, was sent to all those who had not responded after three weeks. Respondents were asked to identify their personal priorities for change by allocating a total of 100 points among the ten factors. They were also asked to suggest, in their own words, strategies by which change might be brought about for their top three priorities. They were asked to do this under the headings; what kind of change do you envisage?; who should be involved in the change process?; how might change be achieved?; what are the potential forces in favour of change?; what are the potential barriers to change?

Response rates

From the 116 first round respondents contacted, 72 usable replies were obtained. We were advised by a practice manager that one other doctor was on maternity leave. The response rate of 62.6% provided a substantive panel of "expert" replies from which to synthesise a consensus. 64.7% of all Northumberland practices were represented. There was no significant difference in response rates across the range of practice settings or among doctors from practices with different referral rates. Nor did practice list size, fund holding or vocational training status have a significant effect on response rates.

Findings

Priorities for change

Three criteria were considered in assessing overall priorities for change:

(i)   The total number of respondents allocating points to each factor.
(ii) The total number of points allocated to each factor.
(iii) The number of points that the factor was rated as the respondent's top priority; in other words, ranked 1st or joint 1st.

A scoring system was derived which allowed us to combine the information provided by each criterion. In this system, the ten factors were ranked separately on each criterion; ten marks were then allocated for first place, nine for second and so on. The marks were summed across all criteria and the five factors with the highest totals (18 or more) were selected for further consideration. Suggestions for strategies for change for the five factors selected in this way were coded and synthesised to provide a basis for discussion in the in-depth interviews. The highest priority for change thus identified was "the length of hospital waiting lists", where waiting times for orthopaedics and ophthalmology (and, to a lesser extent, for dermatology and ENT) were seen to be a particular problem. The "range of open access services available to me" was a fairly clear second; the emphasis was on increased direct access to investigative procedures, especially endoscopy. "Medical knowledge and training" was identified as the third priority, closely followed by "perceptions of the benefits of what is available in secondary care". The latter, and the fifth priority - "knowledge of and relationship with consultants" - reflected concerns about the flow of information from the secondary to the primary sector.

This determination of the top five priorities was reasonably consistent with a choice based on any individual criterion; this high degree of stability allows us to be confident that the factors identified represent a consensus view.

Strategies for change

The suggested strategies for change are summarised in Table 3. As might be expected, the two main parties to change were seen to be general practitioners and consultants, though it was not always clear from which side the initiative for change should come. For example, although hospital consultants were seen as having a major role in influencing the length of hospital waiting lists (69.8% of respondents mentioning this), the role of the general practitioner was also seen as important (mentioned by 62.3% of respondents).

Table 3. Round II Delphi Questionnaire Results: Strategies for Change

	Length of hospital waiting lists	Range of open access services	Medical knowledge and training	Perceptions of benefits of secondary care	Knowledge of and relationship with consultants
What?	Shorter lists especially for orthopaedics and ophthalmology	Increase access especially to endoscopy	Increase in knowledge and expertise	Better information about services available	More direct and personal contact with consultants
Who?	Consultants General practitioners Hospital managers	General practitioners Consultants Service providers	General practitioners Educationalists	Consultants General practitioners	Consultants General practitioners
How?	Increase resources Referral protocols Decrease hospital follow-up	Consultation / negotiation over appropriate access	Protected study time Courses / meetings Hands-on train.	Meetings Improved communication Referral protocols	Meetings Outreach clinics Guides to services
Forces?	Patient pressure GP pressure	Financial arguments GP demand	GP motivation	GP attitude	NHS reforms including fund-holding, trust status hospitals, contracting
Barriers?	Resources Inertia	Consultants' attitudes Money	Time	Time Inertia	Time GP attitudes Consultants' attitudes

Increased resources - both in terms of consultants' numbers and in the number of outpatient sessions provided - were seen as the major key to reducing hospital waiting lists. However, it was also recognised that "unnecessary" referrals might be reduced, perhaps by the agreement of guidelines on when a referral to secondary care was appropriate. Other suggestions for reducing waiting lists included a decrease in hospital follow-up, with earlier discharge to general practice. The range of open access services currently available depended on the location of the practice; it was felt that increased access might be negotiated locally, while recognising that some controls might need to be imposed to avoid over-use or abuse. Time to attend courses and for keeping abreast of the medical literature was seen as a key factor in improving medical knowledge. Some respondents expressed an interest in courses and seminars, while others indicated a preference for "hands-on" training, perhaps by sitting-in on a consultant's clinic. Improved communication and more detailed and timely information were identified as means of increasing awareness of the benefits of what is available in secondary care and of fostering a good relationship with consultants.

Not surprisingly, general practitioners' attitudes were frequently cited as a force for change, particularly their demand for shorter waiting lists and for increased access to open access services and their desire to increase their own knowledge and expertise. It was also suggested that increased open access might be more cost-effective. NHS reforms were also mentioned as a potential factor in favour of change, especially with respect to improved communication and information about service availability.

The most frequently cited barriers to change were resource constraints. Time, money and shortage of consultants were mentioned as problems with respect to the waiting list factor. Money was also identified as a barrier to increased direct access to services, while time was frequently seen as the major barrier to general practitioners and consultants coming together more frequently for educational initiatives or information exchange. Inertia - also expressed as "lack of will" and "easier to maintain status quo" - was also seen as a potential problem; possibly this relates to the lack of consensus over who should initiate change.

INTERVIEWS WITH SELECTED PRACTICES

Methods

The third phase of the study consisted of visits to a small but representative sample of practices to feed back information on the first two phases of the study and to explore the implications of these findings for referral given the particular circumstances of the practices in the sample. Practice details obtained from the FHSA was used to stratify practices by list size (> 8000, 4000-8000, < 4000) and referral rates (grouped into 'high', 'medium', 'low' tertiles). Two samples were randomly selected from the strata; the second to act as a 'reserve' should any of the practices in the first sample decline to participate. Participation in the questionnaire phase was not a pre-requisite for inclusion. In July 1992, a letter was sent to the senior partner in each of the selected practices requesting the practice's co-operation in the interview phase of the study. It was pointed out that the practice had been randomly selected and that the researchers would like to discuss the results of the questionnaire phases and how this related to the practice's current referral patterns. Meetings were arranged to take place at the practices between mid-September and early October 1992. Two members of the research team attended each meeting; one recorded brief notes of the discussion. One researcher introduced the meeting by outlining the purpose of the project as a whole and the current phase in particular. There followed a short presentation of the results of the questionnaire phases, concentrating on the five priorities for change identified in phase 2. At the beginning of the discussion general practitioners were asked how the general findings affected them; in other words whether the suggested changes would influence their referral patterns in any way. After that the conversation followed no pre-determined plan, except to ensure that each of the main areas of potential change was covered at some point.

Response rates

Eight of the nine practices initially invited agreed to take part. The first practice selected from the reserve sample also agreed to participate. Attendance of general practitioners at the meetings was high. Out of a total of 30 principals in the nine practices, 23 (77%) attended the meeting. In four of the nine practices (excluding the two single handed practices) attendance was 80% or above. The practice manager attended the meetings in four of the practices.

Findings

Waiting lists

It was generally felt that long waiting lists in some specialities did affect referral behaviour. General practitioners sometimes referred to hospitals with shorter waiting lists, so long as this was suitable for the patient. They might also refer patients at the earliest signs of some condition (e.g. cataracts) knowing that the waiting time would probably coincide with the time taken for the condition to develop. A minority of doctors felt that long waiting lists created pressures to advise patients about private referrals, but with the realisation that this may further deplete the availability of consultants for NHS work. The interviews identified three other strategies for coping with long waiting lists. First, using the term "urgent" on a referral letter was common practice but, this was seen as a device with uncertain outcomes. If it were to be used more effectively there would have to be a greater degree of consensus amongst clinicians about the meaning of the term and agreement about the circumstances where it was appropriate to use it. Second, telephoning consultants in order to arrange an earlier appointment for a patient was seen as a possible ploy, but depended on knowing the consultant, and was self-disapprovingly seen as "playing the system". Third, use could be made of waiting list data supplied by the Regional Health Authority. Only a minority of practices made active use of this information and several comments were made about the accuracy and timeliness of the data.

Open Access

In contrast to the results from the questionnaire phases of the study, general practitioners in the practices visited did not seem so keen for open access facilities to be extended. Practices were satisfied with the existing arrangements both for open access and for access to facilities available only through an outpatient appointment. A view mentioned on more than one occasion was that unregulated access can result in a large number of inappropriate referrals. Any increase in open access facilities, therefore, ought to be prefaced by some form of joint guideline development on appropriate referrals.

Knowledge and training

General practitioners saw continuing education as essential to their practice, but were critical of existing arrangements surrounding its provision. In spite of the perceived difficulties, however, a number of initiatives were suggested. Doctors from three practices said that they would like to gain some "hands-on" experience of clinical procedures by sitting-in at consultant clinics. Such sessions might not necessarily result in general practitioners doing this work themselves but it would give them insights into new techniques and developments. Small multidisciplinary group discussions were also mentioned on a number of occasions. What was lacking, it was felt, was someone to take the lead. One practice suggested that a systematic review of general practitioners' training and development needs should be undertaken.

Awareness of services

Normally general practitioners acquire their knowledge of what is available in secondary care through routine referrals and circulars distributed at the time of new consultant appointments. If they do not know what services are provided by a department they can telephone, but this can be a time consuming process. A much more efficient way of increasing awareness, it was suggested, would be to provide local directories of services. Such directories would include basic data about each department at a provider unit; the services available, staffs' special interests, and procedures for referrals, admissions and domiciliary visits. This kind of directory has been developed elsewhere and has found favour with consultants and general practitioners alike.

Relationship with consultants

Research studies have established that the referral process is felt to operate more smoothly when general practitioners and consultants know each other (Newton *et al.*, 1991). A close working relationship is seen as productive of shared understandings about what to refer, when, and how. Most of the general practitioners echoed these views in the interviews but felt that there were a number of barriers - especially time and "attitudes" - which made it difficult to foster such relationships where none exist at the moment. Fund holding was seen as an initiative which has begun to force changes, and the likelihood of more inter-disciplinary work on protocols and guidelines might bring consultants and general practitioners together. A number of practices were interested in being involved in the **development** of protocols, albeit with certain reservations about their **use**.

Referral policy

Referral was seen very much as a personal matter: a decision made between the general practitioner and the patient. The idea of referral being an issue for "policy making" was generally disapproved of and would be seen as an intrusion on doctors' professional autonomy.

Referral rate data

Each of the practices was asked to comment on the usefulness of the comparative feedback data on referral rates supplied by the FHSA (Northumberland Family Health, 1992). None spoke favourably about this: the outcome, if anything, was heightened defensiveness and preparedness to "stand by what we've done". One practitioner argued that such feedback could be counter productive in that it might lead people into radical changes in their referral behaviour in an attempt to get closer to the mean, on the assumption that this was the "right" rate. The majority view, however, was that this data had no influence on subsequent referrals.

Intra-practice referral

Most of the group practices visited practised some form of consultation with colleagues about problem cases. Arrangements varied from the completely ad hoc "having a look" during a surgery to more systematic cross referring to acknowledged specialisms within the practice. There were mixed views about the development of specialisation. Some felt that this would erode the very nature of general practice; whilst others thought that it might avoid some hospital referrals. As with other matters to do with referral there was a general feeling that intra-practice referral should be left to develop at a pace and to an extent decided by practices themselves.

DISCUSSION

Whilst the size of a practice, its proximity to provider units, and its population did influence referral in ways that were predictable, none of these factors appeared to influence attitudes to change. In this respect general practitioners seemed to speak with one voice. They regarded referral as their business and any initiatives designed to change the volume, timing, or destination of referrals, would be commonly interpreted as interference. An important barrier to change, therefore, is the strong sense of professional autonomy amongst doctors.

Other attitudinal barriers were identified in the second round of the Delphi survey. For the most part these attitudes were described as "apathy", "inertia", or "conservatism" without further explanation or elaboration. Where explanations for given attitudes were offered they most commonly referred to inter-professional rivalries and antagonisms stemming from the long standing division of primary and secondary care. The most frequent attribution of attitudes were made by general practitioners of consultants and they typically criticised consultants for their alleged aloofness and unwillingness to change working practices which serve their own interests.

Even so, there were areas where everyone wanted change and where for example, there was enthusiasm to be involved with hospital colleagues in training and educational schemes. The main problem with these professionally-led initiatives was who was going to take the lead. As well as vigorously asserting its independence the medical profession has operated according to an espoused norm of equality. Whilst this may insulate colleagues from the type of performance evaluation found in more hierarchical structures (such as business organisations) it produces difficulty in bringing about change. Even where general practices do operate in an hierarchical fashion (i.e. by way of seniority) this tends to work against innovation and change.

None of the obstacles identified in this study is insurmountable. The level of keenness displayed over a wide range of topics in the first round of the survey and elaborated in the second round provides a solid foundation for change in spite of the attitudinal barriers referred to above. An agency such as the MAAG however may have to act as the catalyst for change. As a group which can liaise with other NHS units and agencies the MAAG is strategically placed to develop a referral initiative.

A number of topics, which could form the basis of a series of mini projects, were identified. First, there was considerable enthusiasm for the production of directories of hospital services, perhaps in the form of a set of user oriented and professionally produced handbooks developed within the framework of existing contracts between the District Health Authority and main provider units. Participants in the development process might include hospital consultants, general practitioners, and representatives of the FHSA and District and Unit management. Second, general practitioners were eager for an opportunity to take part in a defined programme of observation in selected hospital clinics. This idea might be taken forward by those involved in post-graduate education and training. Third, there was interest in forming multidisciplinary task groups to develop an agreed set of guidelines for the general (or specific) use of the term "urgent" in referral letters and how consultants act upon its use. Such an initiative would involve general practitioners and hospital consultants. Fourth, the scope for intra-practice referral was recognised; general practitioners might meet together to exchange views about the opportunities and problems associated with the use of partners' clinical expertise. Finally, concerns about the utility of existing referral rate data suggest that there is scope for the involvement of general practitioners in making recommendations to the FHSA about the usefulness and format of such data. Together, these topics form a useful basis for a referrals action plan, whereby general practitioners, consultants and policy makers could come together to review critically their current practice and to identify opportunities for change. The projects are all of a manageable size and share the burden between the various interested parties. The findings and suggestions have been fed back to Northumberland MAAG. The ultimate effects on referral behaviour remain to be evaluated.

REFERENCES

Acheson, D. (1985),   Variation in GP Referral Rates Still Unexplained,   *General Practitioner*, November 8th.

Bond, S. and Bond, J. (1982), A Delphi Survey of Clinical Nursing Research Priorities, *Journal of Advanced Nursing*, 7, 565-575.

Burns, T.G., Batavia A.I., Smith, Q.W. and DeJong G. (1990), Primary Care Needs of Persons with Physical Disabilities: What are the Research and Service Priorities?, *Archives of Physical Medical Rehabilitation*, 71, 138-143.

Coulter, A., Roland, M. and Wilkin, D. (1991), *GP Referrals to Hospital*, Centre for Primary Care Research, Manchester.

Crombie, D.L. and Fleming, D.M. (1988), General Practitioner Referrals to Hospital: the Financial Implications of Variability, *Health Trends*, 20, 53-56.

Duffield, C. (1988), The Delphi Technique, *Australian Journal of Advanced Nursing*, 6(2), 41-45

Healey, A. and Ryan, M. (1992), *Factors Influencing General Practitioners Decision to Refer: a Preliminary Step Towards Explaining Variation in General Practitioners Referrals.* Discussion Document 06/92, Health Economics Research Unit, Aberdeen.

Hutchinson, A. and Fowler, P. (1992), Outcome Measures for Primary Health Care: What are the Research Priorities? *British Journal of General Practice*, 42, 227-231.

Metcalfe, D. (1991), Referrals: Could We Do Better?, *Update*, 42, 1093-1096).

National Audit Office (1991), *NHS Outpatient Services*, HMSO, London.

Newton, J., Hayes, V., and Hutchinson, A. (1991),   Factors Influencing General Practitioners Referral Decisions, *Family Practice*, 8, 308-313.

Noone, A., Goldacre, M., Coulter, A. and Seagroatt, V. (1989), Do Referral Rates Vary Widely Between Practices and Does Supply of Services Affect Demand? A Study in Milton Keynes and the Oxford region, *Journal of the Royal College of General Practitioners*, 39, 404-407.

Northumberland Family Health (1992), *GP Annual Reports 1990-1992. Hospital Referral Data*, Northumberland Family Health, Morpeth.

Pill, J. (1971), The Delphi Method: Substance, Context, a Critique and an Annotated Bibliography, *Socio-Economic Planning Science*, 5, 57-71.

Quade, E.S. (1967), *Cost Effectiveness: Some Trends in Analysis*, RAND Corporation, Santa Monica.

Reynolds, G.A., Chitnis, J.G., and Roland, M.O. (1991), General Practitioner Outpatient Referrals: Do Good Doctors Refer More Patients to Hospital?, *British Medical Journal*, 302, 1250-1251.

Stocking, B. (1992), Promoting Change in Clinical Care, *Quality in Health Care*, 1(1), 56-60.

Wilkin, D and Smith, A.G. (1987a), Variation in General Practitioners Referral Rates to Consultants, *Journal of the Royal College of General Practitioners*, 37, 350-353.

Wilkin, D. and Smith A. (1987b), Explaining Variation in General practitioners Referral Rates to Hospital, *Family Practice*, 4, 160-169.

14 Setting Priorities in Public Hospitals - The Paradoxes of Strategic Planning

JEAN-LOUIS DENIS[1], ANN LANGLEY[1,2] & DANIEL LOZEAU[2]

[1] Université de Montréal
[2] Université du Québec à Montréal

INTRODUCTION

In recent years, formal strategic planning methods originally developed for private business have been widely adopted by public hospitals. In a context of resource constraints and changing environmental demands, these techniques have been promoted as a "rational" means of establishing strategic priorities — bringing order and discipline to what might otherwise be a haphazard political process (see for example, Peters [1985]). It is hoped that through the use of systematic environmental analysis and a detailed assessment of internal strengths and weaknesses, strategic planning can help hospitals become more responsive to changing public needs.

At the same time, proponents of public sector and hospital planning have recognized that strategic planning methods originally conceived for private business must often be adapted in order to be acceptable in this context (Bryson, 1988; Champagne et al., 1987). Indeed, it can be argued that public hospitals have several characteristics that might lead one to question the appropriateness of formal planning methods. For example, these organizations are "professional bureaucracies" according to Mintzberg's (1979) typology of organizational structures. This means that the organization's orientation is strongly influenced by the activities and aspirations of autonomous professionals who are uniquely qualified to determine how work should be carried out. Thus, a formal strategic planning exercise initiated from above may seem, at first sight, to run counter to the natural bottom-up flow of decisions in these organizations (Mintzberg, 1979; Hardy et al., 1983; Cohen and March, 1974). Moreover, the implementation of planned decisions may be rather problematic, especially when this requires that autonomous professionals change their

Setting Priorities in Health Care. Edited by M. Malek
© John Wiley & Sons Ltd

behaviour. Also, because these organizations are publicly funded, they often have limited room to manoeuvre strategically, as government agencies attempt their own more global planning at national, provincial or regional levels (Baker *et al.*, 1990; Evans, 1985). Thus, it is fair to ask how proactive strategic planning on the part of individual organizations fits into this context, and whether it can ultimately make any difference. John Bryson (1988) claims that unlike older and somewhat discredited technocratic management tools (e.g. cost-benefit analysis, planning-programming-budgeting systems, zero-based budgeting, etc.), the strategic planning process he proposes *"builds on the nature of political decision making"*   rather than trying vainly to displace it. Yet, while several authors have attempted to adapt formal strategic planning methods to the public hospital setting (e.g., Champagne *et al.*, 1987; Files, 1983), there has been relatively little empirical research on the use and impact of different strategic management processes in this context (see also Shortell *et al.*, 1985; Pitts and Wood, 1985; Topping and Hernandez, 1991; Blair *et al.*, 1991). Our own research suggests that the successful application of these techniques in the public hospital context may be difficult. Hospital planners confront several paradoxes whose resolution is far from easy. We describe these paradoxes below along with their implications for planning practitioners and public sector managers.

The ideas presented in this paper are derived from three empirical studies of strategic planning (see also Langley, 1988; Denis *et al.*, 1991; 1992) The first study involved the in-depth investigation of the roles of formal strategic planning in three very different public sector organizations: a public service firm, a hospital and an arts organization. The second study involved the content analysis of strategic plans from 66 hospitals across Canada. Finally, the third study was an interview survey with administrators and medical staff in 33 Quebec hospitals.

We have structured our discussion of the paradoxes of strategic planning under three main headings, labelled "paradoxes of purpose," "paradoxes of process" and "paradoxes of performance."   Each deals with a different group of issues and apparent contradictions. Under the heading, "paradoxes of purpose," we note that while strategic planning has often been promoted as a means of introducing an element of rationality into the strategic decision making process, in practice, political and symbolic motives often lie behind it, affecting the kinds of results that may be obtained. Then under the heading "paradoxes of process," we describe the dilemmas confronting managers wishing to design a planning process that will simultaneously produce a focused strategy and organizational consensus around that strategy. Finally, under the heading "paradoxes of performance," we examine the outcomes of strategic planning efforts in the hospital sector, noting that while the plans produced by hospitals often seem to lack the kind of integration, realism, and clarity an outsider would associate with a well-defined strategy, and while the outcomes in terms of concrete action are often limited, most hospital administrators feel that the process is beneficial. To explain this last contradiction, we attempt to identify the underlying forces driving interest in formal strategic planning. We conclude with a number of tentative recommendations for hospital administrators wishing to improve the productivity of their strategic management processes.

PARADOXES OF PURPOSE

As indicated above, in the literature, strategic planning is seen mainly as a rational process aimed at improving the quality of strategic decisions. However our interviews with managers in hospitals and other public sector organizations showed that in practice, planning plays a variety of other roles as well. While *instrumental* motives for planning (such as the need to adapt to a changing or environment, or the need to rationally allocate limited resources) were mentioned to us fairly frequently, *political* and *symbolic* motives for planning were also extremely prevalent. All three types of reasons for planning could have an internal or external focus. This is illustrated in Figure 1 which maps the stimuli for strategic planning reported to us by administrators and medical staff in our hospital survey.

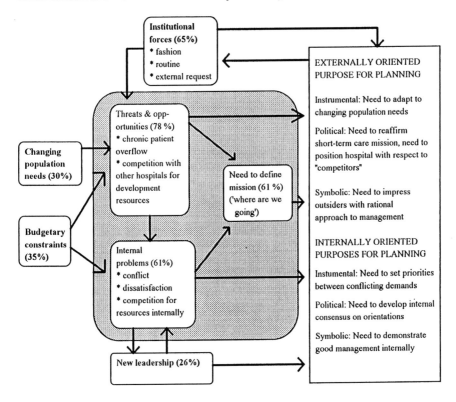

Figure 1. The stimuli for planning in Quebec hospitals

Rounded rectangles show different groups of stimuli identified by respondents. Numbers in parentheses indicate the percentage of hospitals noting this type of stimulus ("strategic planners" only, n=23).

The first two stimuli to the left of the diagram (changing population needs and budgetary constraints) represent key external influences on the Quebec hospital system that have often been cited as substantive justifications for more rational planning. However, only about one third of our hospitals mentioned these factors directly. Far more salient to most hospitals were the problems and threats that these changing conditions later generated internally (shown in the central shaded box). For example, with an ageing population and a lack of alternative resources, many acute care hospital beds were filled by chronic care patients. In several cases, this threatened the hospital's short-term care vocation and created great dissatisfaction among members of the medical staff (whose remuneration was affected). Simultaneously, budgetary constraints increased competition for resources both between and within hospitals. This in turn generated conflict within the organization. Planning was seen to contribute in a multi-dimensional way to the solution of these problems (as summarized in the large box to the right of Figure 1). At an instrumental level, it could help the hospital determine the services required to satisfy population needs and rationally allocate resources to priority areas. This use of planning corresponds well with the "rational" model.

But its use as a political tool was just as if not more significant to respondents. For example, it was often seen as a means of influencing outsiders and defending the integrity of the hospital's current mission:

"We said that with the plan we'd stop rumours of becoming a chronic care hospital."

"We wanted to have our short-term care mission recognized by the ministry.."

Of course, in order for a hospital to show the seriousness of its intention to retain its mission, it will also have to demonstrate some dynamism in its plans to renew its human and physical resources, possibly generating a fairly ambitious program of development. The paradox here is that when used politically and defensively in this way, planning can sometimes seem more concerned with preservation of the status quo, rather than adaptation to the environment! Few really substantive changes can be expected from such a plan — indeed, no change may well be interpreted as success from the hospital's point of view. It is important to note that there is nothing particularly illegitimate about this type of use of planning. In a context where various organizations compete for financial resources and public support, each individual organization must present the best case it can. Problems arise however, if the dynamics and incentives inherent in the system are such that the population needs consistently take second place over parochial interests. Planning in itself cannot be expected to solve this type of problem.

In a different political role, this time oriented internally rather than externally, strategic planning was often perceived as a way of generating a certain level of consensus, legitimacy and support around chosen priorities:

"The new CEO wanted to mobilize the medical staff..."

"We needed to achieve greater adherence..."

However, this type of use of planning also has some potentially paradoxical consequences because the need to achieve agreement among a diverse group of people may make it very difficult to produce genuine strategic choices. To maintain harmony (or at least the appearance of it), the organization may be driven to generate a highly ambitious strategic plan that is not very precise but provides something for everyone, rather than a realistic blueprint for the future.

Finally, it is important to note that planning has become fashionable. Because of the aura of "rationality" surrounding it, well-managed hospitals are expected to have strategic plans:

"There was a "kick" for this new technique..."

"We wouldn't look good if we didn't plan..."

This means that a large number of organizations may be doing strategic plans for purely *symbolic* reasons: for example, managers may have been directly pressured into carrying out planning by external agencies (government, accreditation bodies etc.), or they may simply decide that they can use it to impress insiders and outsiders with their rational, progressive and dynamic approach to management. The paradox here is that in our studies, whenever this type of motive was cited as predominant, people were often remarkably unimpressed! Clearly, if planning does not eventually produce some substantively desirable results for organization members, cynicism will eventually set in. It seems unwise for an organization to embark on a planning process if top managers' hearts are not really in it.

To summarize this section, the popular image of planning in the literature is of a "rational" process of decision making that will enable the organization to rise above politics. Yet in fact, political concerns permeate the context for strategic planning, affecting its ability to produce "rational" strategies. Planning may become a political tool to promote a specific position externally or to achieve guided compromise internally. In addition, because of its "rational" aura, planning may also be used symbolically — simply to create a good impression. We now examine how these same phenomena also affect the design and operation of planning processes.

PARADOXES OF PROCESS

Most of the planning literature focuses on process, with considerable attention being devoted to the steps that should be followed, the people who should be involved at each step and the techniques that should be used (e.g., Peters, 1985; Bryson, 1988) One key feature of planning process design is the emphasis on *formal analysis* of external and internal environments. For many, the essence of strategic planning *is* analysis — the bringing to bear of systematic procedures and objective data to an otherwise arbitrary process. In theory, detailed information concerning the role of the organization and its environment is expected to provide a rational means of selecting between strategic alternatives while the absence of analysis seems likely to inhibit the objective evaluation of new orientations.

At the same time, if the decisions to be made are truly strategic, the opinions of a wide variety of organizational influencers often have to be taken into account. If it is to be taken seriously, strategic planning in hospitals often requires broader and more heterogeneous *participation* than private business planning. In particular, the literature has stressed the need for strong representation of the medical staff on planning committees as well as the use of other means of consultation such as interviews and questionnaire surveys (Champagne *et al.*, 1987; Stacey and Leggat, 1987) Clearly, with their highly specialized knowledge and direct contact with the public, professionals are often uniquely placed to identify key trends and new strategic opportunities. Also, implementation will be facilitated if people feel they were involved in decisions, while it may well be blocked if key players are excluded from the process.

Thus in these organizations, the strategic planning process tends to be organized to simultaneously allow both broad participation and extensive analysis. In a large hospital, it can become a major operation consuming large quantities of time and resources. In our study, hospital strategic plans took an average of 16 months to complete, involved 45% of the medical staff in some way, and required the formation of several committees. Consultants were frequently used to coordinate the complex work (68% of cases), bringing with them analytical tools generally associated with orthodox strategic planning — including extensive analyses of external and internal environments. Even when consultants were not used, environmental analysis was usually considered to be an essential part of the planning process.

The first interesting question that arises is what happens to these analytical elements when they are confronted with a highly participative process. We directly asked our respondents to evaluate the relative importance of analytical data versus informal discussions in determining the content of the plan. In our interviews, 54% of respondents said that opinions counted more than analysis, 31% said analysis and opinions were given about the same weight and only 14% felt that analysis predominated. These figures may be interpreted either positively or negatively depending on one's personal beliefs about the relative usefulness of both types information. However, we found no significant statistical relationships in our data between the use of analysis and the performance of the planning process.

When asked more specifically *how* environmental analyses contributed, two-thirds of respondents suggested that statistical information did not provide new knowledge, but merely confirmed what most people already knew, offering an objective structured basis for discussion and sometimes support for recommendations. The analytical element of formal planning could also be a useful tool for challenging the views of people with vested interests:

> These statistics forced people to think.. they realized that their service was in danger.

However, as the same respondent put it:

> Officially, quantitative data dominate... but in practice, it was the qualitative data. (...) I think it was mainly peoples' reflections, perhaps influenced by the data, that led to decisions.. and then in the two hospitals where I was involved, there were political games that influenced choices at the end that were not necessarily in complete agreement with the objective data.

In one or two cases we observed more closely, it almost seemed as though formal analysis was done so that the "external environment" box of the textbook planning process could be satisfactorily filled. The "orientations" or "recommendations" box was then treated as a totally separate matter whose content was established through somewhat disconnected informal negotiations. In summary, although analysis may be potentially useful to those hospitals willing and able to integrate it into their thinking, paradoxically, the mere collection of information certainly does not guarantee this. A certain amount of analytic data collection was clearly ritualistic.

We also found no relationship in our study between the extent of medical staff participation and planning outcomes. High participation did not necessarily guarantee success while low participation did not always result in failure. In fact, deciding on the appropriate level of participation for a strategic planning process seems to involve a complex trade-off between opposing forces. Broad participation can clearly improve the representativity and legitimacy of strategic choices:

> "The plan must be supported by everyone — so they must be involved..."

However, broad participation can also be extremely time-consuming and may accentuate the expression of divergent views, leading to a loss of control of the planning process. Participants may see planning as an open invitation to promote the development of their own areas, generating previously unsuspected demands for resources and diverting attention away from more global strategic issues:

> "The difficult thing to control was people's appetites.. everyone was looking to gain something from it."

If this phenomenon takes hold, the result may either be an unrealistic plan — or many dissatisfied people.

Thus, the real paradox of process in hospital strategic planning is that there is no perfect solution — whichever option is chosen, problems may be encountered. Limiting participation and increasing the role of analysis may allow management to produce a focused strategic orientation based on objective data that apparently provides a clear guide for action. However, such a plan may suffer from its neglect of softer data provided by professionals closer to operations. Moreover, given the power structure in these organizations, the plan will lack legitimacy and is likely to run into trouble at the implementation stage, if not before. Very broad participation and less reliance on objective analysis on the other hand will tend to generate a vague, unrealistic and unfocused set of proposals that are both unimplementable and strategically incoherent. In other words, you may be damned if you do and damned if you don't!

PARADOXES OF PERFORMANCE

Throughout the previous discussion, we have suggested that for a variety of reasons, hospitals may have some difficulty in producing realistic, clear and focused strategies in the face of the many conflicting influences on strategic decisions. Political and symbolic motives behind strategic planning as well as the political nature of participative planning processes are likely to be reflected in the types of plans generated. This supposition is in good part confirmed by our empirical analysis of 66 strategic planning documents from hospitals across Canada (as well as in the smaller sample of Quebec hospitals contacted for our interview survey).

In fact, we found that on average, the 66 plans in our Canadian sample contained over 22 recommendations each. In spite of resource constraints, 46% of these recommendations were oriented towards developments requiring new resources. At the same time, while the general orientation to expansion was partly offset by an obvious concern for the efficiency of continuing operations (27% of recommendations), only 1% of recommendations proposed any form of down-sizing of services. Several hospitals put forward extraordinarily ambitious development programs. A significant minority of plans (10 out of 66 or 15%) contained twenty or more different recommendations for expansion, showing clear evidence of what might be called a "shopping list" syndrome. Many plans were also extremely vague — 55% of recommendations were classified as being of low precision (i.e. they were expressed in terms of general objectives rather than specific actions, and they were largely unquantified). Often, the language of the recommendations was itself ambiguous (e.g.: using expressions such as "*become more proactive in promoting...*," "*consolidate*," "*consider the possibility of...*"). Clearly, there was considerable variation among the 66 plans examined. There were some cases where the strategies defined appeared realistic, clear and integrated. However, the overall picture was much less encouraging. What in the end had been gained by going through this often very laborious process?

This brings us to the results of our interview survey and the heart of what we call the "performance paradox." This is that in spite of the apparently unrealistic, vague and unfocused nature of many strategic plans, most of the managers and professionals we met were generally positive about the outcomes of their planning processes. In our analysis of outcomes, we divided the benefits and problems mentioned into three major categories called "process" outcomes, "plan" outcomes and "operational" outcomes (see Table 1).

"Process" outcomes concern the benefits and problems directly associated with the activity of going through the planning process. Benefits of this type were perceived to be very important by most of our respondents. It was felt that the activity of planning helped people to work together, created a feeling of belonging and generally improved the level of mutual understanding. These benefits correspond well with the internal political motives for planning we described earlier. "Plan" outcomes concern the benefits and problems associated with the planning document itself. Such benefits included the possession of a "clear" statement of mission which could guide the organization's future decisions, as well as the usefulness of the document as a promotional device with government and accreditation bodies. Finally, "operational" outcomes concern the concrete strategic actions that were implemented as a result of the planning process. In our study, implementation rates claimed by respondents were quite variable, but reached 54% on average. However, a distinction should be made that places these quantitative results in perspective. This is that although the "implementation rate" of a plan may look fairly good, respondents often had difficulty in imputing all the action produced strictly to the planning process:

> "Even if we hadn't planned, we would have done the same things..."

> "75% of it would been done, even without the plan..."

Table 1. The impact of hospital strategic planning

	Process Outcomes	Plan outcomes		Operational outcomes
POSITIVE OUTCOMES	Benefits of consensus and understanding	Clarity of mission, vision future direction	Positioning and promotion outside hospital	Actions taken or results achieved because of plan
Qualitative data (examples)	•"It created a great spirit..." •"We speak the same language..." •"Intellectual stimulation"	•"A sense of long term direction..." •"A uniform and realistic vision..." •"The plan is our bible..."	•"It gave us credibility with the ministry..." •"It helped us to get accreditation"	•"We added 75 chronic care beds..." •"We settled our budgetary deficit..." •"Recruitment and technology..." •"Increase of 12 % in emergency volume"
Frequency mentioned interviews •% of admissions •% of mds •% of hospitals	75% 42% 86%	71% 32% 77%	38% 26% 59%	42% 32% 59%
NEGATIVE OUTCOMES	Process problems (e.g., conflict, workload, etc.)	Problems with plan (e.g., failure to generate clear direction, inadequate document, lack of influence externally)		Inability to generate action, problems with implementation
Qualitative data (examples)	•"The process was too heavy..." •"Too many expectations raised" •"It can turn into a battle..."	•"Document was too detailed..." •"Difficulty of setting aside daily problems and thinking globally" •"No link between strategies proposed and our financial and physical resources"		•"No implementation..." •"Little impact in relation to effort" •"There was no pressure for implementation..." •"It remained theoretical..."
Frequency mentioned interviews •% of adms •% of mds •% of hospitals	75% 63% 91%	21% 32% 45%		42% 74% 73%
QUALITATIVE SCALES	Process benefits (1 = low; 5 = high)	Strategic focus (0 = low; 1 = high)	Promotional usefulness (1 = low; 5 = high)	% of proposals implemented Influence on action (1 = low; 5 = high)
•Overall mean •Std. deviation •Mean (adms) •Mean (mds)	3.73 0.77 4.05 3.34	0.56 0.18 N/A N/A	3.53 1.08 3.89 3.20	54% 3.59 23% 1.00 N/A 3.93 N/A 3.21

In other words, many plans tended to formalize and confirm trends that were already in progress. In addition, 74% of all the physicians interviewed expressed some degree of disappointment concerning the impact of planning on action.

Despite this, and despite the lack of clarity of many hospital strategic plans to an outside observer most interviewees (administrators more than medical staff) viewed planning as beneficial. One explanation for this is that there is more to some strategic plans than meets the eye of an outside observer.   In fact, in our discussions with certain managers, we came to realize that even some apparently all-encompassing plans had not been produced without a struggle.   Paradoxically (again), the real strategic choices in these plans were often hidden in subtle nuances of wording and sometimes in omissions from the plans that indicated implicitly in what directions the organization would probably *not*   develop.   In a context with powerful interest groups where consensus was highly valued, more explicit references were impossible. However, even these subtle indications could give managers the hard-won right to occasionally say "No."   The plan served as an imperfect but useful filter in several instances.

A second possible explanation is that several hospitals used planning to reaffirm their short-term care mission, avoiding the threat of transformation to long-term care status.   The strategy apparently worked in all cases — none of the hospitals examined experienced a change in mission.   Thus satisfaction may have been high partly for this reason.

Finally, process benefits associated with consensus and mutual understanding seemed particularly important to many respondents.   However, even here, we suspect that in some cases, the consensus achieved was sometimes constructed around resistance to an undesirable change in mission rather than around a shared positive vision of the future.   Of course, unrealistically ambitious plans may also generate the illusion of consensus, but this seems likely to dissipate over time as the hospital finds itself unable to deliver on all fronts at once.

In summary, it appears that the main benefits of formal strategic planning in public professional service organizations may lie in directions somewhat different from those that might be expected from a reading of the normative literature.   The following quotation from an article by Allaire and Firsirotu clearly overstates the case, but certainly echoes some of the impressions we obtained from our data:

> Many participants come to believe that the benefits of planning lie not in the product but in the process.   Planning becomes like jogging: it is not an efficient way to get anywhere, nor is it intended to be — but if practised regularly, it will make us feel better. (Allaire and Firsirotu, 1989).

CONFRONTING THE PARADOXES

So far, our analysis of the use of hospital strategic planning may have appeared somewhat pessimistic.   As we have seen, the dynamics of decision making in these complex organizations are not transformed overnight by the mere imposition of a formal technique. On the contrary, formal strategic planning is easily absorbed into the incremental and political decision making processes usually associated with these organizations.   Political and symbolic motives often drive the initiation of planning and the processes themselves usually require participation from multiple groups, each with its own axe to grind.   In some cases, planning may stimulate conflict as opposing interests are exposed, while systematic analysis is often subordinated to the opinions of powerful players when orientations are defined.   The nature of many plans themselves confirms the importance of political processes: in the search for participation and consensus, strategic orientations tend to be wide-ranging, heavily oriented towards development, vague and loosely integrated. Moreover, while respondents claim a wide variety of social benefits from these exercises, their influence on action often seems limited compared with the investment required. In their study of leadership in universities, Cohen and March (1974), with tongue only partly in cheek, recommend strategic planning as the ideal "garbage can" providing a perfect arena for disgruntled professionals to let off steam, while allowing administrators to get on with their jobs undisturbed! We do not feel that this is adequate justification for embarking on what is often an extremely demanding process. However, it must be recognized that voluntarily or not, formal strategic planning in the public hospitals can quite easily turn into a "garbage can" (though not one that administrators can ignore).

And yet, as we noted above, many managers felt that strategic planning was beneficial, at least partly. In this section, we look at what appears to be its real potential and we suggest a number of ways in which hospital administrators and planners can improve its productivity and alleviate some of its problems.

First, what is the real attraction of strategic planning for hospital managers over an above enthusiasm for a passing fad, and the need to impress others with their use of "rational" procedures? In our view, it is the opportunity for administrators to take some kind of proactive role in the orientation and control of their organizations. It is clear that in the hospital sector, in the past, strategic orientations tended to emerge implicitly as independent groups of professionals took initiatives in their daily practice. Managers were expected to ensure that adequate resources were provided but had a very limited role to play in strategic decision making:

> [The medical staff felt that] what's important is that we have the scientific superstars.. they will decide what their priorities are. It's for the professional physicians to say. The strategy of the hospital is just the sum of the strategies of these people. The institution has no business getting mixed up in that

However, increasingly stringent resource constraints changed the situation, giving managers the theoretical power to make choices, but insufficient knowledge and legitimacy to make them on their own. Enter strategic planning as a means of exerting some form of legitimate leadership through a formal collective process:

> One of the objectives of the planning exercise was to avoid the situation where the initiatives of just anybody determines the orientation — in other words, they get their foot in the door and its a battle of the strongest. If you don't take the leadership, someone else will....

At the same time, resource constraints also resulted in increasing competition for funds between organizations. Thus, each individual unit's position needed to be more forcefully defended externally — another place where an approved strategic plan could be very helpful. In fact, in many ways, strategic planning represents a means for leaders of public sector organizations to ensure their direct participation in both internal and external strategic decisions which previously tended to pass them by. The trend is part of what Hinings and Greenwood (1988) have called the increasing "corporatization" of public services: the move away from fragmented service offerings controlled by divergent groups of professionals and towards much greater managerial integration and control. Current interest in information systems and program management form part of the same trend. However, as Hinings and Greenwood note, this type of change is a very difficult one to achieve because it requires transformations of both structures and value systems. It is perhaps not surprising that in initial attempts at strategic planning, the patterns associated with old structures and values still tend to dominate. It will be interesting to see whether the corporatization trend accentuates over time and what roles (if any) strategic planning will eventually come to play.

For it is important to note that other ways of making strategy may often be more appropriate for certain types of organizations. For example, Mintzberg and JØrgensen (1987) have lauded the emergent strategy processes described above for their ability to "grow" innovative ideas and to profit from the deep knowledge of people in close contact with operations. They suggest that if the top-down "rational" strategic planning model comes to dominate completely, it may kill this potential for "active learning." The potential usefulness of strategic planning in hospitals may be inherently limited: e.g., to set very broad "umbrella" strategies that allow scope for creative development within general guidelines.

In this spirit, we make a number of tentative suggestions as to how hospital administrators and planners might attempt to make their planning processes more manageable, and potentially more fruitful. These recommendations stress the need to avoid treating strategic planning as a process set apart from other organizational activities. Part of the problem with the notion of strategic planning is that it has become a canned technique — a ritual that an organization goes through but that it does not connect to ongoing operations. The intensive use of consultants to coordinate these processes has probably accentuated this phenomenon. Our recommendations emphasize the need for direct hands-on involvement, the creative adaptation of decision making approaches to specific organizational needs, and the role of continuity in linking decision making to action.

RECOMMENDATION 1: ADAPT THE PROCESS TO ITS PURPOSE — MANAGE PARTICIPATION AND ANALYSIS.

A great deal of emphasis has been placed in the literature on the importance of a participative process for strategic planning in hospitals. Yet we found that more participation, more analysis and more resources invested in planning was not necessarily better. Perhaps there are general optimal levels lying somewhere between the extremes (i.e., U-shaped relationships). But more probably, each organization must find its own optimum by selecting participants, modes of consultation and analytical studies to suit its own context (i.e., the objectives it is pursuing, the personalities and power relationships in place, and the issues to be tackled). It seems clear that the active involvement of professionals is necessary to ensure their commitment to the decisions made during planning. However, the more people are invited to participate freely, the more they will expect to see their proposals appear in planning documents, and the greater the danger of inflation, fragmentation, confusion, and later, disappointment and disillusionment as expectations cannot be met. Participation is necessary, but must be managed appropriately. For example, in an organization where the main purpose of planning is to begin to develop stronger collaboration, trust and cohesion between people around some broad principles, free and elaborate participative process may be appropriate. But when planning is aimed at substantive strategic decision making, participation may need to be more selective, both in terms of the number, timing and type of people who are consulted, and in terms of the content of the consultations. For example, a narrow mandate to participate in a task force on a specific issue of primary concern may be more likely to produce realistic proposals than a broad invitation to air one's views on the future of the entire organization. This brings us to our next recommendation:

RECOMMENDATION 2: ORIENT ATTENTION TOWARDS A FEW KEY ISSUES

A planning process which tries to tackle too much is almost bound to produce fragmented and loosely integrated strategies. Based on our research, we have become convinced that planning tends to be more successful when it is deliberately oriented to focus on a limited number of key issues, and when top management develops a reasonable idea of the types of strategies to be promoted fairly early in the process. This focuses attention and discussion, directs participation and attenuates the forces of fragmentation. In fact, the term "strategic planning" should probably be avoided where possible because it implicitly opens up far too many issues at once.

RECOMMENDATION 3: USE EXTERNAL ENVIRONMENTAL INFORMATION WHERE APPROPRIATE TO ASSIST IN ACHIEVING FOCUS

In a context where individuals' personal aspirations have an important influence on decision making, and where public needs are usually perceived only through the eyes of professionals under pressure, it is difficult to know whose story to believe. A planning process provides the opportunity to bring to bear environmental data from external sources that may assist in providing a focus for strategic decisions. Such data may be quantitative (e.g. demographic statistics) or qualitative (e.g., a statement of government priorities for the next several years). But in all cases, it constitutes an independent view of the organization's position that is rather difficult to refute. It may therefore provide a legitimate basis for choice and a possible rallying point for consensus on a more focused strategic orientation. However, as shown by our research, the forces for fragmentation remain very strong, and considerable determination may be required to profit fully from this opportunity.

RECOMMENDATION 4: LINK PLANNING TO ACTION.

In our study of strategic planning processes, direct links to action were often very fuzzy or absent altogether. However, the greater the number of specific measures taken to implement plans, the more the overall planning process was perceived to be successful. Links to action are not necessarily easy to achieve in organizations like hospitals where professionals cannot be directed from above. While, control methods such as management-by-objectives may be applied in administrative areas, more subtle "umbrella-strategy" mechanisms are needed for areas where professionals are dominant. A good strategic plan in this context would provide legitimate criteria on which senior managers can base their decisions of whether or not to accept development proposals. This creates a "favourable prejudice" towards certain areas and encourages people to gravitate towards them in the knowledge that resources will be forthcoming. It also forewarns people in unfavoured areas that their proposals will not be accepted. However, such an approach requires determination and consistency on the part of senior management, and the planning process will be immediately discredited if managers themselves show no continuity in their decisions.

RECOMMENDATION 5: BEWARE OF PLANNING IN A LEADERSHIP VACUUM

As we carried out our research, we noticed that leadership issues often became inextricably intertwined with formal strategic planning. When an organization appears to lack direction, leadership or vision, someone is almost sure to call for a strategic plan. Accreditation agencies and government bodies impose it on hospitals that seem to be poorly managed, while leaders under threat often see it as a way of enhancing their credibility:

> Sometimes, the CEO who approaches a consultant is a CEO who is threatened.. and is looking for a solution to his problem through strategic planning. He often doesn't quite realize it or admit it. The consultant discovers this en route and planning becomes a pretext to ensure his future and to direct the energies of people towards other preoccupations. At the end of it, he has a plan for the next five years.. and he is saved.

Yet, if hospital administrators are unable to develop their own visions, manage conflict and negotiate with others to make real choices, it is difficult to see how a mere formal process will really solve the problem. In such conditions, the planning process itself is likely to reflect the same lack of direction and purpose, enabling politics to take over with a vengeance, and generating quite unworkable plans. The only saving grace of the use of formal strategic planning in such circumstances is that it may sometimes be the last straw that eventually forces a change in leadership (this actually happened in several cases in our research). However, there are surely more direct, and less resource-consuming ways of achieving the same result.

And this brings us to yet another paradox. This is that strategic planning is perhaps most likely to produce genuine strategic choices when leadership is strong and credible, and when healthy collaborative relationships have already been established within the organization and with key outsiders, — i.e., in circumstances where formal strategic planning may seem least needed (see also Bryson and Roering, 1988). If strong management capabilities are present, formal strategic planning may be rather irrelevant — an epiphenomenon that some leaders choose to incorporate into their management arsenal, but which may not in itself essential to achieving their goals. This is not to suggest that information on the environment cannot help in focusing organizational decisions or that managers do not need to sit down with their professional staff from time to time to talk about strategic issues. However, lighter and less ritualistic mechanisms than full blown orthodox strategic planning may well be sufficient.

Finally, the ultimate paradox is that in spite of its name, its history and some of the claims made on its behalf, strategic planning on its own cannot produce strategy. The formal process offers no more than peripheral aids to human strategists by feeding in information, by structuring interactions, by providing a forum for the articulation of strategic decisions and by conferring them with a certain legitimacy. A good deal of time may be wasted and considerable emotional energy may be expended for very little reward if strategic planning is expected to substitute for a lack of strategic vision on the part of the organization's principal actors.

ACKNOWLEDGEMENT

The authors thank the Social Sciences and Humanities Research Council of Canada, the National Health Research and Development Program and the Quebec Fonds FCAR for their financial support.

NOTE

This paper has been adapted from the paper: Paradoxes of Strategic Planning in the Public Sector published in the journal *Optimum* (produced by Consulting and Audit Canada), Summer 1993, (31-41) with the permission of the Minister of Supply and Services Canada, 1993.

REFERENCES

Allaire, Y. and Firsirotu, M. (1989). Coping with strategic uncertainty, *Sloan Management Review*, 30(3): 7-16.

Backoff, R.W. and Nutt, P.C. (1990). *Organization Publicness and its Implications for Strategic Management.* Paper presented at the 1990 Academy of Management meeting, August 12-15, 1990.

Baker, G.R., Charles, C., Cockerill, R. and Voelker, C. (1990). *Regulation and Hospital Strategic Planning in Canada*, University of Toronto, Health Service Research Discussion Paper no. 90-03.

Blair, J.D. and Boal, K.B. (1991). Strategy formation processes in health care organizations: a context-specific examination of context-free strategy issues. *Journal of Management*, 17(2): 305-344.

Bryson, J.M. (1988). *Strategic Planning for Public and Nonprofit Organizations*, San-Francisco: Jossey-Bass.

Bryson, J.M. and Roering, W.D. (1988). Initiation of strategic planning by governments. *Public Administration Review*, 48: 995-1004.

Champagne, F., Contandriopoulos, A.-P., Larouche, D., Clemenhagen, C. and Barbir, C. (1987). Strategic planning in hospitals—a health needs approach. *Long range Planning*, 20(3): 77-83.

Cohen, M.D. and March, J.G. (1974). *Leadership and Ambiguity*, Boston: Harvard Business School Press.

Denis, J.-L., Langley, A. and Lozeau, D. (1991). Formal strategy in public hospitals. *Long Range Planning*, 24(1): 71-82.

Denis, J.-L., Langley, A. and Lozeau, D. (1992) *The role and impact of formal strategic planning in public hospitals*, UQAM, Centre de recherche en gestion, Working paper #92-13.

Evans, T. (1985). Strategic response to environmental turbulence. In Parston, G. (ed.) *Managers as Strategists*. Ottawa: Canadian Hospital Association: 11-31.

Files, L.A. (1983). Strategy formulation and strategic planning in hospitals: application of an industrial model. *Hospital and Health Services Administration*, 28(6): 9-20.

Hardy, C., Langley, A., Mintzberg, H. and Rose, J. (1983). Strategy formation in the university setting. *Review of Higher Education*, 6(4): 407-433.

Hinings, R. and Greenwood, R. (1988). *The Dynamics of Strategic Change*, Oxford: Blackwell.

Langley. A. (1988). The roles of formal strategic planning. *Long Range Planning*, 21(3): 40-50.

Mintzberg, H. (1979). *The Structuring of Organizations*, Englewood Cliffs, NJ: Prentice-Hall.

Mintzberg, H. and JØrgensen, J. (1987). Emergent strategy for public policy, *Canadian Public Administration*, 30(2): 214-229.

Peters, J.P. (1985). *A strategic planning process for hospitals*, Chicago, IL: American Hospital Publishing Inc.

Pitts, M.W. and Wood, D.R. (1985). A review and critique of the strategic management literature on not-for-profit community hospitals. *Health Care Strategic Management*, June: 4-12.

Shortell, S.M., Morrison, E.M. and Robbins, S. (1985). Strategy making in health care organizations: a framework and agenda for research. *Medical Care Review*, 42(2): 219-233.

Stacey, S. and Leggat, S. (1987). Strategic planning: a practical guide. *Health Management Forum*, 7(2): 41-51.

Topping, S. and Hernandez, S.R. (1991). Health care strategy research, 1985-1990: a critical review. *Medical Care Review*, 48(1): 47-90.

15 Tools for Use of Societal Criteria in Priority Setting in Evaluation of Medical Technology in the Netherlands — Development and Testing of a Checklist

WIJA OORTWIJN,[1] ANDRÉ AMENT[1] &
HINDRIK VONDELING[1,2]

[1] *University of Limburg, the Netherlands*
[2] *Free University of Amsterdam, the Netherlands*

INTRODUCTION

Health care costs are rising in many industrialized nations. Many government seek to limit expenditures in health care. The rising health care costs, and the recognition that medical technology is a significant contributor to these costs, have provided the stimulus to develop medical technology assessment programmes in the Netherlands. The most important programme in this field is the Investigational Medicine Programme of the Dutch Sick Funds Council. The aim of this research programme is to evaluate both new and established medical technologies, with respect to their medical efficacy, cost-effectiveness, and their social, ethical and legal implications. So far, priority setting for evaluation of medical technologies in this programme has only been based on the scientific merits of individual research proposals. This paper presents the development of a checklist on which priorities can be set concerning both new and existing medical technology based on societal criteria. The checklist was tested, using a random selection of eight granted research proposals in the context of the Investigational Medicine Programme. The paper concludes with some suggestions to improve the methodology of the priority setting process and to widen the scope of the potential applications of the checklist.

Setting Priorities in Health Care. Edited by M. Malek
© 1994 John Wiley & Sons Ltd

POLICIES TOWARDS TECHNOLOGY IN THE NETHERLANDS

The health care system in the Netherlands is pluralistic. Diagnosis and treatment services are usually provided privately. The government has the primary responsibility for providing preventive care services and for giving general guidance, mainly through the Ministry of Welfare, Health and Cultural Affairs (WVC). In clinical care, the government sees its role as encouraging appropriate private actions.

Between 1973 and 1977 health care costs rose by 11 to 18 percent per year and by 1980 health care expenditures accounted for 8.4% of the Dutch gross national product (GNP). The percentage of GNP for health expenditures in the Netherlands was 8.3% in 1991, according to OECD (The reform of health care, 1992).

An important instrument for governmental control over technology is authorized by Article 18 of the Hospital Provisions Act, which gives the government the authority to license high technology services. About 15 technologies are regulated by this law, for example coronary artery bypass graft (CABG), treatment for end stage renal disease and in vitro fertilisation (IVF). Additional methods to control the diffusion of technology, for example by enhancing competition between insurers, are being considered.

Health care technology is a significant contributor to health care costs in the Netherlands (Financieel Overzicht Zorg 1993, 1992). Therefore, increases in health care costs were also a stimulus to the development of health care technology assessment activities. In 1984, a government White Paper stated that technology assessment should be part of policy making in all areas of science and technology (Vondeling, 1993). The Dutch Health Council (Gezondheidsraad) has an important role in advising the government on issues concerning science and technology and the Council has been active in doing assessments. Several academic programs have also developed. Perhaps the most important institution in the field of technology assessment is the Sick Funds Council (Ziekenfondsraad), which began to support technology assessments in the mid-eighties following discussions about whether or not to reimburse heart transplantation, liver transplantation and in vitro fertilisation under the insurance system. Subsequently, the Sick Funds Council took the initiative to develop the most important programme, the Investigational Medicine Fund (Fonds Ontwikkelingsgeneeskunde), jointly supported by the Sick Funds Council, the Ministry of Education, Science and Technology (O&W) and the Ministry of WVC. The aim of this research programme is to evaluate both new and established medical technologies, regarding medical efficacy, cost-effectiveness, and, when applicable social, ethical and legal implications. The Committee for Investigational Medicine began to support technology assessments in 1989 and has 36 million guilders a year available in a three-year revolving fund to support studies (including development and care costs).

Until 1993, more than 80 projects have been funded (Bos, 1993). Results of these studies influence decisions such as to whether a new technology is covered in the benefit package of the sick funds or not.

PROCEDURE FOR SELECTING RESEARCH PROPOSALS FOR EVALUATION OF HEALTH CARE TECHNOLOGIES

The procedure by which the Committee for Investigational Medicine operates is one in which researchers, mainly in the university hospitals, are invited to submit research proposals for approval. The Committee for Investigational Medicine collaborates with the Dutch Organisation for Scientific Research (NWO) to judge the proposals. NWO evaluates the scientific quality of the proposed projects (research criteria). The Committee then advises the Minister of WVC and the Minister of O&W on the basis of the recommendations of NWO and the policy plan of Investigational Medicine. The ultimate decisions are made through a political process (policy criteria). For a number of reasons this investigator initiated or 'bottom-up' procedure does not lead to optimal allocation of scarce resources:

- many research proposals have methodological deficiencies;
- the distribution of research proposals over different specialties is disproportionate;
- there is a general lack of good proposals, so all scientifically acceptable proposals are being funded;
- the proposals reflect the interest of the researchers for specific technologies instead of the needs of health care system (Huisjes, 1992).

To counter these problems, in 1993 the Sick Funds Council decided to spend a maximum of 10 percent of its annual budget through a self-initiated or 'top-down' procedure. In this approach the Committee for Investigational Medicine selects a number of subjects to be evaluated. Then specific investigators are invited to submit a proposal. An invitation for proposals is also published in several Dutch medical journals. Three subjects were selected for evaluation, diagnostic testing, treatment of urine incontinence of nursing home patients and treatment of psycho geriatric patients. One can imagine that societal criteria, besides being used to select specific subjects, can also be used as a complementary criterion to the judgement of the scientific merits of the proposals that are submitted to the Committee in the context of the bottom-up procedure. As such one can pose the question:

> How can societal criteria be used to set priorities with regard to the evaluation of health care technologies?

The aim here would be to improve the priority setting process by taking into account the societal needs for new technologies. Nevertheless, scientific and policy criteria are also important in making decisions because priority setting in the end is a political process. Priority setting cannot be done by a technocratic algorithm or checklist alone. However, the development of our criteria list may lead to an improvement of the decision making process already taking place. The introduction of an explicit procedure, that pays attention to the societal needs, may increase the rationality of the current priority setting process.

DEVELOPING A CHECKLIST

A literature study was performed to gather societal criteria relevant for priority setting in health care. The literature study was based on a Medline search from the years 1984 to 1992. The Medline search was complemented by recent Dutch publications (Raad voor Gezondheidsonderzoek, 1991; Janssens, 1992). A few of the resulting criteria were well-defined. The other criteria were described in other sources (Musschenga, 1987; Bouter, 1988; Heyink, 1988; Commissie Keuzen in de zorg, 1991; Koopmanschap, 1991; Nationale Ziekenhuis Raad, 1991).

The resulting 43 societal criteria were classified in six categories. These categories are:

- burden of disease;
- potential effectiveness of the technology;
- potential costs of the technology;
- uncertainty of applying the technology ;
- the meaning of the technology for research;
- the meaning of the technology for policy.

The Institute of Medicine in the United States has developed a similar method of classifying societal criteria (Donaldson, 1992).

The question that should be answered is which, if any of these criteria are already used in the current judgement procedure of Investigational Medicine. As stated before, NWO evaluates the proposed projects on the basis of research criteria. Regarding the ultimate decisions about medical technologies, policy criteria are taken into account. Political criteria are relevant issues for the study's objective, but they are omitted because are difficult to identify and to quantify. Therefore, so far as the objective of the present study is concerned, only the first four categories of criteria have been worked out in more detail.

LITERATURE SURVEY

In 18 publications (see Appendix 1), 43 societal criteria were mentioned. These criteria were classified in six categories (see Table 1).

Table 1. Societal criteria based on the literature study

BURDEN OF DISEASE	1. epidemiological criteria
	2. volume of patients for which the technology is appropriate
	3. (medical) need
	4. public/professional demand
	5. burden of disease
	6. quality-of-life
	7. public values towards disability
	8. cost-of-illness
	9. frequency of use
	10. public interest
POTENTIAL EFFECTIVENESS	11. efficacy
	12. potential impact on outcome
	13. effectiveness
POTENTIAL COSTS OF THE TECHNOLOGY	14. costs
UNCERTAINTY OF APPLYING THE TECHNOLOGY	15. uncertainty with regard to use of a technology
	16. use of technology coincides with current knowledge
	17. controversy
	18. susceptibility of physicians to new knowledge
	19. obstructing developments
	20. agreement about indication region
	21. variance in use
	22. geographic variations
	23. ethical and social implications
RESEARCH	24. availability of data
	25. improvement of assessment capacity
	26. place of an assessment in the life-cycle of a technology
	27. duration of an assessment
	28. variance in time
	29. alternative strategies
	30. research experience
	31. reason to execute research study in the country
	32. stimulation of research
	33. enlarging medical knowledge
	34. scientific breakthrough
POLICY	35. prevention
	36. equity
	37. effect on policy decisions
	38. preventing needless medicalization
	39. aspects of research policy
	40. priorities of policy
	41. effect on organization and/or staff
	42. quality of care
	43. costs and benefits (ratio)

As stated before, only the first four categories of criteria have been worked out in more detail. The four categories contain 23 of the original 43 criteria (see Table 2).

Table 2. Societal criteria

1. epidemiological criteria	12. potential impact on outcome
2. volume of patients for which the technology is appropriate	13. effectiveness
3. (medical) need	14. costs
4. public/professional demand	15. uncertainty with regard to use of a technology
5. burden of disease	16. use of technology coincides with current knowledge
6. quality-of-life	17. controversy
7. public values towards disability	18. susceptibility of physicians to new knowledge
8. cost-of-illness	19. obstructing developments
9. frequency of use	20. agreement about indication region
10. public interest	21. variance in use
11. efficacy	22. geographic variations
	23. ethical and social implications

The 23 criteria were reduced to 10 criteria on the basis of coherence and/or overlap. These ten societal criteria are: *epidemiological criteria, quality of life, cost-of-illness, frequency of use, effectiveness, costs of an intervention, controversy, susceptibility of physicians to new knowledge, indication region, and ethical and social implications.*

The ten criteria are classified in four categories and described in the following section. To link priority setting with these criteria a statement is made for each category of criteria to determine when technology should get priority for evaluation.

Societal criteria

Burden of disease

The following criteria and their descriptions give an indication of the burden of a disease:

- Epidemiological criteria can be described with the help of prevalence, incidence and mortality of the relevant disease.
- The quality of life or health status can be measured with (a combination of) disease-specific and generic questionnaires, possibly followed by a utility-measurement (Habbema, 1989).
- A cost-of-illness study can be used to determine the societal costs of a disease. The costs can be divided into direct and indirect costs.
- The (potential) frequency of use of the technology is defined as: number of treatments in a certain period of time and/or geographic area (for example, a health region).

Statement: the higher the burden of disease, the higher the priority for evaluating the technology.

Potential effectiveness of the technology

- The effectiveness of an intervention can be described in various ways. The effectiveness of an intervention under optimal circumstances, as in a randomized study, is called 'efficacy'. 'Community effectiveness' is the effect of an intervention when applied in the community. 'Community effectiveness' is determined by five factors: efficacy, screening and diagnostic accuracy, health provider compliance, patient compliance and coverage. Coverage refers to the extent to which the efficacious intervention is being appropriately utilized by all those who could benefit from it (Tugwell, 1985). 'Community effectiveness' indicates that the ultimate impact of a (new) medical technology on the burden of disease can be much smaller than suggested by clinical efficacy studies (Doorslaer, 1990). The effectiveness of an intervention, in terms of efficacy, can be determined by comparing epidemiological criteria and quality of life measurements before and after the intervention.

Statement: the higher the potential effectiveness, the higher the priority for evaluating the technology.

Potential costs of the technology

- Costs of a particular medical technology can be determined with a cost analysis. Prior estimates can be made based on tariffs or, preferably, based on real cost estimates. The quality of the description of alternative strategies and data on costs of the alternative treatments have been chosen to describe this criterion.

Statement: the higher the potential costs, the higher the priority for evaluating the technology.

Uncertainty of applying the technology

Uncertainty with regard to use of a technology can be uncertainty of the mechanism and/or the effects of the technology. Uncertainty is indicated by such observations as controversy, variations in use, or lack of agreement among physicians concerning indications for use.

- Controversy can be described by means of different judgements in a profession of a particular intervention. This is often expressed in terms of disagreement about the use of the intervention concerned.
- The susceptibility of physicians for new knowledge can be described by means of the extent to which physicians differ in adoption of medical technologies. Indications for the existence of differences in this respect are, for example, the professional age of the doctor, the number of subscriptions to scientific journals and belief in scientific knowledge (Burt, 1987).

- Agreement about the potential indication region can be described by a clear definition (in literature) of the indication region.
- Sometimes uncertainty exists with regard to ethical and social implications of a technology.

Statement: the higher the uncertainty, the higher the priority for evaluating the technology.

If quantitative information about the criteria described is unavailable, the criteria can be described qualitatively. Of course, for the purpose of improving the rationality of the decision making process quantitative data are to be preferred.

Table 3 represents a summary of these findings in form of a checklist. As described above the checklist contains 25 descriptions of the 10 societal criteria, divided in four categories.

Table 3. Checklist for Evaluating Medical Technologies

criterion	description
BURDEN OF DISEASE	
epidemiological criteria	1. prevalence 2. incidence 3. mortality 4. qualitative description
quality of life	5. generic questionnaire 6. disease-specific questionnaire 7. utility measurement 8. qualitative description
cost-of-illness	9. direct costs 10. indirect costs 11. qualitative description
frequency of use	12. number of treatments in a period and/or geographic area
POTENTIAL EFFECTIVENESS	
efficacy	13. morbidity 14. mortality 15. generic questionnaire 16. disease-specific questionnaire 17. utility - measurement 18. qualitative description
POTENTIAL COSTS OF THE TECHNOLOGY	
costs	19. costs of treatment
UNCERTAINTY OF APPLYING THE TECHNOLOGY	
controversy	20. different judgements in a profession
susceptibility of physicians to new knowledge	21. differences between physicians
indication region	22. definition
ethical & social implications	23. initial questions 24. application questions 25. regulation questions

APPLICATION OF THE CHECKLIST

This checklist has been used to evaluate (anonymously for confidentially reasons) a random sample of eight Investigational Medicine proposals out of the more than 80 that already had been approved. The proposals were checked on the extent to which descriptions of societal criteria are mentioned and the place of the description (which paragraph) in the proposal. One question of the application form of Investigational Medicine explicitly refers to the implication of the intervention for the health care system. In that section ('implication for health care') all available information with regard to the societal relevance of the intervention should be gathered.

First the societal criteria relevant for each proposal were examined. Not all criteria are relevant for each individual proposal. For example, the description 'mortality' is not relevant for evaluation if a reduction in mortality is not a consequence of the intervention to be studied. To take account of this phenomenon, as a first step, for each proposal the relevant set of descriptions of societal criteria was determined. Second, a scoring system was created with three possible options per description of a criterion:

- description(s) of a criterion is not mentioned in the research proposal (zero points);
- description(s) of a criterion is mentioned in the research proposal but not in the section 'implication for health care' (one point);
- description(s) of a criterion is mentioned in the section 'implication for health care' (two points).

If, for example, eight out of ten relevant descriptions of criteria are mentioned on the right place in a proposal this would result in an absolute score of 16 points and a score of 80%. This proposal will be judged better than a proposal in which six out of nine relevant descriptions of criteria are mentioned, while only three descriptions of criteria are to be found in the right place. This would result in an absolute score of 9 points and a score of 50%. Obviously, it is the percentage score that matters. Third, a relative comparison between the proposals was made based on the maximum percentage score of each proposal.

In summary, this rather uncomplicated method of evaluating proposals is based on the presence and position of the description of relevant societal criteria in a research proposal.

Evaluating Investigational Medicine research proposals

The eight proposals varied in their attention to the 25 categories of societal criteria. The total number of relevant descriptions of criteria for the eight proposals varies from a minimum of 20 to a maximum of 25 (see Table 4).

Table 4. Number and Place of Relevant Descriptions of Societal Criteria in Research Proposals

research proposal →	A	B	C	D	E	F	G	H
number of descriptions of criteria ↓								
number of descriptions of societal criteria not mentioned in the research proposal	5	5	13	11	12	13	13	12
number of descriptions of societal criteria mentioned in the research proposal, but not in the paragraph 'meaning for health care'	11	14	9	7	6	3	8	9
number of descriptions of societal criteria mentioned in the paragraph 'meaning for health care' of the research proposal	7	6	3	5	2	4	4	4
total number of descriptions of societal criteria relevant for the research proposal	23	25	25	23	20	20	25	25

From Table 4 it appears that the number of descriptions of societal criteria described in the section 'implication for health care' varies from two (10%) to seven (30%). This means that, despite the inclusion of a specific question about the implication of the intervention for health care, this issue is hardly dealt with.

Relevant descriptions of societal criteria which are described elsewhere in the proposal varies from three (15%) to 14 (56%). Table 5 represents the relative comparison of the research proposals.

Table 5. Scores of the Research Proposals (percentage of the maximum score)

research proposal →	A	B	C	D	E	F	G	H
categories of criteria ↓								
burden of disease	55%	58%	17%	41%	17%	22%	38%	46%
effectiveness	60%	33%	42%	10%	25%	13%	42%	17%
costs	50%	50%	50%	50%	50%	100%	50%	50%
uncertainty	50%	58%	42%	50%	33%	33%	8%	25%
total score	54%	52%	30%	37%	25%	28%	32%	34%

Table 5 shows that in only one research proposal (F) one of the categories of societal criteria ('the potential costs of a technology') is adequately described. This is possible because this category contains only one description. The total scores of the research proposals vary from 25% to 54%. This means that a relatively large variance exists between the research proposals. Only two out of the eight research proposals have total scores of more than 50%.

DISCUSSION

This project has developed a checklist for the evaluation of the societal relevance of research proposals with regard to medical technologies. The results of the study show that in the present practice of Investigational Medicine societal criteria are either not described, or are described qualitatively and/or in a fragmentated way. Also relatively few societal criteria are described in the paragraph 'meaning for health care' of the application form of Investigational Medicine.

In the context of Investigational Medicine the checklist could work in two ways: if resources are limited in the bottom-up procedure, societal criteria could be used as an additional tool for selection. In the top-down procedure, societal criteria could be used to iteratively select health care issues that most urgently need to be evaluated.

The validity of the societal criteria used in this study are supported by the US Institute of Medicine (IOM) (Donaldson and Sox) However, does this mean that societal criteria for evaluating medical technologies are the same in all countries? This question has not been studied although they probably are more or less similar in all countries.

Another issue that needs to be studied is the relative weighing of societal criteria. The IOM described a model that can be used to set priorities with regard to evaluation of medical technologies. The IOM suggests 'weighing' societal criteria. In principle, weighting individual criteria offers a possibility to adjust the set of criteria to the mission of the funding body. A disadvantage may be that weights can be chosen arbitrarily and can lead to controversy. Another problem is who should weight the criteria. For example, IOM suggests strong input from the general public. However, this could be a complicated issue.

In a few cases the societal criteria are described by means of more than one variable. Nevertheless, not all descriptions of one criterion are necessary to get an impression of the criterion concerned. For example, the quality of life can be measured with disease-specific questionnaires, generic questionnaires or a combination of these questionnaires. One could either select one of the options or weight the relevance of the different descriptions.

Research and policy criteria have not been used in the checklist. However, one or more of these criteria can be added to the checklist, depending on the aim of individual subsidy givers.

CONCLUSION

Setting priorities in health care was first mentioned in the mid-eighties (Leenen, 1984). Although the necessity of setting priorities in health care is obvious, use of societal criteria with regard to setting priorities has received little attention. Using one or a combination of the propositions stated above we hope that the checklist can be adapted and further developed in order to be helpful in priority setting processes of a variety of funding bodies in different countries on both a national and regional level of decision-making.

REFERENCES

Bos, M.A. (1993), *Health Care Technology in The Netherlands*, Health Council of The Netherlands, The Hague (in press).

Bouter, L.M. and Dongen van, M.C.J.M. (1988), *Epidemiologisch onderzoek*, Bohn, Scheltema en Holkema, Utrecht/Antwerpen.

Burt, R.S. (1987), 'Social Contagion and innovation; Cohesion versus structural equivalence', *American Journal of Sociology*, 92, 1319.

Commissie Keuzen in de zorg. (1991), *Kiezen en delen*, Albani, 's-Gravenhage.

Donaldson, M.S. and Sox, H.C. (eds.) (1992), *Setting priorities for health technology assessment; A model process*, National Academy Press, Washington, D.C.

Doorslaer van, E.K.A. and Rutten F.F.H. (1990), 'Medische technology assessment', Maarse, J.A.M. and Mur-Veeman, I.M. (eds.), *Beleid en Beheer in de Gezondheidszorg*, Van Gorcum, Assen/Maastricht, 246-247.

Minister en de Staatssecretaris van Welzijn, Volksgezondheid en Cultuur. (1992), *Financieel Overzicht Zorg 1993, Tweede Kamer, vergaderjaar 1992-1993, 22 808, nrs. 1-2*, Sdu Uitgeverij, 's-Gravenhage.

Habbema, J.D.F., Casparie, A.F., Mulder, J.H. and Rutten, F.F.H. (eds.) (1989), *Medische Technology Assessment en gezondheidsbeleid*, Samsom Stafleu, Alphen aan den Rijn.

Heyink, J.W., Roorda, J. and Tijmstra, Tj. (1988), *Levertransplantatie: psycho-sociale aspecten*. Koninklijke Bibliotheek, 's-Gravenhage.

Huisjes, H.J. (1992), 'Ontwikkelingsgeneeskunde onderweg', *Tijdschrift voor Sociale Gezondheidszorg*, 70, 484-486.

Janssens, M.B.J.A. (1992), 'Prioriteiten voor onderzoek chronische ziekten', *Medisch Contact* 46, 167-170.

Koopmanschap, M.A., Roijen van, L. and Bonneux, L. (1991), *Kosten van ziekten in Nederland*, Instituut Maatschappelijke Gezondheidszorg, Instituut Medische Technology Assessment, Rotterdam.

Leenen, H.J.J. (1984), 'Prioriteiten stellen in de gezondheidszorg', *Medisch Contact* 38, 1323-1324.

Musschenga, A.W. and Neeling de, J.N.D. (1987), *Verdeling van schaarse middelen in de gezondheidszorg*, VU uitgeverij, Amsterdam.

Nationale Ziekenhuis Raad. (1991), *Ethisch aspectenonderzoek inzake gezondheidszorgtechnologie en de rol van het instellingsmanagement*, Utrecht.

Raad voor Gezondheidsonderzoek. (1991), *Advies chronische aandoeningen: prioriteiten voor onderzoek*, Raad voor Gezondheidsonderzoek, 's-Gravenhage.

The reform of health care; a comparative analysis of seven OECD countries. (1992), *Health Policy Studies No 2*, Paris.

Tugwell, P., Bennett, B., Sackett, D. and Haynes, R. (1985), 'The measurement iterative loop: a framework for the critical appraisal of need, benefits and costs of health interventions', *Journal of Chronic Diseases*, 38, 339-351.

Vondeling, H., Haerkens, E., Wit de, A., Bos, M. and Banta, H.D. (1993), 'Diffusion of minimally invasive therapy in the Netherlands', *Health Policy* 23, 67-81.

APPENDIX 1 PUBLICATIONS IN WHICH SOCIETAL CRITERIA FOR ASSESSING MEDICAL TECHNOLOGIES ARE MENTIONED

Bock de, D.E. (1990), Ontwikkelingsgeneeskunde: verwikkelingen rond een beleid, Afstudeerscriptie Rijksuniversiteit Limburg, Maastricht.

Busschbach van, J.J., Hessing, D.J. and Charro de, F.Th. (1991), De kwaliteiten van qaly's, Medisch Contact, 45, 1353-1355.

Dixon, J. and Welch, H.G. (1991), Priority setting: lessons from Oregon, The Lancet, 337, 891-894.

Donaldson, C. and Mooney, G. (1991), Needs assessment, priority setting, and contracts for health care: an economic view. Health Economics Research Unit, University of Aberdeen. Discussion paper 12/91.

Eddy, D.M. (1989), Selecting technologies for assessment, International Journal of Technology Assessment in Health Care, 5, 484-501.

Golenski, J.D. and Thompson, S.M. (1991), A history of Oregon's basic health care services act: an insider account, Quality Review Bulletin, 144-149.

Habbema, J.D.F., Casparie, A.F., Mulder, J.H. and Rutten, F.F.H. (eds.) (1988), Medische Technology Assessment en gezondheidsbeleid, Samsom Stafleu, Alphen aan den Rijn.

Janssens, M.B.J.A. (1992), Prioriteiten voor onderzoek chronische ziekten, Medisch Contact, 46, 167-170.

Jessop, E.G. (1991), Doctors and priorities, The Lancet, 337, 1464.

Johnsson, M., Lundvall, O. and Jarhult, J. (1989), Medical Technologies in need of assessment, SBU, Stockholm.

Lange de, S.A. (1984), Prioriteiten en medische ethiek, Medisch Contact, 38, 1324-1326.

Lara, M.E. and Goodman, C. (1990), National priorities for the assessment of clinical conditions and medical technologies, National Academy Press, Washinghton, D.C.

Leenen, H.J.J. (1984), Prioriteiten stellen in de gezondheidszorg, Medisch Contact 38, 1323-1324.

Loomes, G. and McKenzie, L. (1989), The use of qaly's in health care decision-making, Social Science and Medicine, 4, 299-308.

Peckham, M. (1991), Central research and development committee for the NHS.

Raad voor Gezondheidsonderzoek. (1991), Advies chronische aandoeningen: prioriteiten voor onderzoek, 's-Gravenhage.

Schaapveld, K., Bergsma, E.W., Ginneken van, J.K.S. and Water van de, H.P.A. (1990), Setting priorities in prevention, Koninklijke Bibliotheek, 's-Gravenhage.

Williams, A. (1991), Is the qaly a technical solution to a political problem? Of course not! International Journal of Health Services, 21, 365-369.

16 Assisted Conception Techniques - On What Basis Do Health Technologies Become Routinely Available When They Have Been Assessed as Effective?

NICK FREEMANTLE & IAN WATT

University of York

THE POLITICS OF INFERTILITY

Introduction

The technological possibility of restoring fertility among some couples who otherwise would be unable or unlikely to conceive has led to important political questions about the terms under which such treatments should be made available both in Britain and abroad. Currently there is considerable variation in the availability of these treatments under the UK National Health Service (NHS).

The new managerial structures which have created a form of internal market in health care are technocratically based; it is perceived that the health care needs of a population can be measured, and then resources allocated to effective treatments to maximise the health status of that population. The reality of health care is quite different from this, and there is considerable evidence at a theoretical and empirical level that health care under the NHS discriminates against the needs of minority groups (Lancet, 1993).

Priority setting depends upon a perception of a desired outcome. For example, whether reduced pain and disability as a result of a successful hip replacement is more desirable than reducing psychological pain from infertility. One of the difficulties presented by such a dilemma is that health services are primarily concerned with the health of populations, and maximising the health of a population given limited resources for health care may prove disastrous for an individual who

Setting Priorities in Health Care. Edited by M. Malek
© 1994 John Wiley & Sons Ltd

does not receive available and effective treatment for their condition. However, a more fundamental difficulty is that there does not exist a viable technical solution to the question of prioritization (rationing), which means that questions about the allocation of resources to different areas lead to value based political decisions. This is well illustrated by the following two quotes:

> Friends and family can never possibly know the pain that I feel every time I see a woman walking down the street with a big belly. How could anyone capable of having children understand.
>
> (Phillips and Rakusen: pp 4220)

Or:

> In my view there is no justification for the introduction of treatments for infertility under the National Health Service when there are already so many children in the world.
>
> (Director of Public Health)

This paper examines the politics of infertility, which exist at an individual, organisational and societal level. While interesting on its own, the politics of infertility also provides important insights in to the wider dilemmas which health care systems face, in particular the role of the medical profession and the absence of genuine public accountability in the NHS.

Are Treatments for Infertile Couples Effective?

It remains the case that the majority of health care interventions have never been formally evaluated (Light, 1991). Even where interventions have been adequately assessed there is often a considerable gap before the findings of research are implemented, for example there was sufficient evidence in the 1960s to indicate that the routine use of clot busting thrombolytic therapy in patients immediately following a heart attack would dramatically reduce death rates, and yet this was not generally accepted until further (and unnecessary) major clinical trials had been conducted. Earlier introduction of routine thrombolytic therapy would have led to a considerable reduction in deaths (Antman *et al.*, 1992). Even after the acceptance that a treatment is effective there are often considerable delays in the incorporation of treatments into routine practice (Stocking, 1992).

One essential part of the tool-kit for evaluating the effectiveness of treatments is a set of techniques known broadly as *systematic review* (e.g. Mulrow, 1987). Systematic review entails examining all the available pieces of evidence on the effectiveness of interventions, where appropriate combining them statistically to provide a more accurate estimate of treatment effectiveness (Thompson and Pocock 1991), and then presenting the results of this scrutiny in an accessible form. It is of particular importance given the contradictory opinions of many leading clinical experts, a factor highlighted by the differing conclusions found in many traditional non systematic review articles in the medical literature (Antman *et al.*, 1992).

One of us (NF) has recently been involved in a systematic review of the effectiveness of treatments for infertile couples, and this work provides the technical basis for the discussion of the politics of infertility which will follow (Effective Health Care, 1992).

The systematic review found that there was considerable evidence to demonstrate that a number of treatments were effective in the treatment of infertile couples, though treatment effectiveness was dependent upon the underlying cause of the condition. Some treatments were impressive. Drug treatment restores near normal fertility among many women with ammenohrea (failure to ovulate). This treatment is reasonably cheap (the drug costs are around £35 per month) but requires expertise and high technical facilities to reduce the risk of side effects or multiple pregnancies.

Some surgical interventions for tubal dysfunction are also effective, in well selected groups of patients, though there is considerable evidence that surgery is being offered in the NHS when there is little likelihood that this will increase the possibility of pregnancy (Lilford and Watson, 1990). This occurs at least in part because it is often the only treatment available and is recommended on the questionable basis that some treatment, even ineffective treatment, is preferable to nothing.

Assisted conception techniques, such as *in vitro fertilization* (IVF) and gamete intrafallopian transfer (GIFT) are also effective in well chosen groups, and reports of around 50% maternity rates after 3 cycles of treatment have been published. All assisted conception techniques in some form replicate the natural processes of conception outside the body, and in the case of IVF one or more embryo is introduced into the uterus thus bypassing the fallopian tubes.

GIFT is a less technical procedure which involves the reintroduction of sperm and eggs in the fallopian tubes, leading to a raised rate of ectopic pregnancy, a potentially dangerous condition. Because of the lower level of technical expertise and facilities required, it has come to be described as *the poor man's IVF* by some commentators. Since IVF and GIFT are both performed on women this description provides an interesting insight into the value attached to infertility treatments by their largely male perpetrators. Given that GIFT does not provide additional diagnostic information on fertility (which is gained in IVF), it is inappropriate for the many conditions in which the fallopian tubes are not viable.

The national maternity rate as a result of IVF is around 12% per cycle, but this masks large scale discrepancies between the higher success rates of some larger centres which are performing many treatments when compared with smaller ones performing only a few. In fact in one study of IVF, in which the women were under 40 years old and the men had apparently normal sperm a pregnancy rate of 30% per cycle was achieved (Hull *et al.*, 1992).

Another important, and effective, treatment option is donor insemination. This involves the use of donor sperm, eggs or both and can lead to maternity in many women. It is particularly useful where the cause of infertility has been established. Currently Donor eggs are not generally available in this country, but the collection of a number of eggs during IVF which later prove surplus to requirements may lead to more general availability of this option in the future.

Infertility Treatments on the NHS

Since 1991 the NHS has been managed under new terms (Secretaries of State, 1989). The intention, which was heavily influenced by developments in America, was to create an *internal market* for health care services (Enthoven, 1985). This was perceived to offer a number of advantages.

The central theme is that the responsibility of those who specify care, the purchasers, is separated from the responsibility to implement that care (the providers). New organisations were formed which were responsible for purchasing care, based upon the district health authorities but with responsibilities for operational management gradually hived off as the majority of hospitals, community units and even ambulance services became self managing NHS trusts.

There are three main forms of contract placed by purchasing authorities. *Block* contracts are an arrangement by which the purchasing authority buys a service from a provider. At its most straightforward, a *block* contract may merely transfer the specification of the service to the providers. However increasingly specific criteria (such as exclusions of specific interventions) aimed at controlling activity or improving quality are included. *Cost and volume* contracts are more sophisticated, with alterations in price at different levels of activity acting as sanctions upon provider units. *Cost and volume* contracts may also contain quality criteria and specific exclusion causes and the difference between a *block* contract with exclusions, quality criteria and ceilings and floors for activity and a *cost and volume* contract may be semantic. The third type of contract, *cost per case*, is where an individual price is negotiated for an individual procedure. This tends to be reserved for single high cost procedures or discrete series of work such as work directed at reducing waiting lists.

NHS trusts were a new form of organisation, attractive to many managers (Freemantle *et al.*, 1993), and considerable responsibility is devolved to the trust board for the planning and management of care.

Purchasing authorities place contracts with providers for the provision of care to the resident population. Many patients enter NHS hospital care via accident and emergency departments, but the majority of patients are referred to the secondary care tier via their general practitioner (GP).

Ever since the inception of the NHS, GPs have been self employed contractors rather than NHS employees. New arrangements for larger GP practices have allowed them to opt to develop a new degree of independence as fund holding practices. This means that they are allocated a budget in order that they may place contracts directly for certain elective (i.e. non urgent) procedures.

While fundholding is an interesting development and there is a clear political intention to develop aspects of the fundholding process for all GPs (such as extending drug budgets to all general practitioners) fundholding is only of passing interest here as fundholding GPs are not permitted to use their budgets to buy assisted conception procedures for their patients. Contracts for assisted conception treatments can only be placed by purchasing authorities.

There is considerable diversity in the prioritization for assisted conception treatments among purchasing authorities, which is reflected in the variation in contractual arrangements for these services. A recent poll demonstrated individuals have access to specialist fertility treatments in only around half of authorities (*British Medical Journal*, 1993).

However, all GPs are free to refer patients to any NHS consultant for any treatment regardless of whether or not the purchasing authority has a contract with that provider. If the treatment is considered to be *urgent* the consultant provides appropriate treatment, and then bills the purchasing authority. However if the treatment is considered *non urgent* the purchasing authority assesses the referral and decides whether or not it is appropriate to fund it. These *extra contractual referrals* (ECR) are important since they represent expressed needs at least as they are perceived by GPs, and may indicate gaps in the existing contract or apply to important but rare procedures. Clearly a GP who does not feel sympathetic towards an infertile couple is less likely to agree to place this referral. A GP may also be reluctant to refer if they do not think that the purchasing authority will authorise the treatment. At least one health authority has elected not to purchase assisted conception treatments on false belief that these are 'ineffective' (Harrison and Wistow, 1992). Although *tertiary* referrals, from one consultant to another, could technically lead to health authorities paying for assisted conception techniques on an extra contractural basis without the opportunity to separately assess the merits of the referral, we are aware of no cases where this has occurred.

The NHS Management Executive provides explicit advice on the authorization of non urgent *extra contractual referrals*. The message is clear; effective treatment may not be denied through the refusal of authorization of an ECR which is correctly (bureaucratically) applied for purely on the basis of cost, see Box 1 (NHS Management Executive, 1992).

The advice from the NHSME is clear cut, and yet there is evidence based upon data from 8 purchasing authorities that ECRs for IVF, are currently being refused by some purchasing authorities (Redmayne and Klein, 1993). Given that there is good evidence that these treatments are effective when made available to carefully selected (most hopeful) cases (*Effective Health Care*, 1992), there clearly must be other grounds upon which these decisions are taken.

National Health Service Management Executive:
Guidelines for *Extra Contractual Referral Authorization*

Refusal of ECRs

<u>The grounds on which an ECR can be refused are very limited</u>

Purchasers should respect the clinical judgement of GPs and other clinicians who decide on individual referrals. Occasions on which a clinician's choice of provider can be judged to be unwarranted are likely to be very rare. The only grounds on which refusal may be acceptable are as follows:

a)   the patient is not the purchaser's responsibility, i.e. the patient is not a district resident or the patient is, for the treatment planned, a responsibility of a GPFH.

b)   where prior authorization for the ECR was not sought where it was medically reasonable to expect the provider to have done so.

c)   the referral is not justified on clinical grounds. In making such judgements the DHA would be expected to ensure that it takes appropriate clinical advice. This would include instances where such clinical advice has led to the development and agreement of clear referral protocols and the threshold has not been met.

d)   an alternative referral would be equally efficacious for the patient, taking account of the patient's wishes.

It is not acceptable for a purchaser to refuse authorization solely on the grounds of the proposed cost of the treatment in relation to contracted services.

Where funding for a particular ECR is refused, it is the responsibility of the purchaser to inform the patient, as well as the provider, of their decision. Reasons for the refusal should be made clear...

... purchasers should recognise that they have a responsibility to fund appropriate self-referrals. Clearly they may wish to obtain clinical advice on the case, but requests for authorization of ECRs resulting from the patient's self-referral should be considered in the same way as those resulting from referral by a GP or other clinician.

NHS Management Executive 1992.

Prioritization in Health Care

Since 1976 the NHS has been subjected to centralized global budget setting, with a total budget allocated to the service (Glennester, 1992). The system is very effective, and planned budgets prove to be very similar to eventual outturn expenditure. When new resources appear to be granted to areas perceived to be of particular importance, such as bailing out the provision of drug treatment for AIDS patients, this normally means resources reallocated from within the total budget rather than real new cash (Small, 1988). Therefore, some patients gain while others inevitably lose out.

There is little public accountability in the modern day NHS. The district health authorities. The purchasing authorities, are accountable to a board of directors who are picked not as representative of the local population, but on the basis of their particular skills and business acumen. Trust hospitals have similar arrangements. The majority of board members in NHS Trusts and purchasing authorities are white, middle class, and have the benefits of a university education (Ashburner and Cairncross, 1993).

As discussed above, the purchasing process in the NHS is perceived in a technocratic manner. In essence, the purchasing authority is charged with the responsibility for *measuring* the health needs of their population, and then purchasing the best combination of treatments likely to maximise health status. Competition is intended to provide increased efficiency.

Given that the relative effectiveness of different treatments, especially across specialities, is unknown, and technocratic methods intended to provide comparisons between the utilities gained from different treatments (such as the QALY or quality adjusted life year) are flawed (Carr-Hill, 1989; Drummond *et al.*, 1993), the processes of assessing need and allocating resources are somewhat arbitrary and involve value judgements (Freemantle *et al.*, 1993). Also, rationing decisions are probably being made on a different basis, with an increasing preoccupation with the limited financial resources with which to address key decisions (Freemantle and Harrison, 1993/4). This is illustrated by the following quote from a chief executive of a purchasing authority, describing the decision on whether or not to fund an additional intensive care bed:

> In the end it was a judgement... I looked at the curves and made a decision... I guess it wasn't really very scientific, but in the old days it would just have happened.

(Freemantle *et al.*, 1993)

QALYs attempt to combine information on the effectiveness of procedures with the value put upon that outcome from population surveys expressed in terms of the cost (in monetary terms) of each quality adjusted life year gained from the procedure (Williams, 1985). There are considerable difficulties in the technical derivation of QALY scores for different procedures, but as described below, the attempt to weight them by the mean value given to procedures in population surveys is also highly questionable.

An assessment of the development of purchasing authorities conducted by the Audit Commission proclaimed Directors of Public Health, community physicians employed in purchasing authorities, to be 'the guardians of the public's health' (Audit Commission, 1993). Attempts to prioritise treatments have preoccupied this group, and the recent attempt to extend coverage to the very poor under the *Medicaid* scheme in the US state of Oregon have provided one potential model for this process (Dixon and Welch, 1991).

The Oregon experiment attempted to produce an acceptable list of condition/treatment pairs, based on effectiveness information where this was available, advice from expert clinicians, and extensive public consultation. The result was a list of over 700 condition/treatment pairs in which treatments for infertility were given low priority, allocated to the bottom 16% of treatments. IVF for tubal disfunction fared particularly badly, placed 701st out of the 714 condition/treatment pairs. Small scale attempts in Britain to replicate this process have brought similar results (Bowling *et al.*, 1993), and have proven controversial (Pfeffer and Pollock, 1993).

The Oregon type approach is not a problem free solution to the problem of resource allocation to different treatments. Such prioritization exercises ignore the perceived needs of minority groups, a situation compounded when clinical experts take a moral position favouring or censuring particular treatments.

Prioritizing health services on the basis of public opinion creates a form of moral tyranny of the majority. The Rawlsian attempt to rank health care interventions on the basis of the values of a representative cross-section of the population fails not least because none of us have the information necessary to take in the big picture from behind a veil of secrecy encloaking our health status, economic and social situation (Rawls, 1973).

When, as in Oregon, not all treatments are made available but only those above a certain arbitrary cut off - in this case all the state calculated it could afford - a systematic bias is added to the prejudices of the *average* population. As Klein argues:

> Any argument about rationing that ignores those who are excluded, or... groups who are systematically neglected in the resource-distribution process, will be an exercise in public self-deception.

(Klein, 1992)

Or as the US Office of Technology Assessment report into the Oregon initiative stated:

> In fact, any comprehensive ranking system would, like Oregon's, need to rely on judgement and value-based decision making.

(Office of Technology Assessment, 1992)

The very fact that reasonably effective treatments for many causes of infertility are now available changes the politics of reproduction for couples who are experiencing difficulties in becoming parents. Variations exist in the provision of services in the NHS, and purchasing authorities are ill-equipped to develop strategies for resource use which adequately reflect the complexities of the political processes involved in collectively deciding the value to be placed on a particular treatment option. As Phillips and Rakusen persuasively contend:

> We must guard against doctors playing god - not just in terms of wanting to produce babies themselves (consciously or unconsciously) but also in terms of deciding who 'deserves' their treatment. Doctor's 'power-tripping' over women is linked to all reproductive issues, not just infertility. The difference is that, with infertility, it can be harder to see what's happening because of the intensity and complexity of the emotional pain.

(Phillips and Rakusen: pp 432)

Should Purchasing Authorities Provide a Range of Infertility Treatments on the NHS?

The fact that infertility treatments are available has changed the focus of responsibility for the conditions which may lead to involuntary childlessness, the result of which is all too obvious to childless couples and those around them. The proscription of women from infertility treatments because they have children from previous relationships, live in circumstances other than a traditional nuclear relationship or in other ways offend the traditional social mores, reflects dominant social values. This *social* decision is often justified on the basis that the *outcome* is unlikely to be in the 'best interests of the [unborn] child' (Daniels and Taylor, 1993).

Guidance on the appropriateness of making infertility treatments available is also lacking from supra national bodies. The World Health Organisation has recently produced 2 contradictory reports, from their World and European Offices, which appear both to recommend that IVF be made available, but also to put limits on its availability (Stephenson and Wagner, 1993). The circumstances are further confused by the fact that Clomiphene Citrate, an ovulation inducer which has indications only for use in cases of infertility, is included on the WHO list of essential drugs (Lancet, 1993). However this drug is of limited availability in the UK, and is subject to criteria other than its technical effectiveness on availability (i.e. couples have to be perceived to be appropriate parents).

There are enormous vested interests in the treatment of infertility as in many areas of medical technology. One pharmaceutical company, Serono, manufactures and distributes the majority of drugs used in infertility treatments. There is also a thriving private practice, and many cycles of treatment undertaken in the UK are among patients whose visit to the UK is expressly for that purpose (Pfeffer, 1993).

Health care resources are of course limited, and demands upon those resources are effectively limitless given the activities of health care providers (supplier induced demand) and the uncertainty on the effectiveness of many interventions (i.e. 'it might just help, or 'it is worth a try'). Any additional intervention undertaken is at the cost of all others forgone as a consequence, and economists would claim that decisions about resource allocation should take place at the margin where the return from different interventions is equal. However, given the enormous uncertainty on the effectiveness of health interventions it is not possible to inform the creation of such a margin, or to understand the value of what may be forgone from particular choices.

It is by no means axiomatic that the NHS should provide resources for infertility services, and any decisions in this area will be taken at the expense of some patients or potential patients. The current paradigm, where decisions are increasingly taken on the basis of research evidence, rather than on the basis of the opinion of the doctor leaves such questions unanswered. This example suggests that we are moving away from the situation, described by Foucault, of:

> ...two great myths with opposing themes and polarities: the myth of a nationalized medical profession, organized like the clergy, and invested, at the level of the man's bodily health, with powers similar to those exercised by the clergy over men's souls; and the myth of a total disappearance of disease in an untroubled, dispassionate society restored to its original state of health.
>
> (Foucault, 1973: pp 31-2)

towards one in which other solutions to the prioritization of health care resources are required in a circumstance of accepted scarcity. It is vital that these decisions should be informed not just by dominant social groups, but also by those with minority needs. In fact, the social problems faced in the health care arena in Britain increasingly mirror the inequalities of the wider society. A striking finding of the early years of the reforms in the NHS is the inability of market based health care systems to provide answers to dilemmas around the allocation of resources to different health interventions on a basis which might be considered to be rational, representative of the breadth of views in society, or to adequately reflect notions of equity.

REFERENCES

Antman, E.M., Lau, J., Kupelnick, B., Mosteller, F., and Chalmers, T.C. (1992), A Comparison of Results of Meta-Analyses of Randomized Control Trials and Recommendations of Clinical Experts, *Journal of the American Medical Association*, 268, 240-8.

Ashburner, L., and Cairncross, L. (1993), Membership of the 'New Style' Health Authorities: Continuity or Change?, *Public Administration*, 71, 357-75.

Audit Commission (1993), *Their Health, Your Business: The New Role of the District Health Authority*, London: HMSO.

Bowling, A., Jacobson, B., and Soutgate, L. (1993), Health Service Priorities: Explorations in Consultation of the Public and Health Professionals on Priority Setting in an Inner London Health District, *Social Science and Medicine*, 37, 851-7.

Carr-Hill, R. (1989), Background Material for the Workshop on QALYs: Assumptions of the QALY Methodology, *Social Science and Medicine*, 29, 469-77.

Daniels, K., and Taylor, K. (1993), Formulating Selection Policies for Assisted Reproduction, *Social Science and Medicine*, 37, 1473-80.

Dixon, J., and Welch, H.G. (1991), Priority Setting: Lessons from Oregon, *Lancet*, 337, 891-4.

Drummond, M., Torrance, G., and Mason, J. (1993), Cost Effectiveness League Tables: More Harm Than Good, *Social Science and Medicine*, 37, 33-40.

Effective Health Care (1992), *The Management of Subfertility*, Bulletin No 3, Leeds: University of Leeds.

Enthoven, A. (1985), *Reflections on the Management of the National Health Service: An American Looks at the Incentives for Efficiency in Health Services Management in the UK*, London: Nuffield Provincial Hospitals Trust.

Foucault, M. (1973), The Birth of the Clinic: An Archaeology of Medical Perception, London: Tavistock.

Freemantle, N., Watt, I., and Mason, J. (1993), Developments in the Purchasing Process in the NHS. Towards an Explicit Politics of Rationing?, *Public Administration*, 71, 535-548.

Freemantle, N., and Harrison, S. (1993/4), Interleukin 2: the Public and Professional face of Rationing in the NHS, *Critical Social Policy*, Issue 39: Winter, 3, 94-117.

Glennester, H. (1992), *Paying for Welfare*, Hemel Hempstead: Harvester.

Harrison, S., Wistow, G. (1992), The Purchaser/Provider Split in English Health Care: Towards Explicit Rationing? *Policy and Politics*, 20, 123-30.

Hull, M.G.R., Eddowes, H.A., Fahy, U., *et al.*. (1992), Expectations of Assisted Conception for Infertility, *British Medical Journal*, 304, 1465-9.

Klein, R. (1992), Dilemmas and Decisions, *Health Management Quarterly*, XIV, 2-5.

Lancet (1993), Rationing Infertility Treatments, [Editorial], 342, 251-2.

Light, D.W. (1991), Effectiveness and Efficiency Under Competition: the Cochrane Test, *British Medical Journal*, 303, 1253-4.

Lilford, R.J., and Watson, A.J. (1990), Has In-Vitro Fertilization Made Salpingostomy Obsolete?, *British Journal of Obstetrics and Gynaecology*, 97, 557-60.

Mulrow, C.D. (1987), The Medical Review Article: State of the Science, *Annals of Internal Medicine*, 106, 485-88.

NHS Management Executive (1992), *Guidance on Extra Contractual Referrals*, Leeds: NHSME.

Office of Technology Assessment (1992), *Evaluation of the Oregon Medicaid Proposal*, US Government Printing Office.

Pfeffer, N., (1993), *The Stork and the Syringe: A Political History of Reproductive Medicine.* Cambridge: Polity Press.

Pfeffer, N., and Pollock, A.M., (1993), Public Opinion and the NHS: The Unaccountable in Pursuit of the Uninformed, *British Medical Journal*, 307, 750-1.

Phillips, A., and Rakussen, J. (1989), *The New Our Bodies Ourselves*, London: Penguin.

Rawls, J. (1973), *A Theory of Justice*, London: Oxford University Press.

Redmayne, S., and Klein, R. (1993), Rationing in Practice: The Case of In-Vitro Fertilization, *British Medical Journal*, 306, 1521-4.

Secretaries of State for Health, Scotland, Wales and Northern Ireland (1989), *Working for Patients*, (Cmnd 555) London: HMSO.

Small, N. (1988), Aids and Social Policy, *Critical Social Policy*, 7 (3), 9-29.

Stephenson, P.A., and Wagner, M.G. (1993), WHO Recommendations for IVF: Do They Fit With 'Health for All', *Lancet*, 341, 1648-9.

Stocking, B. (1992), Promoting Change in Clinical Care, *Quality in Health Care*, 1, 56-60.

Thompson, S.G., Pocock, S.J. (1991), Can Meta Analysis be Trusted?, *Lancet*, 338, 1127-30.

Tonks, A. (1993), NHS Infertility is Ruled by Chance, *British Medical Journal*, 306, 290.

Williams, A. (1985), Economics of Coronary Artery Bypass Grafting, *British Medical Journal*, 291, 326-9.

17 Patient-Focused Health Care - Panacea or Pipe-Dream

JAMES SELDON

The University College of the Cariboo

No physician, insofar as he is a physician, considers ... [anything] but the good of his patient

Plato, *The Republic*

INTRODUCTION

Pleas for "patient-focused" health care have a venerable history. Complaints of administrative indifference and practitioner arrogance transcend time, bureaucratic structures, national borders, economic systems and ideological boundaries. From Hippocrates to the WHO, from the high street to the health journals, lip service is paid to providing health care that not only achieves narrowly defined physiological objectives but that also treats consumers with dignity and respect. Quite obviously, there is never enough of it around.

A parallel quest in recent years has been for "accountability" - of practitioners, subsystems and the health system as a whole. This concept often has been left ill-defined by its advocates but the primitive notion at least is clear, particularly in recent calls for reorganization and redirection of Britain's NHS: the wish to constrain a system perceived to be out of control.

The two concerns spring from a common source. The well-recognized nature of health care as 'a commodity unlike any other' generates weaknesses in collective as well as individual control of outputs and costs. Information costs and asymmetries, along with recipient and supplier uncertainties about both *ex ante* and *ex post* causes and effects, ensure that health care production and delivery systems do not fit standard market paradigms. In turn, financing's divorce from consumption under insured payment modes (both private and public) makes assessment of outcomes an aggregation exercise in which there can be no unique right answer. Some calls for accountability are consistent with enhanced patient influence on practitioners; others imply lessened responsiveness to individual wishes. Charles and DeMaio (1992) view

Setting Priorities in Health Care. Edited by M. Malek
© 1994 John Wiley & Sons Ltd

a patient-focused approach as an adjunct to greater lay participation in policy-making, while Starkey and Hodges (1993) see expansion of market and quasi-market transactions within the NHS requiring extended roles for consumers. In contrast, Mooney (1992) stresses the value of increased patient choice and autonomy for its own sake without reference to systemic impacts.

The present paper focuses on individual practitioner control. Analysis proceeds along two related lines. The narrower question deals with the prospect of closing gaps between physician practice and consumer wishes through the use of formal command and control mechanisms. The broader issue concerns the degree to which practitioners should, to achieve the best use of scarce resources, be induced to provide more of the personal touch wanted by patients.

The analysis casts light on both the desirability of and prospects for greater patient influence on health care providers. It suggests that expressions of concern in Britain are consistent with recent developments in both supply and demand conditions, and that increased attention to patient wishes probably would be welfare-improving. However, it argues that change will be more complex than is often assumed. Thus, it seems doubtful that there is any real prospect budgetary and underlying resource constraints will permit substantive near-term changes in the style of care delivered.

PATIENT-PHYSICIAN RELATIONS - SYSTEMIC STRESSES

Provider responsiveness to the wishes of health care consumers, both individually and collectively, clearly is valued by society. More of it is preferred to less. Nevertheless, what is wanted, even wanted very much, is not necessarily what will be chosen when trade-offs must be made against other goods and services. Further, it is only one piece of data relating to what *should* be chosen, and it is vital for policy-makers to recognize that fact when passing judgement on real-world outcomes or agreeing to restructure institutions in response to public pressures.

The question that must be answered concerns the degree to which a more patient-focused health care delivery style is worth the sacrifice of alternatives, and the answer never can be absolute. Even unanimous expression of the wish for a more patient-focused approach falls well short of providing conclusive evidence that society would be better off if current delivery styles were altered. The same group might also agree that better roads are needed, or better schools, or more prisons. Thus, although the underlying principle may seem obvious, it is sufficiently important to bear frequent repetition: only when costs in terms of alternative values foregone are taken into account can correct choices be made.

It may be taken as given that the medical system in general, and physicians-cum-gate-keepers in particular, will display less concern for the wishes of patients than the latter would desire if the amenity were available to them for free. The obvious reason, one that would hold even in an ideal world of perfectly altruistic practitioners, is that resources are limited. Although some consumers might be satiated, there is simply no real possibility of affording each and every one the service he or she would judge to be perfect. Even were there no other resource constraints at all, it is unavoidably costly to devote time to patients. Thus, although providers may sometimes appear overly conscious of the ticking clock when they schedule overlapping appointments or treat patients brusquely, they should not be faulted for recognizing that time spent with one cannot be devoted to others.

This source of friction will be strongest when patients pay zero point of service prices for health care. In particular, if patients wish to consume the techno/physiological aspects of care in more or less fixed proportion with social amenity and accountability, systems that fund the former without explicitly recognizing and remunerating the latter always will generate dissatisfaction. When providers are paid according to the number of services performed rather than the time they spend with patients (such as when U.S. hospitals are funded under Medicare according to DRG schedules, HMO's are remunerated via capitation, or physicians bill according to fixed fee schedules) the latter will be forced to signal the wish for more 'quality' time by public protest and exit rather than market voice. Non-price competition for patients can fill a part of the gap. However, it will be ineffective in cases where entry of new producers is restricted and there are queues for service even from practitioners whose bedside manner is deficient.

In the ideal world of perfectly competitive markets peopled by informed buyers and atomistic sellers carrying out transactions in a frictionless world, consumers of a commodity - more precisely, those at the margin - get what they pay for and pay for what they get. Similarly, producers in such an environment supply exactly what they are paid for and receive just what their output is worth. If consumers value product durability, freedom from risk, or the warmth of a smile, "the market" impersonally matches offers to pay for each of those attributes against the opportunity cost of supplying them and produces the optimal quantity of each. (Inframarginal consumers are in the fortunate position of paying less than their reservation prices and in effect getting more than they pay for, while inframarginal sellers similarly benefit from exchanging outputs for more than reservation prices. Their existence does not change the above reasoning however, because the key decisions are made 'at the margin').

What is optimal, of course, is that no potential consumer places a higher value on an increment of quality than it would cost to expand supply and no-one is receiving a unit of quality that is worth less to them than the value (s)he places on it. If quality were to be increased (perhaps via regulatory intervention, or changes in legislated fee scales, or tax and subsidy changes) the resources to provide that improvement would have to be taken from uses having values greater than would be added by the quality enhancement. Some consumers no doubt could be made better off by raising standards, but others inevitably would be harmed, and there is no way that the winners could gain enough to pay off the losers and still come out ahead. (Expressed more concisely, the benefit-cost ratio would be less than unity). Similarly, if the quality of care were reduced, the increased output of other commodities made possible by freeing resources would have lower value to consumers than the quality they would be giving up. Again, some could benefit from the adjustment, but only at the expense of others.

In practice, few market environments approach the competitive standard. Some, notably including health care, are very far removed from it. Nonetheless, it is important to avoid the fallacy of assuming that because perfect markets would generate optimal practitioner behaviour, it is a trivial matter to identify or achieve improvements to their imperfect counterparts or to the bureaucratic structures and processes set up to augment or replace them. Even at optimality in a perfectly competitive world, consumers would prefer to be provided with higher quality care than they actually find it worth paying for. Thus, complaints by real-word consumers of health care that practitioners are insufficiently patient-focused do not necessarily indicate that too little attention is being paid to patient wishes, let alone that an attainable alternative would perform better.

An additional reason for the widespread perception of a suboptimal amenity level in health care, noted by Starr (1982), is implicit in the very fact of Plato's dictum: the suspicion of health system clients that providers do not always place patients' welfare first. Corresponding stresses beset all principal-agent relationships precisely because of the information asymmetry that leads to agency in the first place. They tend to be more severe in settings where (as is typical in health care) even the agent may be uncertain about the precise links between his or her actions and impacts on the client. Thus, it seems probable that suspicion would persist even if physicians always behaved as perfect agents. Once again, complaints will not always signal under-supply.

Ascertaining the optimum degree of patient focus in health care is well beyond the scope of this paper. However, there are reasons to believe that current British practice lies below the optimum and that greater focus on the wishes of consumers would yield benefits greater than costs. One set relates to rising standards of living; a second, to technical change.

Rising real incomes have fostered increased demand for the composite commodity health care. Wealthier patients throughout history have shown a willingness to pay for private hospital accommodation and private physicians, not to mention colour televisions and other modern frills. Thus, it is predictable that rising average incomes lead the typical patient to demand -- in the economic sense of being both willing and able to pay for -- better personal care and greater respect as incomes rise.

In a complementary effect, a fall in the relative price of the amenity component of health care, even as its absolute price rises, is likely to generate increased demand for that attribute. (Bertonazzi et al, 1993, provides a more general discussion of this latter effect, sometimes referred to as the third law of demand). It seems clear that advances in technology have clearly outstripped improvements -- to the extent that there have been improvements -- in the amenity components of health care over the last few decades, especially in publicly funded systems where 'frills' have been unaffordable. Thus, these effects taken together leave little doubt that enhancement of amenity levels, *ceteris paribus*, would generate a Pareto improvement.

On the supply side, technological advances in health care have led to increasingly capital-intensive procedures. One effect has been to raise the relative cost of having professionals as providers of 'caring' rather than as sources of technical expertise. In concert, practitioners in the course of their training have been conditioned to view authority as flowing from expert knowledge of medicine's technical aspects, not superior bedside manners. The result is that there has been a decline in the importance of practitioners' roles as sympathetic companions and confidantes over a period when broader socioeconomic changes -- such as increased participation of women in the labour force, increased mobility, and the weakening of the church and the nuclear family -- have served to dilute support for patients emanating from other sources. Again, since there is no evidence to suggest that consumer tastes have changed to offset this alteration in the health care attribute mix, the implication is that social welfare has suffered.

PATIENT-PHYSICIAN RELATIONS - INTERPERSONAL CONFLICT

Keeping in mind the qualifications raised in the previous section, the analysis to follow takes as its starting point the proposition that social welfare would be improved if NHS practitioners were more patient-focused. It considers sources of deviation from the ideal at the individual practice level and examines possible initiatives designed to move the system closer to optimality.

In choosing practice styles, providers can be presumed to weigh the costs and benefits associated with alternative courses of action and to select the pattern they anticipate will best serve their interests. They may misjudge costs or benefits. They may fail to anticipate changes in their environment. They may make choices that in hindsight they regret because their own valuations have changed. However, in each case, they will have chosen options they (at the time) believed would have greater value than cost, and will have eschewed those expected to have higher costs than benefits. The range of possible behaviours is virtually infinite. If providers embody a large measure of altruism, their interests and those of patients may be reasonably close, at least at the margin. If they do not, that outcome is less probable. In each case, neither we nor they may be able to specify the exact functional relationship - or wish to attempt the task - but in each instance we can for convenience describe them as utility maximizers.

The utility maximizing choice of style at the individual practice level - treating patients with as much attention and respect (real or feigned) as they desire, ignoring their personal wishes entirely, or adopting any stance between the extremes, emerges as an outcome influenced by the practitioner's background and personality, training, non-professional relationship with the patient, financial incentives, and so on. Whatever the influences and whatever the behaviour, the presumption must be that were perceived benefits higher or costs lower, there would be a tendency to supply more of what patients desire.   Similarly, with benefits lower or costs higher, we would anticipate less of the amenity being provided.

At a more aggregate level, Wolinsky (1993) has investigated the effects of information asymmetries on industry outcomes and has shown that customer search activity combined with supplier reputation effects may give rise to an equilibrium in which experts specialize in different qualities of service.   In such a setting, patients placing higher value on amenities will be able to find providers willing to supply care matching those wants.   Still, each consumer will have reason to be suspicious that the experts are performing their personalized agency roles with less than perfect diligence.

The logic of the argument that individual physicians should be more sympathetic to their patients' wishes raises issues similar to those appearing in long-standing debates concerning Leibenstein's (1973) conception of X-inefficiency within firms. (Sappington, 1991 provides a useful survey of recent literature).   In each case, the essential point is that the quantity or quality of labour effort is less than a level identified as its potential. The fact that a health care firm's owner and residual claimant in many cases also is the primary supplier of labour and capital to the enterprise complicates the picture but does not fundamentally alter the analysis.

A first possibility is that a practitioner fails to perform at an externally-identified optimum for what are unpredictable and uncontrollable reasons.   Agents do make mistakes in pursuing the interests of their principals, and foresight is far from perfect. The deviation then is a part of the environment, much like friction, and the real problem is one of inappropriate expectations, not failure to hit appropriate targets. Like friction or traffic accidents or violent crime, these deviations from the ideal could be reduced.   However, the test of whether they *should* be reduced is whether the *ex ante*, anticipated, benefits of the reduction exceed the *ex ante* costs.

A related possibility is that perceived gaps between actual and desirable performance of agents might reflect failure of external observers to distinguish clearly between efficacy and effectiveness, between best-case scenarios and real-world complexities.   Results obtainable under ideal, experimental conditions often do not emerge when the vagaries of the real world come into play;   but wishful thinking often leads to the belief that they should.

Finally, in another form of misspecification, a practitioner's performance level may be influenced by one or more variables not appearing in the putative health production function.   This third variation warrants further examination.

A standard presumption in agency theory has been that if principals place high value on keeping agents' self-interest in check, they need only - although presumably at a cost - exert high monitoring effort to achieve their goal.   That is, shirking by agents (deviating from ideal performance) is modelled in the same light as negligent behaviour or criminality.   The underlying logic is straightforward.   Holding other factors constant, the lower is the expected punishment cost for engaging in deviant activity (calculated as the probability of detection multiplied by the penalty if detected), the lower is the deterrent effect and the greater the gap between actual and ideal performance. The greater the monitoring intensity and the higher the penalties, the smaller the deviation.

Applied to practitioner styles, the prescription flowing from this model is that bedside manners can be improved by having patients (principals) insist that physicians (agents) pay greater attention to their wishes for courteous treatment, more complete explanations of treatment alternatives, or whatever else they may desire. Conditioned by the implicit threat to find a substitute who will supply the same physiological care accompanied by the desired amenities if the current provider fails to respect the patient's wishes, it follows that eliciting the desired response is only a matter of having each patient apply the appropriate degree of pressure. In effect, we are back to the competitive market paradigm: if patients want a particular attribute badly enough, they need merely pay the price and it will be supplied to them in appropriate quantities.

The logic is impeccable, but the premises may have been misstated and the conclusions rendered of dubious applicability for real world policy-makers. Health care professionals, even those practicing on a fee-for-service basis, fall into a category characterised by Evans (1984) as not-only-for-profit (NOFP) enterprises. For such firms, accounting cost and revenue figures yield a distorted picture of the motivations governing their behaviour. Adjusting incentives to manipulate NOFP performance then will be more complex than for classic profit-seeking counterparts.

Principal-agent relationships are characterized by implicit contracts and understandings. In health care, of particular importance is that in accepting responsibility for care, physicians demand trust from their charges. Thus, if their authority to act on behalf of a patient is challenged - as they interpret matters, and not necessarily as the situation is viewed by the patient - they will perceive themselves confronting the equivalent of a breach of contract. In Frey's (1993, 665) terms, a "norm of reciprocity" may be violated when patients demand greater accountability of physicians. Alternatively, changes in interpersonal relationships may result in a redefinition of fairness and discrete shifts in equilibrium outcomes along the lines of Rabin's (1993) analysis. In either case, determining whether increased monitoring will bring about closer adherence to the wishes of the principal will be more complex than predicting the effects of a change in wages or fee schedules.

As a means of formalizing analysis of efforts designed to generate a more patient-focused style of health care delivery, consider a simple model building on Frey's (1993) discussion of crowding out versus disciplining effects of increased monitoring. Assume that practitioners obtain utility from income (y) and leisure time (L) and experience disutility associated with external monitoring (M) of their workplace activity according to the equation $U = U(y, L, M)$. Since income and leisure both are desirable and being monitored is distasteful, U_y, $U_L > 0$ and $U_M < 0$. Income depends inversely upon leisure (time and effort not spent at work) and directly on the wage rate (w) according to the relation $y = y(L, w)$, where $y_L < 0$ and $y_w > 0$. For simplicity, assume that monitoring does not directly affect the quantity of leisure time but only the practitioner's attitude toward time spent at work.

Conventionally, the practitioner's utility will be at its highest level when, for a given level of monitoring, the marginal rate of substitution of leisure for income (the ratio of U_y to U_L) equals the wage rate.

Consider now the reactions of a physician who has achieved the utility-maximizing mix of leisure and work effort, the latter including choice of practice style, and who is subsequently confronted with an increase in the level of monitoring activity. The model's formal results are set out in detail in the Appendix; more intuitively, two broad impacts can be anticipated. The first is an income effect, stemming from the decline in the physician's maximum attainable wellbeing. The second is a substitution effect, flowing from the rise in the value of leisure time relative to work as the latter becomes more onerous.

In general, reductions in real income lead some workers to increase work effort (decrease leisure) but that reaction is not guaranteed. In agency relationships of the sort considered here, a likely response is what in the cognitive psychology literature is termed a reduction in overjustification flowing from the enhanced monitoring. See McGraw (1978) and Deci and Ryan (1985) for surveys. Thus, work effort is likely to be reduced. Further, even if effort rises, it is conceivable that quantity will be substituted for quality and less attention will be paid to patients' wishes. In addition, the substitution effect definitely will lead to a reduced supply of work effort. Then, the overall effect of closer monitoring will be to crowd out the agent's intrinsic motivation for work unless the income effect on quality is both positive and large enough to offset the substitution effect; and the amenity component of care might fall even if work effort rises.

The implication of these results is that the standard prescription for closer monitoring of practitioner behaviour actually may run counter to patient interests and that a more sophisticated approach to improving practice style may be required. It is arguable that success ultimately can achieved at relatively low cost through socialization of physicians during their medical school training, but that prospect is a long-term one. In the immediate future, with entrenched physician attitudes and expectations, increased monitoring might be combined with adjustments in remuneration to achieve the desired ends. Raising the wage rate would counter the fall in attainable utility levels and enhance the desirability of work relative to leisure. However, since the income and substitution effects generally would mirror those associated with increased monitoring, there is little prospect for bringing about substantive style adjustments by that means.

If fee schedules can be restructured to reward specific styles of interaction with patients (that is, if the wage variable in the above model can be disaggregated) the above prescription can be made more effective for any given cost. However, the practical difficulties with this approach should not be minimized and the task is complicated by the very characteristics that lead to agency relationships in the first instance. It is because judgement and independent initiative are required from practitioners that they are employed as agents and allowed independence in the first place. If the tasks they now perform could have been routinized and payment specified for pre-determined and mutually identifiable outcomes, there would have been no lack of 'patient focus' to be dealt with.

CONCLUSION

Public expressions of desire for more patient-focused health care are widespread. However, this paper cautions against unquestioning acceptance of demands for action, arguing that they constitute less persuasive evidence of potential for welfare gains than their breadth and depth might seem to indicate. One reason is fundamental: in a world of scarce resources, wants always exceed capacities. Particularly when the point-of-service prices they face are near zero and the technological attributes of care are undergoing rapid advance, consumers of health services will tend to perceive deficiencies in amenity levels. Yet, trading substance for style may not be a palatable option, let alone one as desirable as public demands suggest.

Despite these qualifications, reasons from both the demand and supply sides lead to the tentative conclusion that enhanced provider attention to the wishes of patients would augment social welfare. The difficulties are to identify cost-effective means by which to achieve that end, and further — since benefits are greater than costs, but the latter are definitely not zero — to overcome the political obstacles to implementation under current fiscal constraints.

It was argued above that measures designed to pressure physicians and other practitioners into paying more attention to patients' wishes are likely to be less effective and more expensive than suggested by traditional agency theory. Increased monitoring is likely to be seen as breaching an implicit contract between providers and patients, generating discontinuous rather than incremental changes. The analysis shows that in the absence of accompanying adjustments in payment arrangements, such efforts may even provoke reactions opposite to those desired. Thus, although a combination of increased monitoring and selective fee increases can be used to alter practice style in the short term, the cost will be relatively high. Altering the professional training of practitioners may be a means of achieving the same end at substantially lower cost, but that strategy will require considerable time to yield results.

In sum, visions of patient-focused health care delivery are not mere pipe dreams, but increased attention to patient wishes is by no means a panacea for health care system ills. On the one hand, there is substantive evidence that enhancing the amenity component of health care would yield benefits greater than costs. On the other, many expressions of demand for change weaken their own positions by implicitly or explicitly assuming that there would *be* no costs. The case for enhancing amenity levels is particularly strong in publicly-funded systems such as Britain's NHS, where advances in technological capabilities have outstripped additions to 'luxury' elements of care. However, benefits must not be overrated, nor costs overlooked, if practical and political difficulties are to be overcome and the system moved toward an improved performance.

REFERENCES

Bertonazzi, E.P., Maloney, M.T. and McCormick, R.E. (1993) Some Evidence on the Alchian and Allen Theorem: The Third Law of Demand, *Economic Inquiry*, 31 (3), 383-393.

Buchanan, J.M. (1965) The Inconsistencies of the National Health Service, *Occasional Paper No. 7*, The Institute for Economic Affairs, London.

Charles, C. and DeMaio, S. (1992) Lay Participation in Health Care Decision Making: A Conceptual Framework *Working Paper Series No. 92-16*, Centre for Health Economics and Policy Analysis, McMaster University, Hamilton.

Deci, E.L. and Ryan, R.M. (1985) *Intrinsic Motivation and Self-Determination in Human Behavior*, Plenum Press, New York.

Doyle, V., Carson, E. and Sönksen (1993) Customer Supplier Modelling as a Framework for Quality Improvement, Malek, M., Rasquinha, J. and Vacani, P. (eds.), *Strategic Issues in Health Care Management*, John Wiley & Sons, Chichester, 121-127.

Evans, R.G. (1984) *Stained Mercy: The Economics of Canadian Health Care*, Butterworths, Toronto.

Frey, B.S. (1993) Does Monitoring Increase Work Effort? The Rivalry With Trust and Loyalty, *Economic Inquiry*, 31 (4), 663-670.

McGraw, K.O. (1978) The Detrimental Effects of Reward on Performance: A Literature Review and a Prediction Model, Lepper, M.R. and Greene, D. (eds),*The Hidden Costs of Reward: New Perspectives of Human Behaviour*, Erlbaum, New York, 33-60.

Mooney, G. (1992), What Do We Want From Our Health Care Services? What Can We Expect From Our Physicians? *Policy Commentary C92-1*, Centre for Health Economics and Policy Analysis, McMaster University, Hamilton.

Muldoon, J. M. and G. L. Stoddart (1989) Publicly Financed Competition in Health Care Delivery: A Canadian Simulation Model, *Journal of Health Economics*, 8 (3), 313-338.

Rabin, M. (1993) Incorporating Fairness into Game Theory and Economics *American Economic Journal*, 83 (5), 1281-1302.

Seldon, J.R. and Khandker, W. (1990) Quality of Care and Cost-Shifting in the For-Profit Hospital *Atlantic Economic Journal*, 18 (3), 89-95.

Seldon, J.R. (1993) Efficacy, Effectiveness and Efficiency in Human Resource Use: A Primer on the Three Es *International Journal of Public Administration*, 16 (7), 921-943.

Starkey, K. and Hodges, R. (1993) Of Trusts and Markets Ä Accountability and Governance in the New National Health Service, Malek, M., Vacani, P., Rasquinha, J. and Davy, P. (eds.) *Managerial Issues in the Reformed NHS*, John Wiley & Sons, Chichester, 1-16.

Starr, P. (1982) *The Social Transformation of American Medicine*, Basic Books, New York.

Stoddart, G.L. and Seldon, J.R. (1984) Publicly Financed Competition in Canadian Health Care Delivery: A Proposed Alternative to Increased Regulation, Boan, J. A. (ed.), *Proceedings of the Second Canadian Conference on Health Economics*, Boan, Regina, 121-143.

Wolinsky, A. (1993) Competition in a market for informed experts services *Rand Journal of Economics*, 24 (3), 380-398.

APPENDIX

Utility is maximized subject to the income constraint when the value of the Lagrangian expression Λ is maximized.

[1] $\Lambda \equiv U(y, L, M) - \lambda[y - y(L, M)]$

Representing partial derivatives by subscripts, then given an initial value of $M = M_0$, first order (necessary) conditions for a maximum are:

[2] $U_y - \lambda = 0$

[3] $U_L + \lambda \cdot y_L = 0$

[4] $-y + y(L, M_0) = 0$

From [2] and [3], utility maximization requires $U_L / U_Y = -y_L$. Comparative statics are described by the equation system:

[5] $\begin{bmatrix} U_{yy} & U_{yL} & -1 \\ U_{Ly} & (U_{LL} + \lambda \cdot y_{LL}) & y_L \\ -1 & y_L & 0 \end{bmatrix} \begin{bmatrix} dy \\ dL \\ d\lambda \end{bmatrix} = \begin{bmatrix} -U_{yM} \, dM \\ -(U_{LM} + \lambda \cdot y_{LM}) dM \\ -y_M \, dM \end{bmatrix}$

where (given that first order conditions have been satisfied) sufficient conditions for a maximum are that U_{yy} and $(U_{LL} + \lambda y_{LL})$ be negative and the determinant of the coefficient matrix in [5] is positive.

The adjustment in (optimal) L for a given change in monitoring, M, is determined from equation [5] by Cramer's rule as:

[6] $\dfrac{dL}{dM} = \dfrac{\begin{vmatrix} U_{yy} & -U_{yM} & -1 \\ U_{Ly} & -(U_{LM} + \lambda \cdot y_{LM}) & y_L \\ -1 & -y_M & 0 \end{vmatrix}}{D}$

substituting for λ from [2] and reducing yields:

$$[7] \quad \frac{dL}{dM} = \frac{U_{Ly} \cdot y_M + U_{LM} + U_y \cdot y_{LM} + y_L \cdot y_M \cdot U_{yy} + y_L \cdot U_{yM}}{D}$$

where D is the determinant of the coefficient matrix in [5]. It is reasonable to anticipate that U_{yM} and y_{LM} both will be zero. Then, since D must be positive, the sign of dL/dM will be the sign of $\left(U_{Ly} \cdot y_M + U_{LM} + y_L \cdot y_M \cdot U_{yy} \right)$. The final term of this expression always will be negative since the first two of its elements are negative by definition and the last is negative from second order conditions. The first term will be negative as long as the marginal utility of leisure is raised by having greater income. However, since additional monitoring of work effort will raise the relative value of leisure time, the middle term generally will be positive. Then, because the magnitude of that term could be sufficiently large as to outweigh the sum of the first and third, equation [7] cannot be signed in general.

18 Setting Priorities in UK Health Care and the New NHS R&D Strategy

ALA SZCZEPURA[1], KHESH SIDHU[2], BILL COBB[2],
ROB COOPER[2] & ROSIE GELLER[3]

[1] *University of Warwick*
[2] *Solihull Health Authority*
[3] *Shropshire Health Authority*

INTRODUCTION

In 1990, the NHS introduced a purchaser-provider split into UK health care. From that date, each District Health Authority (DHA) was given the major responsibility for commissioning health care for its local residents [HMSO, 1990]. Early guidance from the NHS Management Executive (NHSME) identified one of the main objectives for purchasers as being "to secure measurable improvements in the health of their resident population". In order to do this, they were expected to develop practical methods both for assessing health care needs and then for commissioning or purchasing services to meet those needs. Further guidance from the NHSME in 1991 broke the task down into a number of constituent parts [NHS Management Executive, 1991]. First, in order to effectively assess current and future health care needs, DHAs would need to collect detailed epidemiological data on disease prevalence and demographic trends within their local population. Secondly, provider units which might be able to meet those needs would then have to be compared in terms of their price and quality, so that the "best buy" could be obtained for local residents. Finally, any purchasing strategy developed by the DHA would need to take into account the views of local people, something which was emphasised in a further document from the NHSME [NHS Management Executive, 1992].

The tasks, as outlined above, might be appropriate if a purchaser can assume that the *status quo*, in terms of the pattern of services currently purchased, is suitable and will continue to be so. In this case, a legitimate objective might be to continue to purchase the same or similar packages of care, but at the highest quality and for the lowest price possible. However, if there is a need to set priorities in purchasing in order to maximise health gain then other factors need to be considered. The NHS (like other health care systems) is slowly coming to the realisation that purchasing

Setting Priorities in Health Care. Edited by M. Malek
© 1994 John Wiley & Sons Ltd

strategies may need to consider more than just service quality and price; the question of the cost-effectiveness of health care is increasingly being discussed in Europe [EC Council and Ministers for Health, 1991].

In 1989, such issues were already being tackled in the USA, where the state of Oregon put forward a proposal to alter its Medicaid programme so that more people could be covered within the available budget. In order to do this, Oregon decided it would have to introduce some form of "rationing" [Strosberg *et al.*, 1992]. Only in this way could it increase the *population* covered. The Oregon Project represented an early attempt to put medical services in some sort of objective order of priority by using the best available scientific method [Kitzhaber, 1993]. The methodology used involved a formula which incorporated the duration of beneficial outcome following a procedure, weighted by the quality of life gained as gauged by the general public. Two unusual aspects of the Oregon project were firstly the involvement of the local population in placing a value on various measures of quality of life, and on priority areas for health care provision; and secondly the absence of cost data in the prioritisation process (the initial list was based on effectiveness alone) [Crawshaw *et al.*, 1990; Maynard A, 1993]. The first list was released in May 1990. Following public discussion, numerous refinements, and a change of government, the Department of Health and Human Services (DHHS) finally notified Governor Barbara Roberts in March 1993 that the Oregon Health Plan had been approved subject to a number of final revisions [Oregon Health Services Commission, 1993].

Although the situation in the NHS is not as extreme as that confronted by Oregon, the problems faced by all western health care systems are similar. Demographic changes, technological advances, increased public and professional expectations, and newly discovered diseases such as AIDS have all contributed to increased pressure on health care resources. In common with other services, the NHS is experiencing a period of rapid change with increased accountability and an increased awareness of scarcity and competition for resources. As DHAs continue to purchase health care through their contracting, they will increasingly have to make explicit decisions about what they wish to buy on behalf of their population.

This paper describes two recent UK initiatives, at different levels, which illustrate how the NHS is attempting to tackle this important issue. First, the paper describes a local initiative in one DHA which provides a case-study to demonstrate the practical issues associated with setting priorities at local level. Then, it details the changes currently taking place at national level to develop a research strategy which will support the setting of priorities, both nationally and locally.

At the local level

In 1991, Solihull Health Authority in the heart of England began to consider questions which were similar to those being posed in Oregon, largely because of its new purchasing role. The Solihull Department of Public Health Medicine (DPHM) in the DHA discussed with the Centre for Health Services Studies (CHESS) at the

University of Warwick, the possibility of a pilot project to improve the information available for purchaser decision-making. The proposed project was duly funded by the West Midlands Regional Health Authority through its Research and Development programme and started in 1992, overseen by a Steering Group with members from the DPHM and CHESS.

At national level

Meanwhile, in 1991 at national level, following a government report "Priorities in Medical Research" [House of Lords Select Committee, 1988], the National Health Service launched a new R&D Strategy. The launch marked a shift in emphasis "away from the NHS as a passive recipient of new technologies to a research-based Health Service in which reliable and relevant information will be used for decisions on policy, clinical practice and management of services" [Department of Health, 1991]. The importance of R&D in this respect was indicated by the commitment to move over a five year period to a target expenditure of 1.5% of the NHS budget on research and development (translating the £225 million spent in 1989/90 to £317 million).

SOLIHULL HEALTH OUTCOMES PRIORITIES PROJECT (SHOPP)

The Solihull Health Outcomes Priorities Project (SHOPP) is programmed to run over a 3 year period from 1992 to 1995. The project consists of three phases; the first has been completed, the second is partially complete, and the third has still to be embarked upon. In the initial phase the main focus has been on measuring the local *public view*; a survey of local opinion was carried out using a structured health questionnaire. In the second phase, the emphasis has shifted to establishing what information can be gained from *professionals*; this has involved an examination of published research findings and the canvassing of local professional clinical opinion. Finally, phase 3 will explore the *purchaser* view, and will consolidate the findings from the other two stages.

The aims of the project as described at its outset are:

- to measure the value placed on different *health states* by a representative sample of the local population;
- to identify this public's *priorities* for a number of purchaser options;
- to access available *research findings* on outcomes (especially quality of life and cost-effectiveness) for a selected group of condition/ intervention pairs;
- to obtain supporting *outcomes* information from clinical professionals on these condition/ intervention pairs;
- to *inform* local setting of priorities in health care purchasing using the information obtained.

From its outset, therefore, the project aimed to consider *cost-effectiveness* of services as well as measuring public opinion. Without consideration of costs (as in the original Oregon prioritisation process) one treatment might be given priority because it is 20% more effective than another treatment for the same condition. However, if it is twice as expensive then increased cost may outweigh its increased effectiveness, especially in a cash-limited system. The Solihull project is unique in the UK because of the structured approach it has adopted to public participation and because of the emphasis from the outset on a cost-effectiveness framework [Ham, 1993].

The Public View

An essential requirement in any attempt to identify the cost-effectiveness of health services is some valuation of health outcomes [Wennberg, 1990; Department of Health, 1992]. If a number of outcomes can be defined and a representative sample of the local population values these, then this information can be used to inform the prioritisation debate. SHOPP set out to measure public opinion on health outcomes in as systematic and rigorous a manner as possible. However, before this could be done, the Project had to identify an appropriate outcome or health status measure to use at local level; only then could the practicality of using such a measure be tested. It was also an objective of the study to measure the public's view on the relative priorities of different services; posing questions in a more rigorous manner than had previously been the case elsewhere in the UK [Groves, 1993; Ham, 1993].

Choice of health status instrument

There has been a major increase over the last decade in the number of health status instruments for measuring outcomes of health care interventions [Fletcher *et al.*, 1992]. These fall roughly into two groups; ones which are *specific* to a particular condition or disease, and those which are *generic* and can be applied across a wide range of patient groups. In order to prioritise different interventions or services (the major task facing health care purchasers), an instrument which is generic is required. This can then be combined with the impact of the intervention on survival in order to produce a two-dimensional measure of outcome e.g. quality adjusted life years (QALYs). In the UK, the Rosser Classification of Illness States (developed in the 1970s) has been that most commonly used for QALY calculations [Rosser and Kind, 1978]. A more recent instrument developed for this use in Europe is the Euroqol [Euroqol Group, 1990]. This is a relatively simple instrument to administer and for this reason, among others, was the one chosen to pilot in Solihull. The Euroqol incorporates 5 health domains (mobility, self-care, usual activities, pain/discomfort, anxiety/depression). Health states (represented by different combinations of these) are rated by means of a "thermometer" with end points 0 (worst imaginable state) and 100 (best imaginable state).

Structure of public survey

In order to ensure that responses were representative of local opinion, a random sample (stratified by neighbourhood, age and sex) of 630 Solihull adults was taken from the Family Health Services Authority register. It had been calculated that for a 95% confidence interval, the response level required would be 383 (61%). In Oregon, a telephone survey had only produced a 23% response rate; there were also questions over how representative phone-owners might be in Solihull. A postal survey was therefore chosen as the most effective and also the cheapest method of measuring local opinion. This was conducted between July and November 1992, in conjunction with a systematic follow-up strategy designed to ensure a maximum response rate. Follow-up entailed three postal reminders (each at 3 week intervals) with a further questionnaire enclosed with the second reminder. Following this, contact was then made either by telephone or via a personal visit.

During the 3 weeks after the initial mailing, 210 questionnaires (33% response rate) were returned; the follow-up strategy raised this figure to 429 (68%) which was well above the target response rate. Of the non-responders, 28 (4%) had moved or were not known at the address, and 58 (9%) stated they were unwilling to respond. Respondents were found to be representative of the group surveyed; the overall pattern of responses is detailed in Table 1.

Table 1. Breakdown of Questionnaire Responses

Descriptor	Actual Percentage in Responses (n=429)	Expected Percentage
Age		
Young (18-34 years)	34%	30%
Middle aged (35-64 yrs)	47%	51%
Elderly (65+ years)	19%	19%
Sex		
Male	51%	48%
Female	49%	52%
Location		
North	35%	32%
Central	34%	34%
South	31%	34%

Completion levels for individual questions were excellent in the returned questionnaires. The item for which there were most omissions was self-rating of the state of 'dead'; 57 respondents failed to scored this item (13% of returned questionnaires).

Valuation of health states

Respondents were invited to rate 16 health states based on Euroqol using a "thermometer" or visual analogue scale of 0-100. These 16 health states were numerically coded, using the values of 1, 2, 3 to represent the level of severity for each of the five health domains. This gave a 5 digit code in which '11111' represented 'best imaginable health state', and '33333' represented a state approaching the 'worst imaginable health state'. Table 2 shows the median score for Solihull respondents compared with that for a similar survey undertaken in Frome in the UK [Gudex, 1991]. The Solihull results also compare well with those reported from other parts of Europe, with a higher response rate than achieved elsewhere [Brooks et al., 1991; Essink-Bot and Stouthard, 1991; Nord, 1991]. More detailed analyses of the survey findings are to be published elsewhere.

Table 2. Median Scores for Health States - Solihull and Frome

State (code)	Solihull	Frome
11111	95(a)* 95(b)*	90(a)* 98(b)*
11112	75	85
11121	70	88
11122	56	75
11211	80	65
12111	60	70
21111	70	70
21232	35	35
22233	25	20.5
22323	20	20
32211	30	35
33321	15	19
333333	5(a) 5(b)	4(a) 3(b)
Unconscious	1	5.5
Dead	2(a) 3(b)	5(a) 5(b)

* (a)/ (b)   Questions repeated on each page of the questionnaire; both scores presented separately.

In general, our results confirm that the Euroqol appears to give consistent results across different populations [Williams, 1993]. Also, that surveying a random selection of local people using a postal questionnaire is a practical means of obtaining a measure of public valuation of different health states, although a well-planned follow-up strategy is required to achieve a statistically adequate response rate.

Ranking health services

As well as measuring the public's valuation of different health states, researchers in the UK have recently attempted to obtain the public's view on the relative value of different types of health services [Groves, 1993; Ham, 1993]. However, the questions posed in these instances have generally not incorporated cost or resource-use information; rather the public have been asked to value the service as a whole, without a yardstick of relative cost. SHOPP set out to obtain a more rigorous measure of local public opinion by incorporating information on relative cost; the questions asked were therefore more likely to resemble the prioritising decisions which a purchasing authority might face.

First, eleven different types of health service were all matched in terms of what the DHA considered £50,000 could buy. Numbers of cases or interventions were estimated wherever possible, and otherwise the general change to a service was described. Services were chosen to cover a cross-section of health care in a district. They included preventive services, emergency and non-emergency hospital care, improved access to basic services such as maternity care, care of the elderly, community care for the mental illness, and high tech surgery (see Table 3). Respondents were then invited to rank these 11 health services for two different scenarios. In one case, they were to assume that the DHA had extra funding of £50,000 and the question posed was "where to spend an extra £50,000 first,........eleventh?", and in the second case when a cut in funding of £50,000 was required "which services to cut/ reduce?".

Table 4 shows the public response both for the use of additional funding, and for reduced funding to services. The percentage of respondents placing an item in the upper ranks (i.e. ranked 1-5.5) is presented in both cases. The Table shows that when extra spending was being considered, hospital care for sudden emergency illness was judged most valuable (91% ranked improving the service to people who have suffered heart attacks highly); care for the dying including pain relief was next (75% ranked spending the additional resources on home nursing care for 20 terminally ill patients highly); prevention of infectious disease (a service to try to vaccinate an estimated 200 babies in the district who currently were not vaccinated) came next (72% rated highly); high technology surgery (2 liver transplants) came fourth in priority (68% rated highly); and non-emergency surgery was fifth in the list of priorities (56% ranked using the money to provide 15 additional hip replacement operations highly).

Table 3. Description of Health Service Options which the Local Population Were Asked to Rank

Service	Example given e.g....
Hospital care for sudden emergency illness	Improve the emergency service to people who have suffered heart attacks
	The emergency service to people who have suffered heart attack would be reduced
Care for the dying including pain relief	Nursing care for 20 people at home who are dying
	Nursing care for 20 people at home who are dying would not be provided
Prevention of infectious disease	A service to try to vaccinate the 200 babies in Solihull who currently miss them
	200 babies in Solihull would miss being vaccinated
High technology surgery	2 liver transplants
	2 liver transplants would not be performed
Non emergency surgery	15 hip replacement operations
	15 hip replacement operations would not be performed
Mental Illness services	Improving community care for 40 psychiatric patients
	40 less psychiatric patients would be cared for in the community
Long stay care for the elderly	Caring for 3 additional elderly people in a residential home
	3 fewer elderly people would be cared for in a residential home
Maternity care	Improved quality and accessibility of antenatal clinics
	The quality and accessibility of antenatal clinics would suffer
Waiting lists	Reduce the waiting list by 60 for people with varicose veins and hernia operations
	60 people requiring varicose veins and hernia operations would remain on the waiting list
Preventative services	2,000 people counselled/advised to help them stop smoking
	2,000 people would not be counselled/advised to help them stop smoking
Services for drug abuse	Funding a campaign to reduce drug abuse amongst young people
	A campaign to reduce drug abuse amongst young people would be stopped

Table 4. Local Preferences for Use of Additional Funding* and for Reduced* Funding

Service	More Funding: %** (Rank Order)	Less Funding: %** (Rank Order)
Hospital care for sudden emergency illness	91% (1)	16% (11)
Care for the dying including pain relief	75% (2)	31% (10)
Prevention of infectious disease	72% (3)	32% (9)
High technology surgery	68% (4)	34% (8)
Non-emergency surgery	56% (5)	49% (7)
Mental illness services	40% (=6)	56% (5)
Long stay care for the elderly	40% (=6)	59% (4)
Maternity care	36% (8)	53% (6)
Waiting lists	35% (9)	70% (3)
Services for drug abuse	21% (=10)	75% (2)
Preventive services	21% (=10)	81% (1)

*   Based on additional funding of £50,000 in one year;
       or requirement to reduce expenditure by £50,000 in one year
** % Percentage of respondents ranking this in top half (i.e. ranked 1-5.5)

Certain other services were clearly considered of less value (even with details of the number of cases involved); additional spending on these was ranked high by only 21% to 40% of respondents.   These included preventive services (2,000 people counselled/advised to help them stop smoking); services for drug abuse (funding a campaign to reduce drug abuse amongst young people); waiting lists (reduce the waiting list by 60 people for varicose vein and hernia operations); and maternity care (improved quality and accessibility of ante-natal clinics).

In a scenario of *reduced* funding, the pattern recorded was virtually a mirror-image of that described above. The only discrepancy was maternity care, which was more likely to be preserved from reduced funding than might have been expected based on its rank in terms of increased funding. Support for cuts to services was greatest for preventive services related to smoking, then for drug abuse services, reduction of the waiting list for hip replacement, elderly care (caring for 3 additional elderly people in a residential home), and mental illness services. There clearly was least support for reduced funding to hospital emergency care.

The Solihull results demonstrate that public opinion is internally consistent when identifying relative priorities of different health services, both in terms of which services should be given extra funding and which might be the first to have their funding reduced. Furthermore, the Solihull public priorities might be considered to be better informed than others reported in the UK literature [Groves, 1993; Ham,

1993] because the public were given some indication of relative numbers for different services before being asked to prioritise them.

The Solihull rankings are therefore more directly related to the actual decisions faced by purchasers. Even so, the rank order shown in Table 4 is virtually identical to that found in a public survey carried out in 1992 in City and Hackney Health Authority in which no indication of relative costs was provided [Ham, 1993]. In both cases, emergency care or services for life-threatening conditions are ranked as most important, followed by care of the terminally ill. Also, both groups rank high technology surgery for life-threatening conditions (e.g. liver transplants) above surgery to improve general functioning and reduce pain (e.g. hip replacements); this remains the case even once estimated numbers of patients are provided. Finally, health education (e.g. campaigns to encourage healthy lifestyles) is consistently given the lowest priority by the public.

The findings of a MORI poll of 2000 members of the UK public in 1993 also showed similar views to those measured in Solihull, although there was less overlap in the treatments and services which the public were asked to consider [Groves, 1993]. Smokers came bottom of the list in both, and high tech surgery (heart or liver transplants) came higher than hip replacement operations for the elderly. One explanation given for the high priority placed on high tech surgery was that it "gets lots of publicity without explanation of cost and effectiveness". The Solihull findings show that the public continue to rank high tech surgery higher, even once some indication of cost is provided, suggesting the need for information on effectiveness (i.e. health outcomes) as well as costs. More detailed analysis shows some differences in priorities depending on the health state, age and sex, and lifestyle (e.g. smoking) of respondents. Further analyses of these findings are to be published elsewhere.

Information from professionals

In order to be able to use the valuation of health states provided by the local population to prioritise health care interventions systematically, a DHA would also need to collect information on the effects which the interventions it purchases have on patient health outcomes or quality of life (QoL). Two main sources of QoL data are available to a DHA [Kind and Gudex, 1993]. The first is information from studies carried out by *professionals* and published in peer-reviewed journals [Gudex, 1986; Coast, 1992]; the second is the views of *professional groups* involved in health care, usually doctors, obtained via interviews or questionnaires [Slevin *et al.*, 1988]. SHOPP aims to examine how useful and feasible both these approaches might be in an ordinary NHS purchasing authority.

For the second of these, SHOPP has developed a questionnaire, which is currently being piloted, to measure the consensus between professionals on the impact of selected procedures on health outcomes, in terms of survival and QoL. The QoL questions are phrased so that they fit with the Euroqol health domains valued by the local population in the survey of public opinion.

However, the project first set out to examine published research studies in order to see whether, and how well, these might map against the interventions and services of interest to DHA purchasing. The DHA had on-line access to Medline and this was used as the main source of published research. A literature review of the Medline database (1988 onwards) was undertaken, with a cut-off date of August 1993. This focused on 16 conditions or interventions, which were selected from a list of 110 identified as of potential importance to the district purchaser based on their frequency count in contracts, total cost, and importance to public health. The sample of 16 pilot conditions/ interventions were chosen to cover secondary and primary care, high tech and low tech medicine, emergency and elective work, and prevention and treatment. The final list (in alphabetical order) is shown in Table 5.

Table 5. Conditions/Interventions Used in Literature Search (in alphabetical order)

Acute myocardial infarction	Prostatectomy
Back pain	Renal dialysis
Cataract surgery	Schizophrenia
Cervical screening	Smoking prevention
Hip replacement	Teeth extraction
Hypertension	Threatened abortion
Hysterectomy	Tonsillitis/tonsillectomy/adenoidectomy
Neonatal surgery	Varicose veins

It was anticipated that the literature search would uncover a large number of articles containing information of potential relevance to outcomes and cost-effectiveness for these 16 conditions/ interventions. Therefore, a structured template was developed which could record information key to the DHA's requirements. The development of this template was an iterative process, the content being refined as the literature review progressed. The main objective was to capture outcomes information, but a number of other types of information were also recorded because they were judged to be of potential use to the DHA.

The final template contained details of the specialty, the type of condition (e.g. cancer) and the specific sub-category (e.g. oesophageal), the actual treatment or procedure and its broad use (e.g. preventive, therapeutic, palliative etc.), any outcomes measured (e.g. survival, length of stay, QoL) and the instrument used for the latter (e.g. Rosser Classification, Nottingham Health Profile etc.), all costs measured (e.g. health system, patient, societal), the study design (e.g. literature review, meta-analysis, randomised controlled trial etc.) and country of origin, and the type of patient (e.g. inpatient, day cases, ambulatory etc.) with ages if given and number in sample.

In total some 600 articles were examined and a total of 226 articles summarised using the template. The main "outcomes" identified in these articles were: mortality

21 (9%), morbidity 21 (9%), complications 4 (2%), QoL 3 (1%), QALY 1 (0.5%), recurrence 2 (1%), re-admission 1 (0.5%), more than 1 outcome 15 (7%). Costs were reported in 12 cases (5%). Although these statistics might be expected to vary depending on the conditions or interventions being considered, the findings generally indicate that the available research base in relation to outcomes is sparse and fragmented. Articles currently concentrate primarily on mortality and morbidity as outcome measures and very rarely on the quality of life; they also do not necessarily examine conditions/ interventions of interest to purchasers. Our findings, especially the low incidence of published studies which incorporate outcome measures that combine impact on QoL and survival (e.g. QALYs), are similar to those reported by other authors [Coast, 1992; Neuburger, 1992].

The pilot carried out by SHOPP confirms that the research literature contains information on the efficacy or effectiveness of interventions which may be of use to purchasers, and that this can be extracted based on local needs. However, extraction of this information is a laborious process (approximately 15 working days were required) and, of course, there remains a need to update on a continuous basis. This is therefore a task which cannot sensibly be taken on by a single authority, and which might therefore best be shared on a national basis with individual purchasing authorities taking responsibility for a limited number of conditions or treatments and producing information which is made available to all purchasers. Even so, it is probably not practical to aim to examine an exhaustive list of interventions or conditions; a manageable number may need to be selected and prioritised, perhaps based on local or national interests. Leading on from this, the lack of relevant outcomes information in the literature also shows that there is clearly a need to *prioritise research* so that it better meets the needs of NHS purchasers in the future.

A RESEARCH AND DEVELOPMENT STRATEGY FOR THE NHS

The new NHS R&D Strategy, launched in 1991, represents the first attempt by any country to establish a coherent R&D infrastructure to support the promotion of health and the provision of health care [Szczepura, 1993a]. Following his appointment, the NHS Director of R&D (Professor Michael Peckham) set up a national R&D organisational framework which balances central strategic direction and regional planning and implementation (see Figure 1). The strategic direction is set on the advice of a Central Research and Development Committee (CRDC) supported by expert advisory groups. The executive arm (with the task of implementation) consists of 14 Regional Research and Development Directors (RDRDs) and their directorates, as well as a Research and Development Directorate in the Department of Health. Regional Directors have responsibility for developing regional R&D plans, and for preparing regional registers of research; the first plans were published in 1992, and the Solihull Project is part of this regionally-funded research.

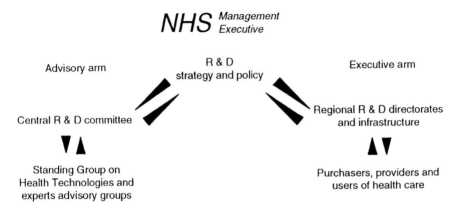

Figure 1. Organisational Framework for NHS R&D Programme (Department of Health (1993), Research for Health, London)

Improved use of existing research findings

The experience in Solihull demonstrates that use of existing research findings by DHAs might be improved; but, that this will require considerable time and effort to gather, analyse, and disseminate existing research results. Furthermore, much existing research appears not to meet the needs of purchasers in terms of usable outcomes and cost-effectiveness information to support prioritisation decisions.

Before any research was commissioned as part of the R&D strategy, therefore, the NHS carried out a central "stock-taking" to identify existing NHS research patterns. This identified a total of 6,185 projects for 1991/92 being carried out within the NHS; of these, one third dealt with evaluation of health interventions, but less than 8% were found to evaluate outcomes or cost-effectiveness [Department of Health, 1993]. Following this initial stock-take, a permanent, co-ordinated system (based on regional registers) is being developed in the NHS. Initially this will only cover R&D funded by the NHS and the Department of Health. However, the intention is then to interface this register with that of the Medical Research Council (MRC) which funds biomedical research in the UK and the major Charities.

Also, in order to improve the information currently available to NHS managers and clinicians, a UK Clearing House was commissioned in 1992 to produce a series of Effectiveness Bulletins detailing the information currently available on the effectiveness of a number of interventions [Department of Health, 1993]. Following this, a Dissemination and Enquiry Unit has been established (at the end of 1993) which will provide continuous access to such information for managers and clinicians.

Finally, because the existing literature on the effectiveness and cost-effectiveness of interventions may require systematic meta-analysis if it is to provide maximum benefit to users in the NHS, the R&D Directorate opened the Cochrane Centre in Oxford in November 1992. Also, because not all research findings are available in a published form, the Cochrane Centre is devoting considerable effort to setting up an efficient *network* so that unpublished, as well as published, work can be reviewed and incorporated in meta-analyses. The first electronically published output, on Effective Care in Pregnancy and Childbirth, was released in May 1993. The collaboration is now to be extended by the opening of a second centre in Canada.

Prioritising future research

The Solihull experience demonstrates that the research results currently available do not necessarily meet the interests or needs of health care purchasers. This is an international problem, and not one confined to the UK [Szczepura, 1993b]. Improved dissemination of existing research findings will not be sufficient in itself; there is a need to prioritise future research. This is one of the most important tasks facing the new NHS R&D Strategy; research priorities need to be identified in such a way as to ensure maximum relevance to the NHS. In order to do this, the strategy has set about identifying key research priorities based on six overlapping perspectives; disease related (e.g. mental health, cardiovascular disease and stroke, cancer, respiratory, dentistry); management and organisation (e.g. interface between primary and secondary care, accident and emergency services); client group (e.g. physical and complex disabilities, mother and child health, elderly people, health of ethnic minorities); consumers (e.g. nature, role and input of users and potential users of NHS); health technologies (i.e. assessment of a range of interventions and services); and finally research methodologies [Department of Health, 1993]. In five of the six areas, a time-limited multidisciplinary group has been convened to identify and prioritise research. The one exception is in the area of health technology, where a Standing Group with a much longer lifetime has been established.

Standing Group on Health Technologies (SGHT)

The term "technology" as defined by the CRDC has a broad meaning; it covers not only drugs and devices, but also medical and surgical procedures, support systems, and organisational and administrative systems within which such care is delivered - these technologies might be located in hospitals, primary care, or the home [Department of Health, 1993]. The importance of technology *assessment* was identified early in the NHS R&D programme. The first discussion paper on R&D to be published focused on the important issue of assessing health technologies [Department of Health, 1992].

Following this paper, a Standing Group on Health Technology (SGHT) was formed in 1993 to advise the NHS Central R&D Committee on assessment of new and existing health technologies. Six Advisory Panels were set up to support the Standing Group (covering pharmaceuticals; diagnostics and imaging; other acute sector technologies; primary and community care; population screening; and HTA methodology). The objective of the SGHT and its Advisory Panels is to identify those technologies which are priorities for assessment in the NHS; the Panels, like the SGHT, are not time-limited.

The Advisory Panels were set up in March 1993 and produced their first report to SGHT on research priorities in October 1993 [CRDC Standing Group on Health Technology, 1993]. A systematic review of technologies was not feasible in the time available, so instead a national postal consultation exercise was chosen as the most appropriate method for identifying priorities. This was carried out in the NHS, the research community, and organisations representing the views of industry, patients and professionals. In total 317 different organisations were contacted, provided with information on the aims of the R&D consultation and the criteria for prioritising research questions, and asked to put forward suggestions. In addition, each of the 14 Regional Directors of R&D was asked to carry out a similar consultation exercise with service staff in their own region (purchasers and providers). The form of these first regional consultations differed; some adopted a similar, systematic approach to that used nationally [Trent Regional Health Authority, 1993; West Midlands Regional Health Authority, 1993]. The UK approach to prioritisation is therefore very different from that adopted in other countries (if any), where often government or political views and requirements prove more relevant to actual patterns of research priorities than the service manager's or clinician's needs.

Once suggestions had been received, each Panel then examined all responses which might be relevant to its own areas of interest. The Panels (supported by a research secretariat) then extracted those suggestions (1,435 in total) which fell within the remit of HTA; numbers per Panel at this stage ranged from 435 for the Primary and Community Care Panel to 65 for the Methodology Panel. The Panels then used a number of techniques (including postal voting and a one-day consensus conference) to reach agreement on a more manageable number of suggestions (24-50) which were judged to be sufficiently important for a formal case justifying the need for assessment to be drafted. These cases were then considered by Panel members and a final "top 20" list agreed. Panels were not necessarily expected to identify whether research (either published or in progress) was already being carried out in these areas; the aim was simply to identify which of the research suggestions received through the national consultation exercise were the highest priority.

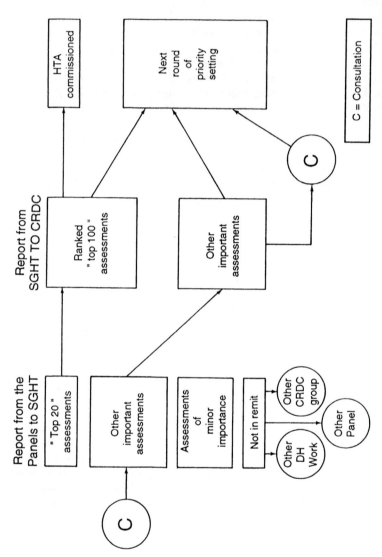

Figure 2. Prioritisation Process for HT Assessments in NHS

"Top 20" lists were then forwarded to the Standing Group by each of the six Advisory Panels. The SGHT went through a similar exercise to select a final set of 26 national priorities for HTA topics; these were endorsed by the CRDC in December 1993. The research finally commissioned may be either primary research (in cases where research is not currently underway), or in other cases, reviews or meta-analyses of existing research findings and dissemination the results.

The sequence of events which constituted the prioritisation process is shown in Figure 2. Potentially valuable assessments which did not manage to get through this process have been redirected to the next round of priority setting to be carried out in 1994.

THE FUTURE

Until recently NHS purchasers have had little information on the impact of most health interventions. As purchasers everywhere become more concerned with the health gains which their money can buy, information on outcomes and cost-effectiveness will become increasingly important to help them plan their purchases better. The new NHS R&D strategy will have an important role to play in supporting purchasers in the NHS in order to improve: setting priorities for resource use; setting contract specifications which evaluate outcomes as well as process; and development of strategic purchasing plans aimed at "securing measurable improvements in the health of the resident population". It will do this firstly through improving the dissemination and use of *existing* research findings; improved "follow-through" is now recognised to be needed internationally [Szczepura, 1993a].

However, the major challenge of prioritising *future* research is one which remains for all health care systems. Once again, the UK initiative is of interest because of the attempt to develop a user-driven approach to setting the research agenda for assessment of health care interventions and services. The importance of involving managers and clinicians in this debate lies in their ability to translate research findings into action, with the ultimate benefit to patients of substituting effective for ineffective services [Szczepura, 1993b]. The R&D reforms currently being introduced in the NHS should help to create an environment in which NHS managers and clinicians are increasingly able to utilise the results of research as a means of improving health.

REFERENCES

Brooks RG, Jendteg S, Lindgren B, Persson U, Bjork S (1991), EuroQol: health-related quality of life measurement: results of the Swedish questionnaire exercise, *Health Policy*; 18: 37-48.

Coast J (1992), Reprocessing data to form QALYs, *British Medical Journal*; 305: 87-90.

Crawshaw R, Garland M, Hines B, Anderson B (1990), Developing Principals for Prudent Health Care association - The continuing Oregon experiment, *Western Journal of Medicine*; 152: 441-446.

CRDC Standing Group on Health Technology (1993), Report of the Advisory Panels to the Standing Group on Health Technology, CRDD, Leeds, October 1993.

Department of Health (1991), *Research for Health: A Research and Development Strategy for the NHS*, Department of Health, London.

Department of Health (1992), *Assessing the Effects of Health Technologies: Principles, Practice, Proposals*, Department of Health, London.

Department of Health (1993), *Research for Health*, Department of Health, London.

EC Council and Ministers for Health (1991), Resolution of the Council, Brussels November 7th, 1991, concerning fundamental health policy choices (91/C 304/05)

EuroQol Group (1990), EuroQol - a new facility for the measurement of health-related quality of life, *Health Policy*; 16: 199-208.

Essink-Bot M, Stouthard MEA (1991), The Rotterdam Survey - Analysis of (non) response. *Euroqol Conference Proceedings*, Lund, October 1991, p31-41.

Fletcher A, Gore S, Jones D, Fitzpatrick R, Spielgelhalter D, Cox D (1992), Quality of life measures in health care. II: Design, analysis and interpretation, *British Medical Journal*; 305: 1145-1148.

Groves T (1993), Public disagrees with professionals over NHS rationing, *British Medical Journal*; 306: 673.

Gudex C (1991), Are we lacking a dimension of energy in the Euroqol Instrument?, *Euroqol Conference Proceedings*, Lund, October 1991, p61-72.

Gudex C (1986), QALYs and their use by the health service, Discussion Paper No 20, Centre for Health Economics, York.

Ham C (1993), Priority setting in the NHS: reports from six districts, *British Medical Journal*; 307: 435-8.

House of Lords Select Committee on Science and Technology (1988), *Priorities in Medical Research*, HMSO, March 1988.

HMSO (1990), *National Health Service and Community Care Act*.

Kind P, Gudex C (1993), The role of QALYs in assessing priorities between health-care interventions, Drummond MF, Maynard A (eds.), *Purchasing and Providing Cost-effective Health Care*, Churchill Livingstone, London.

Kitzhaber JA (1993), Prioritising health services in an era of limits: the Oregon experience, *British Medical Journal*; 307: 373-7.

Maynard A (1993), Future directions for health-care reform, Drummond MF, Maynard A (eds.), *Purchasing and Providing Cost-effective Health Care*, Churchill Livingstone, London.

Neuburger H (1992). Cost-effectiveness register: user guide. Department of Health, London.

NHS Management Executive (1991), *Moving forwards - needs, services and contracts*, DHA Project Paper, March 1991.

NHS Management Executive (1992), *Local voices: the views of local people in purchasing for health*, January 1992.

Nord E (1991), EuroQol: Health-related quality of life measurement: valuations of health states by the general public in Norway, *Health Policy*, 18: 25-36.

Oregon Health Services Commission (1993), Private Communication, Sipes-Metzler PR (Executive Director, Oregon Health Services Commission), June 30 1993.

Rosser R, Kind P (1978), A scale of valuations of states of illness: is there a social consensus?, *International Journal of Epidemiology*, 7 (4): 347-358.

Slevin ML, Plant H, Lynch D, Drinkwater J, Gregory WM (1988), Who should measure quality of life, the doctor or the patient?, *British Journal of Cancer*, 57: 109-112.

Strosberg MA, Weiner JM, Baker R, Fein IA (eds.) (1992), *Rationing America's health care: the Oregon plan and beyond,* Brookings Institute, Washington DC.

Szczepura AK (1993a) , NHS Developments in Health Technology Assessment, Light D, May A (eds.), *Britain's Health System: From Welfare State to Managed Markets*, Faulkner and Gray, Washington DC.

Szczepura AK (1993b), Strategies for Improved Technology Assessment Use in European Health Care, Malek M, Rasquinha J, Vacani P (eds.), *Strategic Issues in Health Care Management*, John Wiley, Chichester.

Trent Regional Health Authority (1993), Private Communication, Cooke P (Regional Director R&D), June 1993.

Wennberg (1990), Outcomes research, cost containment and the fear of health care rationing, *New England Journal of Medicine*, 323 (17): 1202-1204.

West Midlands Regional Health Authority (1993), Private Communication, Stewart J (Regional Deputy Director R&D), June 1993.

Williams A (1993), Private Communication, Centre for Health Economics, University of York, UK.

19 The Impact of 1990 GP Contract on Practice Strategy and Business Organisation

BRENDA LEESE[1] & NICK BOSANQUET[2]

[1]*University of York*
[2]*University of London*

INTRODUCTION

The changes which have taken place in general practice as a result of the 1990 contract (Department of Health, 1989) and the NHS Review (Department of Health 1989a) which led to fundholding (Department of Health, 1989b), as well as the community care changes (Griffiths, 1988, Department of Health, 1990) are far reaching in themselves, but are only a part of wider changes affecting primary care. They are having a major impact, not only on the ways in which GPs organise their practices, but also on the services provided for patients. The family doctor has been given a key role in health promotion, and is having to develop this role under new incentives and relating to new management agencies.

The new contract, implemented in April 1990, changed the way in which GPs are paid for providing general medical services. Greater emphasis was placed on capitation payments which now make up 60% of GP income, one of the aims being to make GPs more "accountable" to their patients. GPs have to produce annual reports on their activities and payment was made for the first time, for health promotion clinics held by the practice. The latter was, however, modified in July 1993 to a "banding" system for preventive work on heart disease and stroke (Department of Health, 1993). Fee for service payments were changed, with some being withdrawn, and others being replaced by target payments. Previously, GPs received a fee for each immunisation or cervical cytology test they carried out. In the new contract, payment is made for childhood immunisation if coverage of 90% of the eligible population is achieved, with a lower payment for 70% coverage. For cervical cytology, the limits are 80% and 50%. If these targets are not reached, no payment is received by the GP.

Setting Priorities in Health Care. Edited by M. Malek

Other fees have been introduced for the first time (for minor surgery, annual health checks for the over 75s, newly registered patients, and those not seen in the previous 3 years). Also, as a result of the NHS Review, greater management responsibilities have been given to the Family Health Service Authorities (FHSAs) which are expected to achieve health targets (Irvine, 1990). In addition, implementation of the new contract has stimulated growth in information technology, and is likely to have further effects on the pharmaceutical and medical equipment industries (Leese and Hutton, 1990).

As well as the changes relating to the new contract, general practice fundholding was introduced in April 1991. (Department of Health 1989b). The details were controversial (Leese and Drummond, 1993). Initially only larger practices (at least 11,000 patients) were eligible for the scheme but this limit was subsequently reduced to 7000. The stated aims of the proposals were to "improve the quality of services to patients", to "stimulate hospitals to be more responsible to the needs of the GP", and for GPs to "develop their own practices for the benefit of their patients". Included in the budget were some hospital (mainly elective) procedures, drugs prescribed and dispensed, and staff and premises currently reimbursed. From April 1993, community health services were also included as a result of the Community Care Act (Department of Health, 1990).

These changes have been controversial, with considerable initial, and lingering, opposition. In 1986/87 a study of general practice structure and organisation was carried out (Bosanquet and Leese 1986, 1988, 1989, Leese and Bosanquet, 1989), to determine how economic considerations influenced practice decisions at the local level. This study showed that practices had developed long term strategies with many showing a willingness to change. They were also prepared to consider more change in the longer term. In 1992/3 a second survey was carried out, returning to the same areas as in the earlier study to look at the effect of the new contract and fundholding changes on practices. This paper reports on the findings of the pilot study in a single FHSA area, carried out in 1992. The views of GPs about the contactual changes and fundholding will be described and the implications for practice management will be discussed.

METHODS

A single FHSA was selected as the pilot area for the study of practice structure and organisation since the 1990 contract changes. This was the same FHSA which had formed the pilot study area for a pre-contract study, carried out in 1986. (Bosanquet and Leese, 1986). A further 6 FHSA areas were selected for the main study both before and after the 1990 contract, representing different socioeconomic regions. The results of this study will be reported elsewhere. The pilot FHSA consisted of a medium sized town and its environs, in the north of England, with a population of approximately 200,000. For the 1992 study, one partner from each practice was asked to take part in an interview during which a structured questionnaire was completed. The interviews were carried out by the authors between September and

December 1992. The single-handed GPs were sent a postal questionnaire. The results of this study will be compared, where appropriate, with the results from the 1986 study in the same FHSA area.

Although both the 1986 and the 1992 studies took place in the same FHSA area, some practices had changed between the two dates. Moreover, some practices which took part in the earlier survey, did not do so in the later study, and vice versa. The study should therefore be regarded as representing GP views in a single FHSA over time, but not necessarily the views of the same GPs.

RESULTS AND DISCUSSION

Response rates and partnership sizes

Partnership sizes and numbers of GPs taking part in the 1986 and 1992 studies are set out in Table 1. The results show an increase in the numbers of single-handed GPs in the study area from 8 to 12, and a reduction in 2 partner practices from 10 to 6. Only 50% of the 8 single handed GPs responded in 1986, and so they were excluded from the study. The response rate in 1992 was much improved, at 92%. The response rate for the 29 partnerships in 1986 was 86%, and for the 28 partnerships in 1992 it was 93%.

Table 1. Response Rates and Partnership Sizes

No. Partners	No. Partners		No. participating Practices		No. Participating GPs	
	1986	1992	1986	1992	1986	1992
	8	12	4	11	4	11
2	10	6	8	6	16	12
3	7	9	6	8	18	24
4	7	8	6	7	24	28
5	3	3	3	3	15	15
6	0	1	0	1	0	6
7	2	1	2	1	14	7
Total	37	40	29	37	91	103

Fundholding

Table 2 shows the fundholding status of participating practices. At the time of the study, there were no fundholdes, but 4 were to take up this option in the third wave

(April 1993). A considerable reluctance was found in the comments made by GPs, to commit themselves to fundholding.

Table 2. Fundholding Status of Participating Practices (1992)

Status	No. (%) Practices	
1st wave fundholder	0	(0)
2nd wave fundholder	0	(0)
Considering 3rd wave	4	(11)
Would consider if size limit removed	4	(11)
None of these	18	(49)
Not asked (single handed)	11	(30)
Total	**37**	**(100)**

One practice was not yet convinced fundholding was a good idea (list size 11,000); two practices were not interested (list sizes 15,100 and 4,300); one practice was against fundholding in principle (4,200); another practice would take part only if they had to (8,500); one practice had applied for the first and second waves, but had no incentive to try again (4,900); in one 2-partner practice, only one partner was keen to combine with another practice, so nothing had been done; one practice would need more space (7,500); and another 2 partner practice would not consider if the size limit were removed. On a more positive note, one practice would participate, but not very enthusiastically (4,200) and another practice was "interested" (9,000).

In the 1986 study, practices were divided into three groups, depending on whether they employed a practice nurse, had taken part in the cost rent scheme or were a training practice. (Bosanquet and Leese, 1986). Practices undertaking 2 or more of the 3 options were known as 'high investors' (later changed to 'innovators'), those which had taken up a single option were 'intermediates' and those which had taken up none were 'low investors' (later changed to 'traditionalists'). Eight practices were 'innovators', 11 were 'intermediates', and 6 were 'traditionalists'. It might have been expected that the 4 practices which were to become third wave fundholders would have been designated 'innovators' in the 1986 survey, although the list size limit for fundholding is a confounding factor. In fact, only one of the 8 innovator practices was to become a thirdwave fundholder, as was one intermediate practice. The third practice to take up fundholding did not participate in the 1986 survey. The fourth practice, although a traditionalist in 1986, had been taken over by 3 new partners on the retirement of the two previous GPs, and the premises had been completely rebuilt using the cost rent scheme. These results probably reflect the acute lack of interest and opposition to fundholding evident in this FHSA area. The results in the other 6 study areas may reveal differences related to socioeconomic factors.

Views on fundholding were strongly held (Table 3). Twenty three (62%) of the interviewed GPs were either opposed or strongly opposed to fundholding, with only 4 (11%) either strongly in favour or in favour. Thirteen GPs opposed fundholding because of concern about its effects, and 6 opposed it on principle. Numerous comments were made about fundholding and its effects. There was concern that it would provide a 2-tier service and would only be effective whilst there were also non-fundholders; that it required more business acumen than possessed by the average GP; it would have an adverse effect on the doctor-patient relationship by setting costs against patient care; that it causes unnecessary administration and increased workload. There was also opposition to fundholding as a concept which is too financially orientated and will not affect outcomes.

Table 3. Views of Respondents about Fundholding

Views	No. (%) GPs	
Strongly in favour	1	(3)
In favour	3	(8)
No strong view	9	(24)
Opposed	11	(30)
Strongly opposed	12	(32)
Don't know	1	(3)
Total	37	(100)

This entrenched opposition to fundholding is significant since it is still very much in evidence some 2 years since the concept was first implemented (April 1991). Whether this a characteristic of this particular deprived area will have to await the results of the similar studies in 6 other areas of England. Thirteen (50%) of the responding partnerships in the study area had list sizes of 7000 or more making them eligible for fundholding, although the option was being taken up, belatedly in the third wave, by only 4 practices.

Much concern has been expressed that fundholding implies a 2-tier service in that patients of fundholding GPs have quicker access to hospital services. The other way in which a 2-tier service can operate, which has been less commented upon, is the location of fundholders in the more affluent areas of the country. If fundholding is seen as a good thing for patients, then those living in areas such as the one in this study will be less likely to have access to the perceived benefits. This is particularly so for inner city areas, served mainly by small or singlehanded practices, but where in many cases, fundholding consortia have been set up. The pilot study area fits into neither of these categories, and may be disadvantaged as a result. Local responses to fundholding suggest that attitudes have become more resistant to change since the earlier study.

Workload and the 1990 contract

Views on workload showed that 8 (22%) GPs could cope with their workload during most weeks, but 16 (43%) were sometimes under pressure and a further 13 (35.1%) were under great pressure and continually short of time (Table 4). These results contrast with those in 1986 where 30 (58%) GPs could cope during most weeks, and 21 (40%) were sometimes under pressure. Of the 23 responding GPs in innovator practices in 1986, 12 (52%) expected that their workload would remain the same in 3 year's time, with 9 (39%) expecting an increased workload and 2 (9%) expecting a workload reduction. (Bosanquet and Leese, 1986). It should be noted that in 1986, all GPs were sent a postal questionnaire, one question of which was about workload. There was a 55% response rate, from 46 GPs. There was some approval for the 1990 contract in that 19 (52%) GPs indicated that the quality of their service had improved or considerably improved since its introduction (Table 5). However, this was paralleled by an increased or considerably increased administrative workload as a result of the contract. This was the view of 36 (97%) respondents (Table 6).

Table 4. Views of Respondents about their workload

Workload	No. (%) GPs	
I am under no pressure at all	0	(0)
I can cope within my working hours in most weeks	8	(22)
I am sometimes under pressure to complete all that needs doing in a week	16	(43)
I am under great pressure and continually short of time	13	(35)
Total	37	(100)

Table 5. Effect of the 1990 contract on the quality of service provided

Quality	No. (%) GPs	
Considerably improved	5	(14)
Improved	14	(38)
No change	13	(35)
Deteriorated	2	(5)
Deteriorated considerably	0	(0)
Cosmetic only	3	(8)
Don't know	0	(0)
Total	37	(100)

Table 6. Effects of the 1990 contract on the administrative workload of the practice

Administration	No. (%) GPs	
Considerably increased	27	(73)
Increased	9	(24)
No change	0	(0)
Decreased	0	(0)
Decreased considerably	1	(3)
Don't know	0	(0)
Total	37	(100)

Moreover, 19 (51%) GPs were either opposed or strongly opposed to the new contract and its provisions (Table 7), with only 8 (22%) in favour. This represented almost as much opposition as that shown to fundholding. The generation of unnecessary paper work and the provision of services, such as clinics, or for 3 yearly health for which there was no demand or health gain were of particular concern. Comments were also made that the provisions of the contract are being continually changed, that they are cosmetic only and that they have been imposed by people who do not understand the problems faced by GPs, particularly in deprived or inner city areas.

The continuing hostility to the 1990 contract changes, evident some 2-3 years after implementation, is partly related to the increased workload, not anticipated in the earlier survey. This hostility, is, however, tempered by the belief of many GPs that services have improved in quality.

Table 7. Personal views on Respondents on the 1990 contract and its provisions

Views	No (%) GPs	
1. Strongly in favour	0	(0)
2. In favour	8	(21.6)
3. No strong view	10	(27.0)
4. Opposed	15	(40.5)
5. Strongly opposed	4	(10.8)
6. Don't know	0	(0)
Total	**37**	**(100)**

Views of respondents about general practice

Table 8 shows the responses of the 37 interviewed GPs to specific statements about general practice. There was a high level of support for the statement that 'too much is being asked of general practices at the present time', with 32 (87%) GPs either agreeing or strongly agreeing. Similarly, 30 (81%) GPs agreed or strongly agreed that "general practice within the NHS is undervalued".

Table 8. GP responses to statements about general practice (n=37)

Statement	Strongly agree	Agree	No strong view	Disagree	Strongly disagree	Don't know/ missing
General practice within the NHS is undervalued	15	15	2	4	0	1
The content of general practice has become too broad	8	14	2	11	1	1
More effort, resources should be directed to health promotion by the NHS	9	11	9	6	1	1
More services should be provided in general practice	4	9	4	16	2	2
Too much is being asked of general practices at the present time	20	12	2	2	1	0
The primary health care team should include a broader range of health professionals	4	17	5	8	1	2

There was some difference of opinion amongst GPs to the statement that "the content of general practice has become too broad", with 22 (60%) agreeing, but 12 (32%) disagreeing or disagreeing strongly. Twenty (54%) GPs agreed or strongly agreed that more effort and resources should be directed to health promotion by the NHS.

However, 18 (49%) GPs disagreed or strongly disagreed that more services should be provided in general practice, with 13 (35.1%) either agreeing or strongly agreeing. By contrast, in 1986, 29(56%) GPs hoped to bring about major changes and improvements in services in the next 3 years. In 1992, there was a high degree of support for the primary health care team to include a broader range of health professions, with 21 (57%) either agreeing or agreeing strongly.

These views again suggest that GPs are experiencing many changes in a relatively short time, which are proving difficult to assimilate. The enthusiasm for change, evident in 1986, has changed to resignation and disillusionment. The support for a broader range of health professionals is an indicator of the increased workload and the desire for others to take over some of this.

Table 9 shows the results of asking the GPs to assess their situation in relation to premises, staffing, workload, practice costs, net income, and services from community nursing staff. Staffing, premises and services from community nursing staff were considered to be satisfactory by 27 (73%), 24 (65%) and 24 (65%) GPs, respectively. However, 32 (87%) GPs thought that their situation with regard to workload had worsened in the last 2 years, as did 28 (76%) GPs for practice costs.

There was a difference of opinion when net income was considered, with 20 (54%) GPs agreeing that the situation had worsened in the past 2 years, and 16 (43%) saying that things were satisfactory.

Table 9. How would you assess your situation in relation to the following items? (n=37)

	Situation worsened in past 2 years		In general satisfactory		Missing	
1. Premises	12	(32)	24	(65)	1	(3)
2. Staffing	10	(27)	65	(73)	0	(0)
3. Workload	32	(87)	5	(14)	0	(0)
4. Practice costs	28	(76)	8	(22)	1	(3)
5. Net income	20	(54)	16	(43)	1	(3)
6. Services from community nursing staff	12	(32)	24	(65)	1	(3)

Table 10 shows the responses to a series of questions about whether specific services would be appropriate at GP surgeries. Services which more than half of the GPs thought should be more widely available were crisis counselling, addiction counselling and physiotherapy. The first two are representative of local social problems, and the latter of restricted access to hospital and community services.

Table 10. Do you think the following services would be appropriate at GP surgeries, assuming adequate resources were made available?

Service	should be more widely available		should not be more widely available		no strong view		already available in my practice		not applicable in general practice		should be available by open access	
Crisis counselling (e.g. bereavement)	21	(57)	2	(5)	4	(11)	6	(16)	2	(5)	2	(5)
Addiction counselling (e.g. drugs)	19	(81)	2	(5)	2	(5)	2	(5)	9	(24)	3	(8)
Hypnotherapy	9	(24)	4	(11)	14	(38)	2	(5)	8	(22)	0	(0)
Homeopathy	6	(16)	6	(16)	14	(38)	0	(0)	10	(27)	0	(0)
Acupuncture	13	(35)	4	(11)	10	(27)	4	(11)	6	(16)	0	(0)
Dietetics	15	(41)	2	(5)	1	(3)	16	(43)	1	(3)	2	(5)
Physiotherapy	22	(59)	1	(3)	0	(0)	9	(24)	2	(5)	3	(8)
Chiropody	13	(35)	1	(3)	2	(5)	13	(35)	3	(8)	5	(14)
Chiropractic	8	(22)	4	(11)	11	(30)	1	(3)	11	(30)	1	(3)
Osteopathy	8	(22)	5	(14)	10	(27)	0	(0)	11	(30)	2	(5)
Laboratory analysis (e.g. pathology)	8	(22)	3	(8)	5	(14)	9	(24)	7	(19)	5	(14)
Full pharmacy service	11	(30)	5	(14)	6	(16)	4	(11)	6	(16)	3	(8)
Optometry	10	(27)	7	(19)	6	(16)	0	(0)	7	(19)	4	(11)
Hospital consultant session	18	(49)	7	(19)	4	(11)	0	(0)	5	(14)	3	(8)
X-ray services	4	(11)	5	(14)	5	(14)	6	(16)	9	(24)	8	(22)
Endoscopy	5	(14)	4	(11)	4	(11)	5	(14)	5	(14)	14	(38)

Retirement

Dissatisfaction with general practice amongst responding GPs was expressed in their desire to retire early. Currently 25 (68%) GPs were planning to retire at 60 or 65 years with only 6 (16%) at 55 years. (Table 11). However, if pension rights were protected 12 (32%) would retire at 55 years, and the number retiring at 65 years would fall from 13 (35%) to 5 (14%). The desire to retire early is another reflection of the disillusionment felt by many GPs to the pace of change in general practice in recent years.

Table 11. Responding GP views on their likely and preferred retirement ages

Age of retirement	At what age do you personally plan to retire from general practice?		Assuming pension rights were protected, what age would you retire?	
70 years	2	(5)	2	(5)
65 years	13	(35)	5	(14)
60 years	12	(32)	13	(35)
55 years	6	(16)	12	(32)
Other	4	(11)	5	(14)
Total	**37**	**(100)**	**37**	**(100)**

SUMMARY

The 1986 study showed that practices had developed long term strategies, with many showing willingness to change. They were also prepared to consider more change in the longer term. The first reactions to fundholding, and particularly to the new contract, were to increase hostility and to create resistance to more change.

This is evident in the opposition expressed by many GPs to both fundholding and the new contract, and the lack of uptake of fundholding by eligible practices. There was also a marked desire to retire early in favourable financial circumstances. This resistance to change is, however, tempered by the acknowledgement, by many GPs, that the quality of services they provide to their patients has improved. The continuing opposition to change which is still evident 2-3 years after implementation may mean that GPs will be less willing to undertake future change and investment because of negative feelings towards existing changes. This may be a localised response in an obviously deprived area generally receiving no deprivation payments, and differential responses may be evident in areas with more advantageous socioeconomic characteristics. It is evident that options for policy development must be found which allow cooperation and co-working between national strategy and local enterprise if the full benefits of the changed strategies are to be seen by patients and GPs alike.

The study shows the problems of planning and organising change within a large organisation in which GPs are independent providers working as decentralised firms. National policy makers set certain aims and targets which have to be translated into local programmes, but success requires a commitment by local practices.

Responses under the Family Doctor Charter were highly variable between areas and they may well continue to be so under the new system. For example, the survey evidence shows a very low take up of fund-holding in an area where fund-holding might have had positive effects on local services. The study points to the need for a more explicit consideration of how to increase incentives to local participation. There also needs to be more evidence on variability in response between areas if a repetition of the inverse care law is to be avoided, with more development in areas of lower health need.

ACKNOWLEDGEMENT

We would like to thank the Economic and Social Research Council for funding this study.

REFERENCES

Bosanquet N and Leese B (1986) Family doctors: their choice of practice strategy, *British Medical Journal,* 293, 667-70.

Bosanquet N and Leese B (1988). Family doctors and innovation in general practice, *British Medical Journal,* 296, 1576-80.

Bosanquet N and Leese B (1989). *Family doctors and economic incentives,* Dartmouth, Gower Publishing Company.

Department of Health (1989). *General Practice in the NHS. A new contract,* February, London, Crown Copyright.

Department of Health (1989a) *Working for Patients.* Cmnd. 555, London, HMSO.

Department of Health (1989b) *Practice budgets for General Medical Practitioners,* Working Paper 3, London, HMSO.

Department of Health (1990); *Community Care in the next decade and beyond.* Policy guidance, London, HMSO.

Department of Health (1993). GP contract health promotion package, Guidance on implementation, NHS Management Executive, *FHSL,* (93) 3, London.

Griffiths R (1988) *Community Care: agenda for action,* London, HMSO.

Irvine D (1990) *Managing for quality in general practice,* Kings Fund Centre, Medical Audit Series, July.

Leese B and Bosanquet N (1989) High and low incomes in general practice, *British Medical Journal,* 298, 932-4.

Leese B and Hutton J (1990). Desk top analysers in general medical practice, how useful are they? *Medical Laboratory Sciences,* 47, 256-62.

Leese B and Drummond M (1993). General practice fundholding; Maverick or Catalyst?, Drummond M and Maynard A (eds), *Purchasing and Providing Cost-Effective Health Care,* Churchill Livingstone, London, 157-168.

20 The Iron Cage Revisited - Technocratic Regulation and Cost Control in Health Care Systems

JEAN-LOUIS DENIS, ANNE LEMAY,
ANDRÉ-PIERRE CONTANDRIOPOULOS,
FRANCOIS CHAMPAGNE, STÉPHANIE DUCROT,
MARC-ANDRÉ FOURNIER & DJONA AVOCKSOUMA
Université de Montréal

INTRODUCTION

The high costs of health care systems and the inflationary pressures that they generate are a matter of concern for governments of all developed countries irrespective of the level of public funding of these systems. Health-related expenditures are just as worrisome to the British government, which has been able to keep the growth of the health sector under control, as they are to the U.S. government. Since almost universal accessibility to health care has been achieved in nearly all developed countries (except the U.S.), concern now focuses on the effectiveness of the system, i.e., the delivery of quality services, to meet the population's need, at minimum cost. In all countries, this concern has given rise to numerous debates on the efficiency of the health care system, on regulatory mechanisms, and on necessary reforms. Inspired by what is being done elsewhere, each country seeks ways to better control health expenditures, but no consensus on an ideal cost-control model has been reached (Contandriopoulos, Champagne, Denis, Lemay, Ducrot, Fournier, Djona, 1993).

In practice, the effectiveness of a regulatory system corresponds to its ability to implement organizational policies that will cause actors and institutions to move towards solving that system's key problems (Crozier & Thoening, 1976; Hult and Walcott, 1989). Effective regulation assumes that structural mechanisms will be mobilized to further politically-defined objectives. In the case of health care, cost containment has been one such important objective in most Western countries since the 1970s.

Setting Priorities in Health Care. Edited by M. Malek
© 1994 John Wiley & Sons Ltd

This paper will attempt to assess the effectiveness of technocratic mechanisms to control health care costs in member countries of the Organization for Economic Co-operation and Development (OECD). More specifically, it will assess the effectiveness of macro and micro organizational instruments characteristic of the technocratic regulatory model, to control health care costs. Research has indicated the effectiveness of these tools in systems where competing interests and objectives coexist.

First, we describe the supporting arguments for policies and management techniques aimed àt controlling health care costs. We then provide a theoretical overview of the technocratic regulatory model and the operational mechanisms associated with that paradigm. Methodology and results follow. The conclusion relates empirical findings to a broader perspective on health care system regulation. The argument is made that regulatory strategies for health care systems must attempt to reconcile the virtues of bureaucratic control with the demand for more dynamic management leaving spaces for the expression of professional freedom and consumerism.

WHY CONTROL HEALTH CARE COSTS?

There are three interrelated arguments in favour of policies and management systems that would achieve the control of health care expenditures.

The first argument is financial. The crisis in public finance resulting from the economic slowdown of the late 1980s and the growing public debt has made it increasingly difficult to maintain the same level of public funding of the health care system without altering fiscal policies. Given the growing burden of debt on public treasuries, and the impractical nature of increased taxation spending, maintaining the status quo in government funding of the health system implies a reduction of other expenditures (e.g., education), which may be detrimental to general socio-economic development and individual well-being.

A second argument is the decreasing returns to health expenditures in terms of the improvement of population health. It is both well known and documented that the level of the health of the population is not associated with an overall level of per capita spending on health. The most significant determinants of a population's health are found outside of the health care system. Policies intended to raise health levels should be aimed at educating and supporting young children, providing employment, achieving reductions in income disparities, raising overall educational achievement, and promoting a healthy lifestyle. Under those conditions, a responsible government must keep the costs of health care under control so as to maintain the capacity to intervene in other areas that affect the population's health (CIAR, 1991).

The third argument is from an economic perspective. It is generally acknowledged that the economic development of a society is linked to its capacity to innovate and to invest in areas that produce wealth. Generally speaking, health-related spending has a low capacity to generate wealth. If, however, in the short term, the health sector supports a significant number of jobs, any responsible society should attempt to limit the expansion of the health system so as to concentrate its efforts on investment that will eventually generate wealth, to the extent that this is socially possible without affecting the population's health and social cohesion. This suggests that not only public spending on health care should be considered, but all health-related expenditures. Policies aimed only at reducing the burden of public health expenditures do not necessarily result in an improvement in the country's economic situation, as recent forecasts for U.S. health reforms show.

THE TECHNOCRATIC REGULATORY MODEL

In this section, we provide a conceptual definition of the technocratic regulatory model and present a set of mechanisms that serve to operationalize this paradigm for a health care system.

The technocratic approach to regulating health care systems is historically rooted in the development of bureaucratic structures in complex societies. In his seminal paper on power and bureaucracy, Weber sees the emergence of bureaucratic structures as an unfolding process of rationalization in so-called modern societies: (Weber, in Gerth and Mills, 1979, p 244). By rationalization, he means the production of systematic coherence in collective life. This systematic coherence is achieved through the implementation of a hierarchical system, based on the formal authority of superior levels over subordinate levels. The purpose of this hierarchy is to increase the predictability of the system and to insure a certain standardization of its process. From a Weberian perspective, authority in a bureaucratic system is supposed to be devoted to the production of rules. Furthermore, bureaucrats regulate the system in an abstract context, without considering the particularities of specific cases or situations. For Weber, this ideal type of bureaucracy emerges from a qualitative shift in the nature of administrative tasks. As societies become more affluent, they must accommodate an increasing diversity of demands: satisfied locally or by a private economy.» (in Gerth and Mills, 1979, p 212). This is a clear argument in support of the need for bureaucratic regulation of different aspects of society. Bureaucracy may, as Weber recognized, coexist with or accommodate other forms of domination in society; however, due to historical development, it also provides the technical means to achieve the fulfilment of a diversity of needs in complex societies. It does so by structuring collective action according to norms or to a set of plausible relationships between ends and means.

The development of bureaucratic structures generally corresponds to a very specific form of regulation of collective life. From a Weberian perspective, it culminates in the disenchantment of the world, coupled with a significant increase in the capacity to expand the production and consumption of goods in society. The bureaucratic form of regulation is antecedent to the expansion of technocracy in our societies. Technocracy can be conceived as the reinforcement of bureaucratic logic based on the use of experts. From an organizational point of view, it corresponds to an increase in the power of a techno-structure in a given system (Mintzberg, 1978). Appointed officials, in a technocratic model, are experts. This model responds to increasing complexities in the regulation of social systems by augmenting expert knowledge of the regulatory process.

In the technocratic approach to regulating health care systems, trained experts guide the system by relying on their specialized knowledge and dominant position within political and economic institutions (Fischer 1990). This regulatory approach, also called the "command and control planning model" (Saltman 1991), is based on normative analyses produced by experts who are responsible for structuring, monitoring, and assessing the activities of the health care system, deciding the extent to which these activities are likely to achieve the system's objectives. Normative analysis thus consists of making judgements on the gap between the system's resources, activities and results, and forecast or planned needs. In the health care sector, the particularities of the health care commodity and the public provision of those services implies direct intervention of the State in the operation of the health care system, to achieve rationalization and to limit shifts in the system's goals caused by the specific behaviours of the system's actors (Fischer 1990). Thus, technocratic intervention is justified by its capacity to present itself as an apolitical and rational action in the public interest. Theoretically, it significantly increases the role of scientific based knowledge in the standardization of production and management processes, also fundamental to the Weberian model of bureaucracy. This model is therefore fundamentally opposed to proposals aimed at encouraging new types of negotiated relationships between policy makers, service providers, and consumers in order to promote transformation in the health care system.

The technocratic approach to regulation may exert pressure on the health care system and, by legislative or regulatory means, force its actors to adopt specific objectives. Therefore, technocratic regulation may contribute to a greater standardization of the health care system's output, thus making this output less unpredictable. For example, it is probably capable of forcing the system to meet a specific short-term cost-control objective. On the other hand, this approach may result in a negative shift in the performance of agents within the system, as the normative pressure imposed by technocratic control, as a rational agent, may generate confusion between the means and the ends of the system. Actors in the health system may emphasize conformity to norms instead of focusing on goal achievement. In such a situation, the system's production rationale is characterized by subservience to norms established by the technocratic authority. The potential of actors to innovate within the system is likely to be superseded by an obligation to conform to bureaucratic norms. Agents learn to circumvent bureaucratic controls and to manipulate information to project a favourable image to the technocratic authority. This dynamic may give rise to a gradual increase in technocratic controls in order to compensate for these dysfunctions. This is the "bureaucratic vicious circle" analyzed by Crozier (1965) in the field of organizational theory.

We may thus expect two possible outcomes of a technocratic regulatory approach. From a Weberian perspective, a technocratic approach must respond to growing societal demands, as the bureaucratic nature of society increases and its complexity deepens. However, from a more contemporary perspective, the implementation of technocratic regulatory mechanisms may increase political domination and generate perverse effects that will compromise the actual achievement of expected benefits. That threat is particularly important in the field of health care, in which the uncertainties associated with diagnosis and treatment remain present even when a technocratic regulatory approach is used. These uncertainties in turn legitimize the importance of professionalism within the health system.

We will now present the macro organizational characteristics and the micro cost control tools associated with the technocratic regulatory model. Through these mechanisms, the State seeks to regulate the health care system by promoting conformity to rules that attempt to make the system more predictable and manageable. Before presenting results regarding their effectiveness to control costs, we will discuss the rationale behind their potential effects on cost control.

MACRO ORGANIZATIONAL CHARACTERISTICS

Macro organizational characteristics are those characteristics which concern the overall health care system. Three interacting macro characteristics of organization and financing of the health care system were considered: centralized management, limitation of the number of financing sources, and limitation of private financing. The rationale is that the State's effectiveness improves as its involvement in the functioning of the health care system broadens; conversely, a large number of actors implies complex management and a possible loss of coherence.

The first macro organizational characteristic is the harmonization and centralization of the management process. The hypothesis is that the more centralized and harmonized the management process is, the easier it is to control the health system's structure and organization, and thus its expenditures. This relationship has been observed for major organizations such as the HMOs in the U.S., and for whole systems, as in the case of medical services in the Canadian provinces as compared to the U.S. (Barer *et al.*, 1988).

The second macro organizational characteristic is the number of different sources of financing of the health care system. The hypothesis is that the smaller is the number of sources of financing, the easiest it is to control costs and to increase management efficiency in the system (Woolhandler and Himmelstein, 1991; Evans, Barer and Hertzman, 1991, Benson, 1975).

The third macro organizational characteristic is the importance of private financing. The more significant the amount of private financing is, the harder it is to control health expenditures. This aspect of health system management is linked to the dimensions covered by the first two: the more significant the amount of private financing is, the more diversified are the sources of financing, through the development of private insurance, and the less harmonized is the management of the system. In a global sense, it is therefore important to control private financing of the health care system. Many policies aimed at regulating the public health care sector, namely the "cut and shift strategies" used in most Canadian provinces and OECD countries, have important consequences in the long term, on the health care sector as a whole. These strategies could be directly linked to the faster growth of pharmaceutical and equipment costs in Canada, many of which were never, or have ceased to be covered by public health insurance plans, as opposed to hospital and medical services (Health and Welfare, 1990).

MICRO COSTS CONTROL TOOLS

Micro mechanisms are tools that concern only one sector of the health care system. (Abel-Smith, 1987 ; Baris *et al.*, 1992). Most of these tools involve the hospital or medical services sector. Services in these two sectors are the main sources of cost for the health care system and, in most Western countries, are almost fully covered by public insurance plans, which is not the case of other sectors such as pharmaceutical, home care, dental and other professional services. Thus, their regulation is extremely important to public agencies.

THE MEDICAL SECTOR

Two types of tools are most commonly used concerning physician services, in order to control the costs of medical services themselves, as well as the functioning and the cost of the health care system as a whole. The first tool is control of the number of physicians. The assumption behind this strategy is that physicians play a central role in the use of the health care resources. It is a well-known fact that medical density plays an important role in explaining the level of health spending, because the physician is responsible for the utilization of almost all resources within the health care sector. Thus, the hypothesis is that the smaller the number of physicians is for a given level of others resources (mainly hospital), the easier it is to control costs.

The second type of tools are the containment of physician income containment. These are caps on physician earnings, control of the quantity of services delivered and control of fees. Physician incomes are linked to payment modalities. Payment modalities of physician services cannot be limited to the method of compensation (fee-for-service, salary) but must also include the organizational context in which payment occurs: price determination methods and payment mechanisms which could affect the quantity of services delivered, the price of services and ultimately overall earnings (Reinhardt, 1985, Contandriopoulos *et al.*, 1993). We have set forth the following hypotheses concerning the ability of the above elements to control health care costs :

- physician remuneration on a per capita basis allows for better cost control than compensation on a salary basis, which in turn permits better cost control than fee for service;
- price determination by administrative decision allows for better control than negotiation, which in turn permits better control than price determination by physicians;

• physician remuneration assumed by the organization allows for better cost control than remuneration by a third-party payer, and much more than when assumed by the patient.

This enables us to establish scores for the capacity to control health care expenditures for each possible combination, (Appendix 1).

The hypotheses concerning compensation method are based on a large body of empirical research which shows that salary or capitation are associated with better cost control than is fee-for-service, mainly due to the absence of incentives to produce unnecessary services (Glaser, 1970; Reinhardt, 1984; Reinhardt 1985; Glaser 1978). Limited efficacy of control over price was also demonstrated by negative elasticity of physician supply (Rochaix, 1990). Physicians reacted to lowered or frozen fees by delivering more services or more complex services (Gabel and Rice, 1985; Barer and al., 1988; Rochaix, 1990, 1991). It is thus necessary to control not only fees, but also quantity of service (Lomas *et al.*, 1989).

Regarding payment mechanism, it can be said that modalities based on fee-for-service, paid by a third party or by an organization, exhibit a high quality of information and transparency in their functioning (Reinhardt, 1984). However, health care systems with these modalities can be complex and costly to administer (U.S. Congress, Office of Technology Assessment, 1986; Glaser, 1976; Babson, 1972). The ability of these systems to plan and evaluate their development, and to anticipate and control expenditures, is limited. In contrast, when physicians are paid by a third party or employed by an organization, and paid by salary or capitation, administration is relatively simpler and less expensive.

Price determination for medical services is easier to control when set by administrative decision rather than through a process of negotiation. This type of modality, however, does not really exist in developed countries, where price or remuneration levels are generally determined by a bargaining process between government agencies or insurance companies and physician associations. Where overbilling is prohibited, a technocratic approach would settle disagreements between the two parties by administrative decision. Where overbilling is allowed, the approach is more like the laissez-faire or market-based model. According to Barer *et al.*, (1988), differences between the U.S. and Canada in the attainment of cost control of medical services are largely due to the presence of a negotiation process in Canada.

THE HOSPITAL SECTOR

Two types of tools are used to control the cost of hospital sector. The first deal with the financing of hospitals. Financing by prospective global budgeting would be more effective for controlling costs than on a per diem basis. Global budgeting considers all hospital costs and not just the price of hospitalization. Financing hospitals by global budgeting gives managers a certain degree of freedom, if their only constraint is the budget. In this respect, global budgeting could be associated with the professional self-regulation model. The introduction of specific criteria in the calculation of the global budget could strengthen professional self-regulation and facilitate a budget increase. In contrast, population-based budgeting criteria do not give the manager much flexibility.

The second tool is control over the utilization of hospital beds. This could be achieved by controlling hospital construction or expansion, or by using alternatives to expensive in-hospital care. Technocratic regulation seeks explicitly to limit hospital bed use. As with controlling the number of physicians, controlling the number of hospital beds is not sufficient to contain costs. Price of hospital days and/or the intensity of bed utilization must also be controlled.

METHODOLOGY

To test empirically the effectiveness of technocratic tools of regulation for controlling health care costs we analyzed OCDE countries.

DEPENDENT VARIABLES

In order to test the impact of management indicators on the level of health care expenditures, we used four dependant variables that measure the level and rate of change in those expenditures. Our aim was to explain longitudinal and cross-sectional variations in health care expenditures by the level of general wealth relative to population size. To achieve this, we conducted regression analyses for OECD countries for the year 1980 and 1987. Using linear regression analysis, we estimated the relationship between the level of per capita health expenditures weighted by purchasing power equivalents (PPE) as a dependent variable, and the level of overall per capita wealth of the countries weighted by PPE as an independent variable. The position of countries in relation to the regression line enabled us to determine the positions of individual health care systems relative to the average for industrialized societies, while controlling for the level of general wealth.

Data were drawn from the 1991 version of the ECO-SANTE database created jointly by OECD and CREDES. Data are lacking, however, for some countries at certain periods (Iceland, Portugal, and Turkey were completely excluded from our analysis because of insufficient data).

The regression equations and the relative positions obtained for 1980 and 1987 are presented in Figures 1 and 2 (see appendice 2). The distance between the position of the country and the regression line was the value of the first dependent variable, "ranking". This value was computed for both 1980 and 1987. For our analysis, however, only the value for 1987 was used as the first dependent variable. The difference between the values obtained for 1987 and 1980 constituted our second dependent variable. The third dependent variable was the share of the total health care expenditures in the GDP in 1987. The fourth dependent variable was the variation in the share of total health expenditures in GDP between 1980 and 1987. Considering these variables for almost all OECD countries, in a longitudinal study covering nearly a decade, shows both relative performance in cost control, as well as the evolution of this indicator over time.

INDEPENDENT VARIABLES

The three macro organizational mechanisms and the seven micro cost control [1] tools were our independent variables. The information was taken from ECO-SANTE, the literature and from national agencies [2].

Centralized management is a dichotomous variable: 1) so-called centralized systems (value=1), where management or organizational responsibility is in the hands of the national agency; and 2) so-called decentralized systems (value=2), where the management system is more fragmented.

Number of financing sources is a continuous variable. For each health care system, we used categories of financing sources that account for 90 percent of health expenditures. This enabled us to eliminate sources deemed to be marginal.

Importance of private financing is a continuous variable. Private financing was measured by the share of private expenditures in total health care expenditures in 1987.

Physician compensation was measured by two continuous variables, one for the ambulatory sector and one for the public hospital sector. We used the score presented in Appendix 1, which corresponds to a combination of the three dimensions of physician compensation. When two or more combinations of compensation coexisted in the same sector, the scores associated with each of them were weighted by the proportion of physicians so compensated.

Payment of hospitals was measured by two dichotomous variables. First, systems were classified according to whether hospital financing was on a per diem basis (value = 1) or on the basis of global budgeting (value = 2). Second, for the case of global budgeting, further classifications were made according to whether historical costs (value = 2) or specific criteria (value = 3) were used.

In testing our hypotheses, we used regression analysis when the dependent variable was continuous, and a t-test for dichotomous variables. From a statistical point of view, attempting linear regressions with fewer than 30 observations leads to distortion. Nevertheless, we felt it would be very interesting to identify certain trends, even if statistical relationships between our variables are not as sound as we would like.

RESULTS

The regression equation and the relative position between the level of per capita health expenditures and the level of per capita wealth of the countries are displayed in

---

[1] Of course, other tools exist that could be used in the technocratic regularoty model, such as limitation of the number of professionals, but these tools could also be used in other regulatory approaches as well. For the moment, our analysis does not enable us to make such a distinction.

[2] See Contandriopoulos et coll., 1983, for a more detailed description of the methodology.

Figure 1 and 2 (see appendix 2. The health care systems that diverge the most from the average - i.e., that spend more than the level predicted by the equation - are, in descending order, the U.S., Sweden, Germany, France, the Netherlands, Austria and Ireland. The systems with the lowest expenditure levels relative to a wealth-related standard are those of the United Kingdom, Denmark, Japan, Luxembourg, Norway, Switzerland. Canada's spending is close to the level predicted by the regression.

The bivariate analysis indicates that macro organizational characteristics seem effective in controlling health care costs.

For centralized management, with a confidence interval of 95 percent, no dependent variable displayed significant average differences between countries (Table 1). Given the low degree of freedom (due to a small sample), it nonetheless seemed important to analyze the differences between the means of the two groups with respect to those dependant variables with significance levels close to 0.5. Thus, countries with centralized management devoted an average of 7.17% of their GDP to the health care sector in 1987; for countries with decentralized systems, the average was 7.93%. The performance of decentralized systems was inferior to that of centralized systems. We observed the same tendency with the dependent variable variation of the share in GDP between 1980-87. While these results are not conclusive in a statistical sense, they do reveal a certain trend.

Results for the two other macro organizational characteristics were more conclusive. Almost all coefficients were significant and we obtained the same form of relationship for the four dependent variables.

The regression performed for "number of financing sources" enabled us to generate a number of significant results (Table 1):

Table 1. Results on the Effectiveness of the Macro Organizational Mechanisms to Costs Control, OECD Countries

	Ranking (1987)	Variation of Ranking (1980-87)	Share % in GDP (1987)	Variation % in GDP (1980-87)
Centralized Management	p= 0.72 (+)	p= 0.75 (+)	p= 0.20 (-)	p= 0.77 (-)
Number of sources of financing	R= 0.54* (+)	R= 0.50* (+)	R= 0.36 (+)	R= 0.38 (+)
Importance of private financing	R= 0.63* (+)	R= 0.45* (+)	R= 0.58* (+)	R= 0.32 (+)

*   Significant at 0.95%
R   Correlation coefficient of simple regression analyses
P   Signification of the difference between the means of the two groups

The greater the number of financing sources available,

- the higher the health care expenditures as measured by ranking and % of GDP; and
- the greater the increase in health care expenditures.

For "importance of private financing":

- The greater the private share in the financing of health care expenditures,
- the greater their increase as measured by the two other dependent variables.

Our bivariate analyses revealed few significant relationships for the micro mechanisms (Table2). Nonetheless, some trends can be observed.

Table 2. Results on the Effectiveness of the Micro Costs Control Tools, OECD Countries

	Ranking (1987)	Variation of ranking (1980-87)	Share % in GDP (1987)	Variation % in GDP (1980-87
Medical Sector				
Physician compensation ambulatory care	R = 0.35 (-)	R = 0.50* (-)	R =0.24 (-)	R = 0.46* (-)
Physician compensation hospital care	R = 0.29 (-)	R = 0.32 (-)	R = 0.47* (-)	R = 0.33 (-)
Hospital Sector				
Global versus per diem budget	p = 0.77 (+)	p = 0.30 (-)	p = 0.15 (+)	p = 0.41 (+)
Historial versus criteria budget	p = 0.22 (-)	p = 0.05 (+)	p = 0.36 (-)	p = 0.08 (+)

* Significant at 0.95%
R Correlation coefficient of simple regression analyses
P Signification of the difference between the means of the two groups

The results of the regression analysis with the independent variable "physician compensation" enabled us to observe the following trends, in spite of low significance.

The more the compensation regimes of physicians in the ambulatory and hospital sectors are revealed by our score index to have a positive effect on cost control,

- the lower the health expenditures and the slower their growth;

- the lower the share of health expenditures in GDP and the less it tends to increase.

We conducted two t-tests for assessing the effects of type of hospital financing. None of the differences were significant, but some trends were identified :

- global budgeting seems more effective than per diem financing in controlling costs;
- health spending, measured by "ranking", in countries with historical-cost budgeting is lower than those with criteria-based budgeting. Similarly, health care accounts for a smaller share of GDP in this group. On the other hand, health care spending tends to increase more rapidly in countries with hospital budgets based on historical costs. This suggests that countries with criteria-based budgets spend more on health care but that the introduction of this budgeting approach has enabled them to improve their situation relative to other countries.

DISCUSSION

Our results show that the technocratic regulatory model seems to work well at the macro level of regulation. Limiting the number of financing sources, the importance of private financing and, to a lesser extent, the centralization of management created a homogenous system and provided potentially powerful cost control tools. These strategies also enabled the use of effective micro mechanisms. For the micro mechanisms associated with technocratic regulation considered in our analyses, prospective global budgeting and type of physician compensation showed potential in controlling costs. It should be noted, however, that the number of observations in our analyses was small, reducing the statistical significance of the results. The 21 countries considered are not a random sample of the population, however, but rather almost the entire population of the OECD countries, which share social, economic, demographic and hygiene characteristics. These results confirm observations in the literature based on smaller samples or less elaborate empirical analysis of regulatory mechanisms.

We are conscious, however, that an outlier observation could influence the relationship observed. The U.S., the "odd man out" of Abel Smith (1985), is the outlier of these analyses. Results on the effectiveness of macro organizational mechanisms indicate that the U.S. approach to managing health care is at the opposite extreme to the solution for controlling health care costs.

Our results seem to indicate that micro level technocratic regulation can work well in the hospital and medical sectors. We conclude that technocratic regulation at this level has some potential to control health care costs, but maintain that macro organizational mechanisms, as we have defined them, seem more effective for attaining this objective.

Our empirical results generally emphasize the need to maintain a technocratic approach at the macro level of health system regulation. The coherence that technocratic mechanisms provide at this level is a basis for cost control. However, the use of technocratic regulatory mechanisms at a more micro level may not be as promising to control health care costs. Macro level technocratic mechanisms seem to fulfil the potential described by Weber with regard to the capacity of bureaucratic structures to regulate collective action in social systems. Establishing broad rules contributes to limiting the nature and diversity of funding. The implementation of a superordinate authority over the system which produces and enforces these rules favours better control of health care costs. If we accept the arguments presented earlier concerning the necessity of such control to achieve broad socio-economic development in a given social system, macro-organizational mechanisms can help a society to control those economic forces which sustain destructive competition between its different institutional domains (education, health, manpower policies, etc.).

These considerations make it clear that the regulatory problem can be defined as the difficulty of finding proper mechanisms to move from macro technocratic regulation to micro regulation of a health system. The fundamental problem is to search for regulatory options that will create new dynamics in the public health care system, based on a broad technocratic framework. In other words, how can the benefits of systematic coherence produced by a broad technocratic framework be obtained without creating the rigidities and perverse effects of bureaucratic mechanisms at a more micro level. Recently, Crozier (1991) argued that the basic problem of the modern State is to maintain a legitimate but modest role in the regulation of collective affairs. The State must preserve its role in the production of the basic rules of a given system and delegate the role of enforcing those rules to more autonomous units. Crozier emphasizes the increasing demand for organization in a context where direct intervention of the State on specific problems is less and less effective. In such a context, simple rules are the best answer to increasing complexity or uncertainty about the proper solutions to social problems. As an alternative to public intervention, he proposes the emergence of a system based on the collaboration and active roles of citizens and professionals in the regulation of social systems. Current suggestions about regulation of the health care system seem to be moving in that direction.

In addition to the technocratic regulatory model, we can define a larger set of theoretical models or archetypes for the regulation of health care systems. These models suggest various approaches for solving problems in the organization and management of health care. They contain incentives and rules that guide decisions made by individuals and organizations within these systems. These incentives and rules may be adapted to address the particular problems encountered within a health care system. Before moving on to a brief description of the different models, it is important to recall that the basic dilemma in regulating health care systems is finding an acceptable balance between the principles of equity, individual freedom, and control of health care expenditures. Different regulatory approaches will obviously respect these principles to varying degrees. In addition , the extent to which a trade-off between these three principles in a particular health care system will be acceptable depends on the social, political and historical context. Thus, regulatory models not only contribute to shaping a system, but also reflect the ideologies and values prevailing in society. Selection of a particular model must therefore be based on both its technical properties (i.e., the likelihood that it will produce desired effects) and its social, political and cultural acceptability.

A health care system is built around three major poles of interest: the State, health care professionals, and the user population. The predominance of these three social forces and their interactions favours the emergence of different approaches to regulation. The State, as we discussed, pushes the system toward a more technocratic form of regulation. Professional self-regulation corresponds to the medico-naive model defined by Evans (1984). It is based on the asymmetry of information between physician and patient concerning diagnosis, treatment and prognosis. In this model, the physician acts as the patient's agent, has access to all information concerning the patient's needs and is expected to provide care based on these needs. The quantity and variety of care being provided is under his control.

Laissez-faire (or market-based) regulation is based on the existence of a market economy where all goods are traded in competitive markets. In contrast with the technocratic and professional self-regulation models, the laissez-faire model does not seem to have received serious consideration as a primary mechanism for regulating the health care system, mainly because the system's characteristics are such that the competitive-market process is unable to achieve an optimal allocation of resources. When viewed as economic goods, health services and health itself have certain characteristics: the uncertainty linked to the incidence of disease or illness; the inherent uncertainty linked to clinical activity both in determining a diagnosis and in forecasting the effectiveness of health services; the asymmetry of knowledge between the consumer patient and the supplier physician; and the presence of externalities and scale economies. As a result, only certain mechanisms associated with the competitive model have been marginally considered in the organization of planned markets. Public-competition and mixed-market models are based on planned markets and have been described at length by Saltman and Von Otter (1987, 1989, 1990, 1991), Enthoven (1985), and Enthoven and Kronick (1989).

The mixed-market (or internal-market) model (Enthoven 1985) is predicated on the coexistence of private and public producers in the same health care system. A mixed market develops when a health system with public insurance seeks tenders from private and public producers in order to offer services. In a mixed market, competition is based on prices evaluated by district or regional managers. They administer a global budget established on the basis of the number and characteristics of the residents of the district or region. In this model, allocational decisions are made by administrators, not by consumers. Thus, this model is closer to the technocratic than to the public-competition model.

The mixed market model places the economics of service production at the core of health regulation. As a result, it is attractive for health systems preoccupied with the efficiency of their output. It is close to the technocratic model and may lead to a heavier regulatory apparatus. In this respect, contract negotiation and enforcement may be costly and may become burdensome.

The professional incentives model is based on a dominant role for health care professionals. It assumes that it is possible to establish standards for medical practice and that doctors, like any other economic group, respond to financial or organizational incentives. It also assumes that the use of incentives by managers and by the State will have an influence on the decisions made by health professionals. These measures can allow for a substantial degree of decentralization in decision making - for example, measures that make doctors responsible for taking an overall amount earmarked for medical staff compensation and allocating it among various activities.

The management incentives model falls between the professional and technocratic models of the health system. In this model, managers play a central role in determining the trade-off between the interests of health professionals and those of the State. Regulation is structured to facilitate convergence between the behaviour of managers and the goals of the health care system (Breton and Wintrobe 1982; Kirkman-Liff and Van de Ven 1989). A system of rules and incentives must be established to encourage innovation among managers while ensuring that objectives are met by rewarding individuals or organizations. In order to maintain a high level of innovation and flexibility, performance standards must be determined *ex post* rather than *ex ante* - that is, the performance of individuals or establishments must be assessed within the context of that organization. Managers are expected to demonstrate the high quality of their performance rather than simply show that they have met pre-established criteria.

The public-competition model described by Saltman and Van Otter (1987, 1989, 1990, 1991) is an interesting approach to revitalizing the public health care system while maintaining its integrity and its funding structure. Fundamentally, the public-competition model seeks to increase the efficiency and effectiveness of the health care system on the basis of consumer preference and choice. In this model, funding of the system is wholly through public sources (i.e., the taxation system). Funding health care establishments is competitive and based on each establishment's ability to attract patients. Users may be called upon periodically to select the institution where they will receive health care. This model forces public service providers to compete for a larger share of an essentially public market. It assumes that control over health care costs will be decentralized, leaves institutions great flexibility in using and managing their assets, and requires them to be accountable for resource utilization. In this model, competition operates on the demand side. The provision of information to health care users and the creation of institutions aimed at supporting consumers in their health care market transactions are the preferred tools of competition in the public-competition model. It has potential for cost control, because it leaves autonomy of decisions regarding resources at the point of delivery. It combines attention to patient needs with cost control mechanisms. The public-competition model is appealing, as it both maintains the integrity of the public health care system and offers the means to make its operation more dynamic.

It is clear that the regulation of health care systems must be multidimensional, combining a proper dosage of technocratic mechanisms with other approaches in favour of more dynamic management, respect of professional autonomy and patient preference. The technocratic approach plays an important and fundamental role in the organization of the health care system's output. To a certain extent, it reflects the State's determination to assume its responsibilities in the organization and management of the system. There is a risk, however, that use of the technocratic model will generate many perverse effects and thus limit its efficiency.

ACKNOWLEDGEMENT

The authors thank the Queen's University of Ottawa Economic Projects for their financial support

REFERENCES

Abel-Smith, B.   Maîtrise des coûts dans 12 pays européens. *World Health Statistics Quarterly*, 1987, 37, : 351-468.

Abel-Smith, B. Who is the odd man out? The experience of Western Europe in containing costs of health care. *Milbank Memorial Fund Quarterly/Health and Society*, 1985; 631 : 1-17.

Babson, J.H. *Health Care Delivery: A Multinational Survey.* London, Pitman Medical, 1972, 128 p.

Barer, M. *et al.*l. Fee controls as Cost Control : Tales from the Frozen North. *The Milbank Quarterly*, 1988; 66 (1) : 1-64.

Baris, E, Contrandiopoulos, A.-P., Champagne, F. *Cost containment in health care : A review of policy options, strategies and tools in selected OECD countries.* Université de Montréal, GRIS, 1992, N92-07, :31 p.

Benson, J.K. The Interorganizational Network as a Political Economy. *Administrative Science Quarterly*, vol. 20, 1975 : 229-249.

Breton, A., Wintrobe, R. *The Logic of Bureaucratic Conduct,* Cambridge University Press, Cambridge, 1982.

Canadian Institute for Advanced Research (CIAR). *The determinants of health,* 1991.

Contandriopoulos, A.-P., Champagne, F., Denis, J.-L., Lemay, A., Ducrot, S., Fournier, M.-A., Avocksouma, D. *Regulatory Mechanisms in the Health Care System of Canada and Other Industrialized Countries : Description and Assessment.* Queen's, University of Ottawa, Economic Projects, 1993, 163 p.

Contandriopoulos, A.-P., Champagne, F., Baris, E. *La rémunération des professionals de santé.* GRIS. (à paraître, été 1993).

Crozier, M. *État modeste, État moderne.* Paris, Seuil, 1991.

Crozier, M. *Le phénomène bureaucratique,* Paris, Seuil, 1965.

Crozier, M., Thoenig, J.C. *The regulation of complex organized systems.* Administrative Science Quarterly, 1976; 21 : 547-70.

Enthoven, A., Kronick, R. A Consumer-choice health plan for the 1990s : universal health insurance in a system designed to promote quality and economy. *New England Journal of Medicine*, 320, 1989 : 29-37, 94-101.

Enthoven, A.C. *Reflections on the Management of the National Health Service.* London, Nuffield Provincial Hospitals Trust, 1985.

Evans, R.G., Barer, M.L., Hertzman, J. The 20-year experiment: accounting for, explaining and evaluating health care cost containment in Canada and the United States. *Annual review of public health*, 1991; 12 : 481-518.

Evans, R.G. Strained Mercy: The Economics of Canadian Health Care. Butterworths, Toronto, 1984, 390 p.

Fischer F. *Technocracy and the Politics of Expertise.* Newbury Park, 1994, Sage.

Gabel, J.R., Rice, T.H. Reducing public expenditures for physicians services : the price of paying less. *Journal of Health politics, policy and law,* 1985; 9 (4) : 595-60.

Glaser, W.A. Controlling Costs through Methods of Paying Doctors : Experiences form Abroad in Stuart O. Schweitzer (ed.) *Policies for the Containment of Health Care Costs and Expenditures,* Washington, D.C., U.S. Government Printing Office, 1978.

Glaser, W.A. Paying the Doctor under National Health Insurance: Foreign Lessons for U.S. Columbia University, Bureau of Applied Research, New York, N.Y., 1976.

Glaser, W.A. *Paying the doctor.* Baltimore, The Johns Hopkins Press, 1970.

Hult, K.M., Walcott, C. Organization design as public policy. *Policy Studies Journal,* 1989; 17 (3) : 469-94.

Kirkman-Liff, B.L., van de Ven, W.P.M.M. "Improving Efficiency in the Dutch Health Care System : Current Innovations and Future Options". *Health Policy,* vol. 13, 1989 : 35-53.

Lomas, J., Fooks, C., Rice, T., Labelle, R. Paying physicians in Canada : Minding our Px and Os. *Health Affairs*, Spring, 1989 : 80-102.

Mintzberg, H. *The structuring of organizations.* Englewood Cliffs, N.J. Prentice Hall; 1978.

Reinhardt, U. The compensation of physician approaches uses in foreign countries. *QRB,* December 1985 : 366-77.

Reinhardt, U.E. The Compensation of Physicians: The Experience Abroad. Paper presented at the 1984 AUPHA Annual Meeting.

Rochaix, L. *Adjustment mechanisms in physician's service market.* Unpublished doctoral thesis, University of York, 1990 : 268.

Saltman, R.B. , von Otter, C. Re-vitalizing Public Health Care Systems : A Proposal for Public Competition in Sweden. *Health Policy,* 1987; 7 : 21-40.

Saltman, R.B., von Otter, C. Public Competition Versus Mixed Markets : An Analytic Comparison. *Health Policy,* 1989; 11 43-55.

Saltman, R.B. Competition and Reform in the Swedish Health System. *The Milbank Quarterly,* 1990; 68 (4) : 597-618.

Saltman, R.B. Emerging Trends in the Swedish Health System. *International Journal of Health Services,* 1991; 21 (4) : 615-623.

U.S. Congress, Office of Technology Assessment. *Payment for Physician Services : Strategies for Medicare,* O.T.A., H-294, Washington, D.C., Government Printing Office, 1986, 273 p.

Weber, M. Bureaucracy in H.H. Gerth and C. Wright Mills (eds.). *From Max Weber : Essays in Sociology,* New York, Oxford University Press, 1979 : 196-265.

Woolhandler S. Himmelstein D.U. The deteriorating administrative efficiency of the U.S. health care system. *The New England Journal of Medicine;* 324 (18) 1991 : 1253-8.

APPENDIX 1 & 2

Table 1. The three dimensions of physician compensation

Price determination		Payment mechanism		Compensation method	
Physician	1	Individual	1	Fee-for-service	1
Negociation	2	Third-Parity	2	Wages	2
Administrative decision	3	Organization	3	Per capita payment	3

Table 2

Price determination		Payment mechanism		Compensation method		Score
Physician	1	Individual	1	Fee for service	1	3
Physician	1	Third party	2	Fee for service	1	4
Negotiation	2	Individual	1	Fee for service	1	4
Negotiation	2	Third party	2	Fee for service	1	5
Negotiation	2	Third party	2	Wages	2	6
Administrative decision	3	Third party	2	Fee for service	1	6
Negotiation	2	Third party	2	Per capita	3	7
Negotiation	2	Organization	3	Wages	2	7
Administrative decision	3	Third party	2	Wages	2	7
Administrative decision	3	Organization	3	Wages	2	8
Administrative decision	3	Organization	3	Per capita	3	9

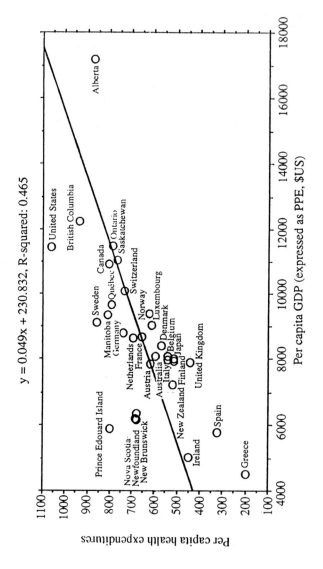

Figure1. Regression Analysis, Health Care Systems, 1980

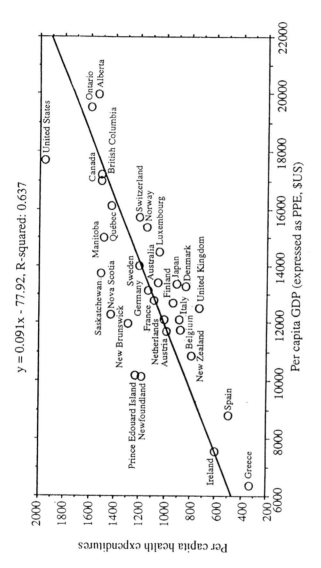

Figure 2. Regression Analysis, Health Care Systems, 1987

21 Identifying and Solving Problems in the Contracting-Out State

KEITH WARD & JULIE QUINLAN

Cranfield University

SCARCE RESOURCES AND THE NHS

Advances in new technologies, developments in drugs and treatments, an increase in life expectancies, an ageing population - all of these factors have resulted in an increased demand by the public for the services that the National Health Service (NHS) provides. Demand now constantly outstrips supply, waiting lists are common and real costs are escalating. In 1993 the NHS cost the British tax payer approximately £33 billion. Such problems led the government to comment in 1989 that:

Today's Health Service is a complex multi-billion pound enterprise. Demand is continuously increasing while resources are inevitably limited (White Paper, 1989:64)

This problem has led to questions about how to prioritise and allocate the resources that are available. The response by the government has been to introduce market forces and private sector processes into the NHS. A number of market force initiatives have been introduced, the most recent and perhaps most radical of these being the introduction of an "internal" or "quasi" market in 1989. This initiative is said to be:

the most far-reaching reform of the National Health Service in its 40 year history
(White Paper, 1989: foreward)

THE INTERNAL MARKET

Based upon the ideas of an American Health Economist, Professor Alain Enthoven (1985), the internal market has introduced the concept of competition between the providers of healthcare. This has been achieved by separating the roles of the purchaser and the provider.

Setting Priorities in Health Care. Edited by M. Malek
© 1994 John Wiley & Sons Ltd

Purchasers

On the purchasing side, GP practices who wish to do so can take control of their own budgets for a limited range of services. Such practices are known as GP Fund Holders (GPFH). They are free to use their budgets to purchase the best service for their customers, be this from the NHS or the private sector. District Health Authorities (DHAs) are also free to purchase services. They can negotiate contracts with the hospitals that they believe will best serve the needs of their residents. The primary task of each DHA is thus to:

> secure the best and most cost-effective services it can for its patients, whether or not those services are provided by the Districts own hospitals
>
> (White Paper, 1989:30)

Providers

The freedom of choice described above has introduced an element of competition amongst providers. Their revenue is no longer guaranteed by a Resource Allocation Working Party formula (RAWP). Instead, it is dependent upon the contracts that they successfully negotiate with the new purchasers in the marketplace. Each hospital now has to compete against its counterparts, including newly formed "Self Governing" Trust hospitals, to convince the purchasers that only they can provide the service that they need. The government claims that this will improve:

> the choice and quality of the services offered and the efficiency with which those services are delivered
>
> (White Paper, 1989:22)

Thus, there is a belief that by introducing competition between suppliers of healthcare and giving freedom of choice to purchasers, the service will be more responsive to consumer needs. Resources will therefore be allocated in line with demand. Those hospitals which provide the required level of services at the lowest cost should attract a larger share of the purchasers' limited resources as money follows the patient to the hospital of their choice. Since those with the most work will in theory be the most efficient, the health of the nation should be optimised with the resources that are available. The internal market is therefore an attempt by the government to address the problem of scarce resources and increasing demand in the NHS.

In this competitive environment, hospitals should be utilising every tool and technique that will give them a competitive advantage. They need to strive for cost-efficient, quality services that meet the needs of the purchasers. Those that refuse to take up the challenge are likely to lose contracts to more efficient service providers in the market.

Obtaining a competitive advantage through market testing and contracting-out

The testing of a hospital's in-house services against external service providers is one route to a sustained competitive advantage and an efficient allocation of resources in the internal market. Comparing services to see which supplier can provide the required level of service and at what cost is a credible method to ensuring that resources are utilised efficiently. Where the external service provider proves to be the most suitable supplier, then the service should normally be contracted-out.

The contracted company then provides the goods or services specified in the contract between itself and the hospital. It is responsible for the operation, maintenance and provision of the specified service. Such companies can often provide services more efficiently than an in-house team because they can capture economies of scale in areas such as new technology, personnel, management, research and development and equipment purchase. Thus, by contracting-out activities which can be provided more efficiently by other service providers, hospital management can concentrate its scarce resources in those areas where the maximum value added can be generated.

The sizeable potential benefits of contracting-out can be demonstrated by the successful usage of the concept in certain areas within the private sector.

Contracting-out in the private sector

Contracting-out has been used extensively by much of manufacturing industry for many years to provide the components it requires for its in-house manufacturing process. The result is that several, previously highly vertically integrated industries, now comprise a limited number of large assembly focused companies whose needs are supplied by a large number of sub-contractors. Success in this area has meant that, more recently, the concept has been applied to other less tangible areas of their operations. Many companies now contract-out functions such as training, recruitment, ancillary services, personnel and information technology. For example, BHS contracts-out its business re-engineering, development of IT links into the supply chain and other similar functions to outside suppliers. Whitbread has recently entered into a £12.5m contract for its systems development and maintenance. IBM contracts-out the handling of its customer requests for information to Manpower Services (Financial Times Survey, 1993).

Increasingly, companies are using the contracting-out concept to improve the running of their operations. In a 1991 survey of 500 CIO's and IS directors (Schwartz, 1992), 53.6% contracted-out in order to obtain knowledge and expertise and 39.8% to relieve labour constraints. Mr John Kerry, head of outsourcing at Ernst and Young, in a recent FT Report (20 Feb., 1992) identified skills shortages, reducing costs and capital investment as some reasons for contracting-out. In a similar report in 1993, the FT identified the need for flexibility, reduced costs, quality of service and the ability to concentrate resources on the core business. Clearly, if these expectations were not being met, this strategy would not be pursued.

Healthcare

The success of contracting-out has also been reported in the provision of healthcare in the USA. A survey of 1090 hospitals by *Hospital* in 1992 (Hard) showed that 90%

of respondents were satisfied with the performance of their hospital management firms. They usually met the hospitals' Total Quality Management and cost goals and provided specialist expertise necessary for the provision of the service. Another study of 4 hospitals in 1991 (Gardner) looked at the contracting-out of information technology. They adopted this strategy for the effective use of capital, personnel issues, the ability to cope with technological change and cost stability. A survey of clinical service contracting also reported similar findings (Lumsdon, 1992). These examples show the benefits that can be obtained by a successful application of the market testing and contracting-out concept.

Contracting-out initiatives in the NHS

The government has realised the benefits that contracting-out can achieve. It has therefore advocated and sometimes enforced the use of market testing and contracting-out on a number of occasions. For example, in 1983 Compulsory Competitive Tendering (CCT) for the provision of domestic, catering and laundry services was established. The aim was to ensure that hospitals test:

> the cost effectiveness of their domestic, catering and laundry services by putting them out to tender in the market

> (HC(83)18:2)

Contracts with external service providers were advocated where this proved to be the most "cost effective way of providing support services" (HC(83)18:1). This message was re-enforced by Kenneth Clark at the study day of the Hospital Caterers Association in September 1983. In his speech there he defined the purpose of competitive tendering as being to ensure:

> the total cost effectiveness of the service to be provided and that costs of the service be reduced to the lowest level that will still enable the excellent standards

> (Clarke, 1983:5)

In the White Paper "Working for Patients" (1989:8) the government's commitment to the benefits of contracting-out are also quite clearly stated:

> [One of] the most important aims behind these changes [is] to contract-out more functions which do not have to be undertaken by health authority staff and which could be provided more cost effectively by the private sector

In a more recent initiative, the Citizens Charter (1991) sets out a programme of change to improve the choice, quality, value and accountability of all public services. The NHS features in this programme. To meet the goals of the charter, public services are once again encouraged to compare the efficiency of their in-house departments with external service providers and to contract with the private sector where this secures a more efficient provision of services. Building on these initiatives, the White Paper "Competing For Quality" (1991:14) also promotes the benefits of market testing and contracting-out as a means to ensuring that:

> resources are used as effectively as possible, for the benefit of patients

These statements clearly illustrate the government's support of the contracting-out concept as a means to securing the efficient and effective provision of services. In fact, it is currently proposing an extension of the concept into the provision of clinical services:

> there is scope for much wider use of competitive tendering beyond the non-clinical support services which have formed the bulk of tendering so far...health authorities and their managers will be expected to consider such opportunities as an option in carrying out their new role
>
> (White Paper, 1989:70)

The viability of this option has been discussed both at the recent National Association of Health Authorities and Trusts (NAHAT) conference and by the Langsland Review. Unfortunately, the problems of previous contracting-out eras suggest that this option should be seriously reviewed before any decision is taken. In the contracting-out of ancillary services these problems have been heavily documented.

The success of contracting-out

There is a substantial amount of evidence which demonstrates the failure of the contracting-out mechanism. For example, a report entitled "More Contractors' Failures" by the Trades Union Congress (TUC, 1986) detailed 42 cases of tendering that had "*gone wrong*", leading to falling standards and high staff turnover. A report by the Institute of Personnel Management (IPM) in 1986 reported adverse effects on industrial relations and conditions for workers. Newbiggings and Lister's research for the Association of London Authorities (1988:6) also concluded that:

> An ever-growing list of scandals and failures; a toll of suffering, inconvenience, hygiene risks ... these are the fruits of the government's policy of putting hospital ancillary services out to tender

Although the political beliefs and ideologies of the authors could have tarnished some of these results, a number of independent studies have also been conducted to support their claim. A study conducted by Warwick Business School (Bach, 1989b) looked at one health authority's decision to contract-out its cleaning. The cleaning function was the first of many that were put out for tender in response to the government's claims of improved efficiency and quality service. Tenders were based on price, mainly of staff, materials and equipment - the result being that other issues, particularly those of quality, were ignored and subsequently found to be unacceptable. The study by Newbigging and Lister (1988:5) of contracting-out in the London region reported on the:

> disastrous effect which competitive tendering and privatisation has had on the London NHS

Other significant contributions in this area include works published by Kakabadse and Chandra (1985), The National Audit Office (1987), The Nuffield Provincial Hospital Trust (1987), The Kings Fund Institute (1988) and HM Treasury (1992).

Such problems appear to have arisen because of a fundamental lack of understanding of the government's "cost-effective" initiatives and a consequent failure to implement the contracting-out concept correctly. "Cost-effectiveness" appears to have been interpreted as "cost efficiency" or "cost reduction" - a flawed interpretation with potentially severe results. The following definitions will illustrate this point:

Definitions

Bowman and Asch (1987:383) define efficiency and effectiveness in the following manner:

> Efficiency usually refers to the utilisation of the means (the resources) whereas effectiveness relates to the goals of the organisation. Thus an organisation could be very efficient but totally ineffective

A more in-depth description is offered by Culyer (1990:3,4). He defines effectiveness and cost-effectiveness in the following manner:

Effectiveness is about *"not using more resources than are necessary to achieve an end"*. The idea is to find all those combinations of resources that meet the organisations objectives. For example, in order to clean a hospital ward to a specified standard, a number of combinations of domestics, supervisors, equipment and procedures could be used.

Cost-effectiveness therefore refers to *"not incurring a higher cost than is necessary to achieve an end"*. It involves choosing from the combination of effective resources that which is least costly.

Efficiency is therefore concerned with "doing things right" and focuses on the relationship between inputs and outputs. Cost efficiency is therefore concerned with the lowest cost combination of inputs and outputs. In contrast, effectiveness relates to how well the objectives of the organisation have been achieved and is concerned with "doing the right things". It refers to how resources can be combined to best meet the goals of the organisation. A cost-effective service is, therefore, one which maximises its contribution to the hospital's goals in the most cost-efficient manner. Clearly, a failure to perform an effectiveness evaluation before a review of efficiency takes place could result in the provision of a service which is 100% efficient but totally ineffective!

The government claims that when market testing ancillary services, the cost savings that are now being achieved are an illustration of its success. For example, the report by the National Audit Office (1987) highlights the annual accumulated savings of £73m that have been achieved. In the White Paper "Working For Patients" (1989), the success of the initiative is demonstrated in terms of the cost savings of £120m/yr. which were obtained over the period 1983-1989. In the White Paper "Competing For Quality" (1991) the falling costs of ancillary services from £514m to £428m between 1984-1985 and 1989-1990 are also heralded as showing the success of the initiative.

Clearly, using the above definitions, the cost savings so freely proclaimed are valid only if the services involved have maximised their contribution towards the objectives and goals of the hospital in the most cost efficient manner. This will only occur if the decision process is broken into stages in which the required level of service is first established by assessing the objectives of the organisation before the most cost-efficient way of achieving this level of service is selected. The management of these stages is encapsulated under the umbrella of "strategic management", defined by Bowman and Asch (1987:4) as being the:

> process of making and implementing strategic decisions

Successful contracting-out and the strategic management process

An illustration of the steps involved in the strategic management process is shown in Figure 1:

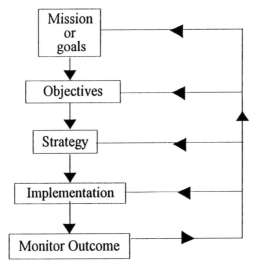

Figure 1. Strategic Management Process

First of all, the mission/goals of the organisation are established. These are usually quite general statements which are not changed every year. They are statements of what the organisation is and what it wants to be. These goals are then translated into strategic objectives which the organisation will aim to achieve in the long term. The methods used to achieve the objectives are then selected and implemented at a functional level. The outcome is then monitored and a feedback process established so that the performance can be measured and any changes in the strategic plan and its implementation made as the environment changes.

Within this model a successful contracting-out decision requires that a series of steps is undertaken. These are shown in Figure 2:

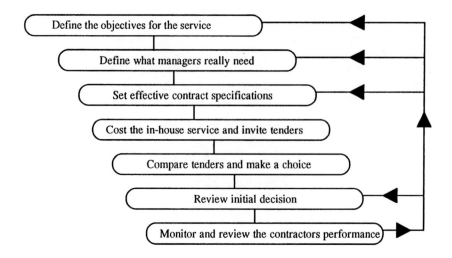

Figure 2. Steps for Successful Contracting-out Decisions

First of all, the objectives for the service should be defined. These should flow from the strategic objectives of the organisation. Then the level of service that is required should be established. This requires the manager to have a clear idea of what service is actually needed, or indeed, if the service is needed at all. Thus, a thorough review of the service should take place at this point. From this review, clear and unambiguous contract specifications should be set. This is a crucial stage. A careful specification of the required service is vital if a valid comparison is to be made between the competing potential internal and external sources. Such a specification should also include measurable performance criteria by which the service will be judged.

The in-house service should then be costed. It is crucial that such costings are based upon the costs that will incurred if the service is outsourced and the savings that would be made if the internal department was closed. These are known as avoidable costs. Any apportioned costs, or long term committed costs which will still be incurred even if that particular department is closed, should be excluded from the comparisons. The tenders should then be compared and the least costly, or most cost-efficient service provider chosen. This provider should then be monitored by the performance criteria that were specified in the tender and the results fed back to the relevant decision makers.

Unfortunately, all of the evidence to date suggests that the strategic management and contracting-out decision making process in the NHS is sometimes flawed. For example, objectives for the service are not always clear which makes defining what is required virtually impossible. The service level is not always reviewed before the service specification is set and monitoring techniques can be inadequate. These flaws can be seen in three major problems that frequently occur. These are:

- Poor staff morale and conditions of employment
- Reviewing services and setting contract specifications
- Measuring standards and monitoring and controlling contractors

These are demonstrated in further detail below:

Staff morale and conditions of employment

Libraries are overflowing with research showing the detrimental effect that market testing and contracting-out can have upon the staff involved. It shows hours, pay and holidays being reduced and overtime and bonus rates cut. It shows part-time employees being used to reduce costs by reducing the number of lunch breaks and national insurance contributions. The IPM (1986), Milne (1987) and Sheffield City Council (1988) all found this to be the case. The Joint Privatisation Research Unit (1990:4) went so far as to say that:

> Competitive tendering in the health service is more about forcing down standards and wages and conditions...than it is about improving services to patients

In fact, even when the service remains in-house, management have often used the tendering process as a means of introducing changes in work practice and tightening their control over staff and trade unions. Although a large amount of this literature could be argued as lacking objectivity and neutrality due to the political interests of the researchers, it does emphasise the drive for cost reduction by reducing the cost of staff. Referring back to our definitions of cost-effectiveness, this reduction in costs is only beneficial if the service the staff provide is still effective and standards have been maintained.

Unfortunately, this does not appear to have been the case. The cost cutting exercise has often been detrimental to the efficient operation of the hospital. The change in employment conditions often causes a decline in staff morale. Where hours have been reduced, Mially (1986) and Bach (1989b) found that this left domestics with less time to spend with the patients, a task which Harrisson (1986) saw as being a crucial ingredient to service quality and patient welfare. The increased use of part-time staff has often reduced the calibre of those employed. According to Griffith, Iliffe and Rayner (1987:168) the contracting-out process has led to:

> lower morale, industrial action, increased exploitation and unemployment and for some districts at least, lower standards

These declining standards of service, a failure to understand the linkage of the service with other functional areas and the detrimental effect on patient well-being are signals of an organisation pursuing a cost reduction strategy at the expense of effectiveness and quality. It implies a lack of fit with the hospital's objectives, a misunderstanding of the government's desire for a cost-effective health service and an inadequate strategic management process.

Reviewing services and setting contract specifications

When management set contract specifications they should be clear and precise - giving full details of the service that is required (see Figure 2). This should flow from the evaluation of the service level that is needed to meet the hospital's strategic goals. It should therefore be a relatively easy task to perform. Unfortunately, many hospitals appear to have experienced substantial problems when attempting to set effective contract specifications. For example, the contracts are sometimes based upon the existing level of service with no investigation to establish if a different level or arrangement of the service would better fit the hospital's strategy. Managers appear to be often unaware of the service that they really need. Even when specifications have been set, they have often been unclear, leading to misunderstandings on the part of the contractor. Numerous studies could be quoted to illustrate this point.

For example, Bach (1989a) cited one example of a region which specified that "the inside windows" of the hospital must be cleaned. The chosen contractor did not interpret this to be the inside face of the external windows, as the hospital had intended. Instead, it was interpreted to be all windows inside the hospital which were not on an outside wall! Problems inevitably arose between the hospital and the service provider. A study by Domberger, Meadowcroft and Thompson (1987) also found that poorly thought out specification led to contractors making their own assessment of the service required. Paine (1984) and The Joint Privatisation Research Unit (1990) reported similar findings.

HC(83)18 forces hospitals to accept the lowest cost tender. This is on the assumption that the service specified in the contract is effective. Clearly, the fact that many NHS managers do not appear to be able to identify and specify all components of the service to be market tested suggests that the effectiveness of the service has not been evaluated. Since they usually accept the lowest cost tender they may therefore be purchasing services which are cost efficient but not necessarily cost effective. Once again, it implies a lack of fit with the strategic objectives of the hospital and suggests that the contracting-out process is not being correctly performed.

Monitoring standards and controlling contractors

Figure 2 shows that if contracted services are to remain "cost-effective", they must be monitored and evaluated to ensure that:

• The service still meets the objectives of the organisation
• The objectives are being satisfied in the most cost-efficient manner

Such monitoring requires appropriate measures against which performance can be evaluated. These measures should be relatively easy to establish. The effectiveness measures should flow from the strategic objectives of the hospital. The cost-efficiency measures should focus on the input-output relationship and should flow from the contract specification. Unfortunately, such measures are frequently missing, inadequate, crude or judgmental. When adequate measures have been established they are usually efficiency rather than effectiveness oriented. Once again, this suggests that an evaluation of the objectives of the hospital and the level of service required is not always undertaken. A number of surveys can illustrate this point.

In the comprehensive survey conducted by the National Audit Office in 1987, of the 27 contracts it examined, 11 were found to contain problems with their monitoring and control systems. In one case, poor quality control mechanisms had led to pests in the kitchen. In another, problems arose because of discrepancies between the quality control results of the authorities monitoring staff and those of the contractor. Such observations led to the conclusion that there are:

> major problems arising on some contracts regarding [the] monitoring of performance
>
> (NAO:22).

Carnaghan and Bracewell-Milnes (1993:143) also noted that the monitoring of services has been "*badly neglected*". In fact, in many cases monitoring is an after thought, arising only when problems occur. The actual measurement tool itself is also often quite crude and judgmental. For example, in one hospital, Bach (1989a) found that the monitoring officers for domestic services took a large number of observations every month and converted these into performance measures. However, the performance would vary depending upon the time of day that the sample was taken and the opinion of the monitoring officer. Crude formulas are often used:

$$\frac{Satisfactory\ observations}{Number\ of\ observations} * 100 \text{ (Bach, 1989: 21)}$$

Once again these incidents point to a fundamental misunderstanding of the government's cost-effectiveness goals and a flawed decision making and strategic management process.

A need for further action

The problems that we have outlined above are not uncommon. They strengthen our belief that cost efficiency may often be pursued to the detriment of cost-effectiveness. However, such problems are by no means universal. The contracting-out initiative has also been heralded as a success in some areas. For example, the Cleaning and Support Services Association (1991:6) quotes the General Manager of the St Helier Hospital, one of the first to adopt the contracting-out concept in response to HC(83)18, as saying that:

> under direct labour, the standards of cleaning were very variable and the quality of management was clearly inferior to that achieved by the company. Now there is a far tighter structure of command and a higher overall standard of service

The Contract Cleaning and Maintenance Association (1990:2) claims that:

> after seven years, substantial savings have been achieved, with improvements in standards and the ability of managers to manage their service

The government clearly believes that the initiative has been a success because it is now promoting its extension beyond the provision of support services. Carnaghan and Bracewell Milnes (1993:125), in their review of the CCT literature to date, also concluded that:

> the overall success of competitive tendering, despite a number of problems particularly in the initial stages, is such that it is now widely accepted

In recent years there has also been a significant decline in the number of reported contract failures. In fact, some hospitals now contract-out all of their support functions to one service provider. This could lead to criticism that the hypothesis posed is outdated and irrelevant. However, to do so would be to show a fundamental misunderstanding of the problem which we have highlighted.

The literature of the early 1980's certainly showed symptoms of a service pursuing a cost-efficient strategy to the detriment of quality and effectiveness. This is highlighted in the number of problems that arose during the first round of tendering. The fact that these problems appear to have been eliminated may simply mean that contractors are fulfilling the terms of their contract; they are providing high quality services with motivated, well paid staff. However, unless the problem of setting effective specifications and controls has been resolved (and there is no reason to suggest that this is the case), then contractors may merely be providing services that are 100% efficient but not at all effective.

Unfortunately, the research that has been conducted to date cannot reject or accept our hypothesis. Further research is required to clarify the situation.

Clinical services and contracting-out

The need for this research has been strengthened by the recent calls for the extension of CCT into the clinical services arena. The Trust Federation's draft submission to the Langslands NHS Review (1993) said that tendering for clinical work would maximise value for money. At the NAHAT conference in June, York Health Services Trust Chief Executive, Peter Kennedy, advocated that tendering for clinical services would reduce the "*scandalous over provision*" of services. He said that it would encourage trusts to adopt 'best practice' methods quickly. In Nottingham a hearing services department regarded as a centre for excellence is currently progressing through the tendering process. Tenders have been received and are currently being evaluated (1/2/94). It is the first time that such a department has been put out to tender (Moore, 1993). Unfortunately, the experience at Nottingham is already revealing some traits of the earlier contracting-out era. Some staff have left, morale is said to be low and there is a fear of a decline in service quality.

Such services have a more direct impact upon the treatment of patients, their welfare and their satisfaction. It is imperative therefore that the problems outlined above do not recur. The process of strategic management and the attainment of cost-effective services must be researched to determine if the initiative is likely to bring the rewards which are acclaimed. It is in light of this development that we are about to embark upon a research project at Cranfield School of Management to explore the process of strategic management and the attainment of cost-effective ancillary services. It will focus upon the establishment of the "fit" between strategic and functional strategies and the implementation, evaluation and control of the service. The research findings should establish whether cost reduction strategies are being pursued to the detriment of effectiveness and quality. If this proves to be the case then suggestions for improvements to both the strategic management and contracting-out processes will be made. Implication for the extension of CCT and contracting-out into the clinical service arena will then be drawn.

CONCLUSIONS

In the new exciting, competitive environment of the internal market, hospitals should be utilising every tool and technique that will enable them to provide a cost-effective service. Contracting-out is one mechanism that can help them to achieve this goal. When a service is contracted-out to an experienced team with clear contract specifications and monitoring mechanisms, a significant contribution towards the provision of cost-effective services can be achieved.

Unfortunately, in the area of ancillary service provision, the rewards of successful contracting-out have not always been achieved. Some of the problems that have contributed towards this lack of success are currently being addressed. For example, information systems are being upgraded to provide better information to management. Consultants are being employed to advise upon the management and implementation of change. Other problems could be easily resolved. For example, service costings could be improved by an adoption of more appropriate management accounting techniques such as transfer pricing, avoidable costings and zero based budgeting. Efficiency monitoring could be improved by the adoption of standard costing.

However, unless the service specified in the original contract is effective, then these measures may only serve to provide services that are 100% efficient but not at all cost-effective. Until strategic and functional objectives are matched, appropriate costings and measures of performance installed and a feedback mechanism established to adapt the service as the needs of the hospital change, then the establishment of cost-effective services cannot be assured. With the government's recent encouragement of the extension of the contracting-out concept into the clinical service arena, the need to ensure that such systems are in place and that cost-effectiveness is not being interpreted as exclusively cost reduction is paramount.

REFERENCES

Bach, S. (1989a) Trading For Health Services: Lessons from the Competitive Tendering Experience, *Journal of Management in Medicine"*, Vol.4, No.3, pp.160-166

Bach, S. (1989b) *Too high a Price to Pay: A Study of Competitive Tendering for Domestic Services in the NHS*, Warwick Papers in Industrial Relations, No. 25, Industrial Relations Research Unit, University of Warwick: School of Industrial and Business Studies

Bowman, C. and Asch, D. (1987) *Strategic Management,* London: Macmillan Education Limited.

Carnaghan, R. and Bracewell-Milnes,B. (1993) *Testing the Market,* Research Monograph No.49, London: Institute of Economic Affairs

Clarke, K.(1983), Hospital Caterers Association, *National Study Day Report Document,* 28 September 1983, Health Caterers Association

Cleaning and Support Services Association (undated- about 1991), *Safe in their hands: the record of private contractors in public services",* London: Cleaning and Support Services Association

Contract Cleaning and Maintenance Association (1990), *The Facts on the NHS Privatisation Experience: a response to 'The NHS Privatisation Experience' by the Joint NHS Privatisation Research Unit,* London: Contract Cleaning and Maintenance Association

Culyer, A.J. (1990) *The Internal Market: An Acceptable Means to a Desirable End,* Discussion Paper 67, University of York: Centre for Health Economics

Department of Health and Social Security (1983), *Competitive Tendering in the provision of Domestic, Catering and Laundry Services,* HC(83)18, London: HMSO

Domberger, S.; Meadowcroft, S.; Thompson, D.(1987) The Impact Of Competitive Tendering on the Cost of Hospital Domestic Services, *Fiscal Studies,* Vol.8, No.4, 1987, pp.39-54

Enthoven, A.C. (1985), *Reflections on the Management of the National Health Service,* Occasional Papers 5, London: Nuffield Provincial Hospitals Trust

Financial Times Survey (1992) Contracted Business Services, *Financial Times,* 20th February 1992

Financial Times Survey (1993) Resource Management: Buying-in Services, *Financial Times,* 28th July, 1993

Gardner, E. (1991) Going on line with outsiders, *Modern Healthcare,* 15 July 1991, pp.35-47

Griffith, B.; Iliffe, S.; Rayner, G.(1987), Banking on Sickness: Commercial Medicine in Britain and the USA, London: Lawrence and Wishart

Hard, R. (1992) Hospitals look to Hospitality Service firms to meet TQM goals, *Hospitals,* 20 May 1992, pp.56-58

Harrisson, S. (1986) A valuable part of the team, *The Health Service Journal,* 96(5029), 11 December 1986, pp.1608-1609

HM Treasury (1992) *Market Testing and Buying In,* London: Public Competition and Purchasing Unit

Institute of Personnel Management and Incomes Data Services (IDS) (1986), *Competitive Tendering in the Public Sector,* London: Public Sector Unit

Kakabadse and Chandra (1985) *Privatisation and the National Health Service,* Hants: Gower Publishing Company Limited

Lumsdon, K. (1992) Clinical Contracting: CEO's see demand for specialized skills, advanced services, *Hospitals,* 20 August 1992, pp.44-46

Mially, R. (1986) Competitive Tendering Approaches Adopted in the NHS, *Health Care Management,* Vol1. No.3, 1986, pp.24-29

Milne, R.G. (1987) Competitive Tendering in the NHS: an economic analysis of the early implementation of HC(83)18, *Public Administration*, Vol. 65, Summer 1987, pp.145-160

Moore, W.(1993) HA calls in private sector to tender for clinical work, *The Health Service Journal*, 2 September 1993, p6

National Audit Office (1987), *Competitive Tendering for Support Services in the National Health Service* London: HMSO

Newbigging, R.; Lister, J. (1988) *The record of private companies in NHS support services*, London: Association of London Authorities

Paine, L. (1984) *Contracting Out In The Bethlem Royal And Maudsley Hospital*, in Contracting Out In The Public Sector, Proceedings of a Conference, London: Royal Institute of Public Administration

Schwartz, J. (1992) Ordering Out for IS, *CIO*, February 1992, p18

Sheffield City Council: Employment and Economic Development Dept (1988) *Competitive Tendering for Support Services in the National Health Service: Who Pays the Price?* Sheffield: Sheffield City Council

The Joint NHS Privatisation Research Unit (1990), *The Privatisation Experience: Competitive Tendering for NHS Support Services*, London: The Joint NHS Privatisation Research Unit

TUC (1986), *More Contractors' Failures*, London:TUC Publications

Weale, A. (1988) Cost and Choice in Health Care, London: *Kings Fund*

White Paper (1989) Working for Patients, *CM 555*, London:HMSO

White Paper (1991) *The Citizens Charter: Raising The Standard* London: HMSO

White Paper (1991) *Competing For Quality: Buying Better Public Services*, London: HM Treasury

22 Evolving a Strategic Planning Philosophy to Reflect the Managerial Environment Confronting the NHS

IAN CHASTON & BERYL BADGER

The University of Plymouth

INTRODUCTION

When the National Health Service was established on July 5th 1948, it was widely expected that once the initial backlog of health problems had been treated, the NHS would face decreasing demand for services as the population became healthier and any unforeseen cost problems would be offset by increased national productivity (Pollard 1969). Subsequent Governments have, however, continually faced demands from the NHS for more resources. Two factors influencing this situation have been the ever increasing rate of technological advances in health care and the changing age demographics of the UK population.

The issue of increased funding for the NHS came to a head in the 1980s when the general economic climate and the UK Government's manifesto to reduce inflation meant that all public sector bodies were placed under pressure to reduce expenditure.

Review of the causes of NHS overspending indicated the fundamental problem that although clinicians were often excluded from providing inputs for the budgeting process, the judgements made by this group (e.g. selection of treatment; adoption of a new drug) had a dramatic impact on actual expenditure. The usual response of managers in the face of lack of control over clinical expenditure was to seek counterbalancing cutbacks in areas such as catering, nurse staffing or laundry services (Perrin 1988).

In an attempt to involve clinicians in the resource allocation process Ian Mills, in his newly appointed capacity as Director of Financial Management to the NHS Management Board, launched the Resource Management Initiative (Department of Health 1986). The concept, which had the stated aim of enabling "the NHS to give better service to its patients by helping clinicians and other managers to make better

Setting Priorities in Health Care. Edited by M. Malek

informed judgements about how the resources they control can be used to the maximum effect" , received the full support of the BMA and the Royal Colleges.

Although the objectives of the Resource Management Initiative were clearly stated, actual processes by which they could be achieved were not specified. Instead the Department of Health identified six hospitals to pilot and develop the concept. The Department of Health's Research Management Division commissioned the Health Economics Research Group at Brunel University to evaluate the progress and methodologies at the pilot sites. In general terms it was found that clinical staff felt the initiative provided greater insights over the resource constraints facing their hospitals and this situation led to operational improvements in areas such as inter-departmental co-operation and intra-organisational communication. There was, however, no statistical evidence to demonstrate that the concept resulted in any quantitative or qualitative improvements in patient care (Health Economics Research Group 1991).

THE ARRIVAL OF THE MARKET FORCES MODEL

Although further reform of the NHS was not contained within the 1987 Conservative Party manifesto, within a few months after the election, the Government embarked on a review to identify a revised NHS structure capable of reducing the costs of health care. The review reflected the prevailing Conservative "market forces" philosophy of using competition to reduce costs. As the transfer of services to the private sector was not seen as an option acceptable to the general public, the selected solution was the creation of an Internal Market which was designed to introduce the concept of competition through the separation of purchasers and providers (Department of Health 1989).

Within the Acute Sector, the reforms permitted hospitals to compete with each other for contracts in relation to their ability to meet the cost, quality and quantity specifications of the purchasers. A further impetus to the concept of competition was the creation of General Fundholder Practices who have the authority to negotiate directly with providers on behalf of their patients.

MANAGERIAL RESPONSE TO THE INTERNAL MARKET

To understand how the reforms might be affecting the Acute Sector, the authors participated in a number of 1:1 and group meetings with NHS staff in Devon and Cornwall. The prevailing view revealed by these discussions was that as handling competitive threats is a fundamental aspect of the management process in commercial organisations, then this is where the NHS should turn for guidance on how to respond to the Internal Market scenario. Many of these NHS managers favoured the adoption of the strategic planning philosophy involving the classic three stage process of answering the questions of "where are we now", "where to we going" and "how do we get there." Our experience, similar to that reported by Common et al (1992), is that such deliberations have usually led to the consideration of the standard Porter (1985) competitive responses of seeking some form of cost leadership or performance superiority strategy. In a limited number of cases, managers had progressed their thinking to encompass alternative planning scenarios. Typically these individuals utilised concepts such as the Ansoff (1984) matrix to examine opportunities for entering new markets, seeking new customers or developing new product/service portfolios.

During these discussions the authors encountered some NHS managers who favour, presumably as a result of the Government's "market forces" terminology, increased emphasis on marketing management to ensure delivery of their Unit's strategic goals. Their conceptual frameworks are usually based upon the classic consumer goods strategic marketing philosophy proposed by writers such as Abel and Hammond (1979) of using the 4Ps to defend and/or increase market share. Some planners feel it is necessary to treat the NHS as a service industry and include the additional "Ps" of process, people and physical assets (Cowell 1984). The competitive analogies used by this latter group tend to be drawn from private sector scenarios such as retailing or financial services. Consequently they point to the importance of Customer Care and/or Total Quality Management as a mechanism for achieving a differentiated market position over other potential health care providers.

REVISITING STRATEGIC THEORY

In recent years, the validity of assuming that strategic planners must always give priority to identifying ways of defeating competitors has been brought into question by studies of actual marketing practice in various industrial sectors. Nystrom (1977), for example, concluded that success in world markets for some leading European firms was a result of a strategy based upon the selection of customers to reflect mutual benefits for both parties in the exchange relationship. Subsequently he has suggested that Western management thinking is too heavily dominated by the views of U.S. academics who have evolved their theories through observations of the extremely competitive climate which faces American fast moving consumer goods companies in their domestic markets(Nystrom 1990). The typical strategic response of this type of firm is to use aggressive price and/or promotional spending to counteract the threats of technically very similar product offerings by their competitors (e.g. coffee, detergents and paper towels).

If one accepts Hughes' (1978) somewhat broader definition that strategic marketing should be viewed as "the activities that relate an organisation successfully to its environment", then planners are offered the freedom to consider the alternative philosophy of relationship marketing in which strategic focus is directed towards using collaboration and co-operation in the buyer-seller relationship as the basis for achieving market success (Speckman and Johnson 1986). There is a now a growing body of evidence from the private sector that relying on aggressive pricing and/or promotional activity can often be much less certain process for optimising long term performance than the alternative of creating exchange relationships in which the seller continually strives to seek ways of "moving closer to the customer" (Peters 1992; Band 1991).

A critical element in the implementation of a   relationship-based marketing strategy is a commitment of the entire organisation to meeting the needs of the external customer. Oakland (1989), for example, states that "for an organisation to be truly effective, every single part must work together... failure to meet the requirements in one part or area creates problems elsewhere." Gronroos (1982) has described this process as "internal marketing" in which the objective is to integrate the multiple functions of the organisation by ensuring employees understand all aspects of business operations and are motivated to act in a service-orientated manner.

Given the growing body of literature which suggests that in certain situations, corporate battles based on aggressive pricing and/or promotional campaigns may not be to the benefit of either the seller or the customer, then possibly there is a need to question the fundamental assumption that the most effective response to the NHS reforms is for Unit managers to base their strategic behaviour on Porterian contending forces models which mimic the warfare scenarios demonstrated in the ongoing battles between brands such as Pepsi Cola versus Coca Cola or Nestle versus Maxwell House.

It is not suggested that NHS managers should reject all concepts originating from the private sector. What is proposed, however, is that health care strategists should exhibit a greater willingness to (a) openly question the validity of the paradigms currently in use and (b) begin to construct planning models which actually contain the capability to effectively respond to the unique problems which confront UK health care community.

In seeking an alternative paradigm for the health care sector, perhaps it is beneficial to revisit the original aims of the Resource Management Initiative; namely better service to patients through informed judgements about how resources can best be used. There are two reasons for offering this suggestion. Firstly it must be assumed that both the purchaser and the provider do share the common goal of wishing to optimise the delivery of cost effective health care to their local community. Under these circumstances there seems little benefit, therefore, (except possibly in cases where providers will not accept major duplication of services exists in a specific geographic area) for either party to perceive any advantage to the patient in seeking to instigate costly marketing wars between NHS Units. Secondly studies of markets where the philosophy of strong supplier-customer chains prevails over the alternative of intense inter-firm rivalry, typically reveal that value added processes are enhanced accompanied by either rising product quality and/or declining product costs (Schonberger 1990).

RESEARCHING THE CAPABILITY OF ACUTE UNITS TO ADOPT A RELATIONSHIP-BASED STRATEGIC PARADIGM

For the purposes of this paper, it is assumed District Health Authorities are progressing their responsibilities to undertake the research necessary to specify patient needs and forecast demand for treatment provision within their local community. The issue of balancing available resources against medical priorities should then become basis for the negotiations between the informed Health Authority representing the needs of the patients and the Acute Unit as the supplier of appropriate treatments.

Effective relationship-based strategic paradigms demand that if customers and suppliers are to successfully build stronger working relationships then this activity has been preceded by actions to optimise and integrate working relationships between all departments within their respective organisation. Hence the start point in any assessment of whether Acute Units have the ability over the longer term to move towards a relationship-based strategic planning philosophy as the basis for working with NHS purchasers should be to determine the current status of the internal marketing processes inside these provider organisations.

Having defined the research objective of wishing to comprehend the status of internal marketing processes in South West Acute Units, the researchers faced the obstacle that although there is extensive mention of the concept in the literature, there appeared to no available descriptions of how to actually undertake an audit of internal customer management practices. It was decided, therefore, to adopt the quasi-ethnographic approach suggested by Morgan and Smirich (1980) of asking managers to describe critical incidents concerning poor working relationships between departments. These examples could then be used to build a paradigm which could be refined through further discussions with NHS staff. In this way it is possible to fulfil the Arygris et al (1985) action science guidelines of building management models which reflect actual situations.

It was decided that a deductive approach of surveying staff in South West Acute Units would be the most appropriate way of gaining further insights on the actual status of internal management practices within this sector of the NHS. To improve the prospects for the generation of reliable data and to permit comparisons to be made with other studies, it was felt the research tool should attempt to replicate an existing, validated methodology. Possibly the most frequently quoted technique for evaluating customer management processes is the SERVQUAL instrument developed by Parasuraman et al (1988). For application in this study, the tool did require some modifications in order to link the survey questions to certain variables in the sector specific internal customer management model which had been developed. Pilot testing also revealed that a 5 point agreement scale was preferred over the 7 point scale commonly used in the SERVQUAL technique.

ASSESSING ACTUAL INTERNAL CUSTOMER MANAGEMENT PRACTICES

On the basis of the critical incident examples, it was possible to identify six major gaps which are barriers to successful integration of inter-departmental working relationships within an Acute Unit. These are:

- Gap 1 reflecting an orientation which is so concerned with priorities and tasks inside a department that no meaningful attempt is made to respond to the needs of other departments.
- Gap 2 caused by an failure to understand the actual needs of other departments.
- Gap 3 which arises because departmental staff are not provided with any formal standards against which to evaluate tasks associated with meeting the needs of others elsewhere in the organisation.
- Gap 4 which arises because departmental staff lack the competencies necessary to provide the outputs required by other departments.
- Gap 5 caused by errors which arise due to the inadequacy of inter-departmental information flows during and/or after the output provision activity.
- Gap 6 reflecting the combined influences of gaps 1 through 5 leading to a significant difference between the inputs required by the internal customer and the actual output delivered by the supplier department.

The survey was mailed to 186 middle managers working in various medical, technical and administrative roles in 9 South West Regional Authority Acute Units. Usable questionnaires were received back from 64 respondents representing a response rate of 34.4%. In the survey, respondents were presented with 34 statements concerning various aspects of internal customer practices within their organisation. A mean rating score of >3 indicates that the majority of respondents tend to agree about the description of a specific situation being applicable to their work situation. A score of <3 will tend to indicate that most individuals do not feel that a specific situation description can be associated with managerial practices inside their department.

The survey presented eight statements concerning internal customer orientation. Appendix 1 shows scores of <3 for six statements and an overall mean score of 2.40. This would tend to indicate that a Gap 1 situation is likely to exist in many Acute Units because the prevailing culture is not strongly orientated to meeting the needs of internal customers.

Of the six statements concerning understanding of customer needs, only three statements scored >3 and the overall mean rating is 2.90. This would indicate that a Gap 2 situation may exist because some staff have only a limited understanding of the needs of other departments within the Unit.

Four statements concerning specification of goals and assessment of performance were rated <3 contributing to a mean overall score of 2.63. Hence there seems a high probability that a Gap 3 situation can occur in respondent Units because staff are provided within insufficient formal guidance on required performance targets for serving the needs of other departments.

All eight statements concerning departmental capability were rated >3 indicating that Gap 4 scenario is unlikely to occur because staff feel they have the necessary competencies to undertake assigned tasks. Five statements about communication were rated <3, yielding a mean overall score of 2.43 and suggesting that Gap 5 situations may occur due to weaknesses in the information flows between departments.

The results of the survey would indicate that the presence of Type1,2,3 and 5 Gaps and the consequent outcome of this situation will be to jointly contribute to the creation of Gap 6 scenarios in the surveyed Acute Units; i.e. there will significant differences between the inputs required by internal customers and those outputs actually delivered by the supplier departments. Hence it appears from these results that within the Acute Units which contributed to this study the prevailing culture in not one which strongly promotes the concept of seeking to build close working relationships between internal customers and their suppliers.

One possible explanation for this situation is that it merely reflects the differences of opinion which have always existed between professionals and administrators about how medical organisations should be managed (Freidson 1970). A view frequently expressed to the researchers during this study, however, was that the introduction of the Internal Market has been accompanied by senior management in many Acute Units assuming absolute control of all decisions concerning planning and allocation of resources. Presumably they feel this is the only effective way of ensuring their Unit can fulfil the performance requirements specified in the contracts negotiated with Health Authority purchasers. Unfortunately evidence from the private sector would tend to suggest that this style of management usually leads a deterioration in the working relationships between departments which over time will be translated into a decline in organisational productivity.

THE FEASIBILITY OF ADOPTING A RELATIONSHIP-BASED STRATEGIC PHILOSOPHY

The scenario facing the NHS for the foreseeable future is that of an ever increasing gap between the demand for healthcare and the capability of the nation to fund these services from the public purse. Under these circumstances it appears the only logical aim is finds better ways of optimising the use of resources which are be made available to the sector. This of course was the intent behind the reforms associated with the establishment of the Internal Market. Unfortunately this study would suggest that these reforms run the risk of achieving exactly the opposite; namely resources may be dissipated by (a) providers embarking on costly marketing battles with each other to build market share and (b) an evolving senior management style which may prevent staff using internal marketing as a technique for optimising the utilisation of scarce resources within Acute Units.

In view of this situation, there be may a need to reconsider how the Internal Market model can be reformulated to ensure optimal utilisation of scarce health care resources. The proven benefits of a strong internal customer culture is that by promoting a sense of common purpose staff will proactively seek new, innovate ways to solve problems, effectively allocate scarce resources to areas of greatest need and exhibit a degree of flexibility which permits a much more rapid response to any changes in the external environment. None if this can occur, however, if organisations are managed using the tightly controlled, hierarchical style (Slevin and Covin 1990) which certainly on the provider side, appears to favoured by many of the present generation of Acute Unit senior managers.

In defence of these senior managers, however, the authors have received the impression that this latter group of individuals are having to contend with purchasers who also seem to favour highly formalised information flows, closely defined operational procedures, tight controls and non-consultative decision making. Thus by the end of the data acquisition phase of this study, the researchers were left with an overall impression that the Department of Health has created an Internal Market in which neither the purchasers or the providers appear to have any awareness of the benefits offered by either (a) establishing a strong internal customer management culture or (b) adopting a relationship-based strategic planning orientation.

Possibly an key influencer of this situation has been the fact that by specifying the composition for the boards of both Acute Units and District Health Authorities must ensure these entities are more "business-like" (Cairncross et al 1991), the roles of clinicians and managers specifically charged with delivering patient care may have excessively marginalised. Other than some restructuring of Regional Authorities and/or mergers of smaller District Authorities, it seem unlikely that the new purchaser-provider model will not be drastically revised in the foreseeable future. Consequently there exists an urgent requirement to identify philosophies and processes which ensure that the paradigms actually being used by managers have the capability to fulfil the objectives stated in the Department of Health's recent documents (1989, 1992a, 1992b) concerning the creation of an NHS capable of meeting the needs of both the individual patient and the nation.

For a genuine partnership to be created between purchaser and provider, it is suggested that both sides must firstly commit to a culture based upon an ethos of a strong internal customer orientation inside their respective organisations. Although this study only examined the provider side of the equation, there is evidence in a 1993 Audit Commission document that purchasers are also encountering operational difficulties due to internal customer gaps emerging between those responsible for identifying the health care needs of the local community and the staff responsible for specifying contracts for negotiation with primary and acute care providers.

One possible starting point for changing the operational philosophies within the Internal Market is to for non-executive Boards members on both the purchaser and provider side to demand that their Chief Executives include in all future strategic plans a section which specifically details:

- The current status of the working relationships which exist between departments at all levels within their organisations.
- Defines how organisational structuring and managerial processes are supportive of the goal for building a strong internal customer orientation.
- Progress in closing any internal customer management gaps which have been identified, especially in the context of those which will have measurable impact on the delivery of the Patients' Charter.

- How the internal customer management concept has been incorporated into the organisation's appraisal and staff development programme.

An understandable reaction of NHS managers is that this additional requirement in the documentation process associated with preparing strategic plans is merely another administrative burden which will further compound the problems they face responding to a growing mountain of rules and regulations associated with the effective operation of the Internal Market. Hopefully, however, these individuals can be persuaded that without the adoption of internal customer management philosophy, then their organisations are unlikely to create the climate of co-operation and collaboration which is critically important to the success of existing initiatives such as clinical audit, T.Q.M. and Patient Care.

Once these organisations have begun to establish a stronger internal customer philosophy, then on the basis of private sector experience, it can be expected that this will soon be followed by a move from an environment of confrontational contracting towards a supplier-customer relationship based upon negotiations aimed at achieving mutual satisfaction for both parties. Creation of a climate of co-operation and collaboration will then enable clinicians and administrators to openly debate issues such as setting realistic targets for standards of patient care and the optimal balance between treatment priorities in relation to available financial resources.

No claims are being made by the authors that relationship-based strategic planning will eventually lead to a situation where staff in the NHS are never again faced with having to favour one treatment and/or patient group over another. The emotive issue of treatment rationing will remain a feature of the health care sector for the foreseeable future. What is offered, however, is a scenario in which purchasers and providers are seen by the general public as working together to create an environment where the common goal is to serve the needs of the patient. Recent reports in the media such as non-executive Boards openly challenging the capabilities of their Chairman and Unit Chief Executives expressing concern about increasing bureaucracy is doing little to persuade the nation that the NHS reforms have made any real contribution to improving quality of health care in the UK. Over time, however, a stronger internal customer orientation and the consequent move towards a relationship-based strategic planning ethos may begin to convince the general public that the Internal Market does have the potential to improve patient care in their local community.

REFERENCES

Abel, D.F. and Hammond, J.S. (1979), *Strategic Market Planning*, Prentice-Hall, Englewood Cliffs.

Argyris, C., Putman, R and Smith, D.M. (1985), *Action Science: Concepts, Methods And Skills For Research And Intervention*, Jocey-Bass, San Francisco.

Ansoff, H.I. (1984), *Implanting Strategic Management*, Prentice-Hall, Englewood Cliffs.

Audit Commission (1993), *Their Health, Your Business*, H.M.S.O., London.

Band, W.A. (1991), *Creating Value For Customers*, Wiley & Sons,Toronto.

Cairncross, L., Ashburner, L. and Pettigrew, A. (1991), Membership and learning needs, *Authorities In The NHS.*, Paper 4, NHSTD, Bristol.

Common, R., Flyn, N. and Mellon, E. (1992), *Managing Public Services: Competition & Decentralization*, Butterworth-Heinemann, Oxford.

Cowell, D. (1984), *The Marketing Of Services*, Heinemann, Oxford.

Department of Health (1986), *Health Notice 34 - Resource Management*, H.M.S.O., London.

Department of Health, (1989), *Working For Patients*, H.M.S.O., London.

Department of Health, (1992a), *The Health Of The Nation*, H.M.S.O., London.

Department of Health, (1992b), *The Patients' Charter*, H.M.S.O., London.

Friedson, E. (1970), *Professional Domination: The Social Structure Of Medical Care*, Atherton Press, New York.

Gronroos, C. (1982), An applied service marketing theory, *European Journal of Marketing*, Vol. 16, No. 7, pp 30 - 41.

Health Economics Research Group (1991), *Resource Management Progress And Process - Final Report*, Brunel University, Uxbridge.

Hughes, D.G. (1978), *Marketing Management: A Planning Approach*, Addison-Wesley, Reading.

Morgan, G. and Smirich, L. (1980), The case for qualitative research, *Academy of Science Review*, Vol. 5, pp 491 - 500.

Nystrom, H. (1922), Market strategy and market structures - learning and adaption in marketing relations, *Marknadsvetande*, Vol. 8, pp 41 - 45.

Nystrom, H. (1990), *Technology And Market Innovation: Strategies For Product And Company Development*, Wiley & Sons, Chichester.

Oakland, J.S. (1990), *Total Quality Management*, Heinemann, Oxford.

Parasuraman, A. Zeithmal, V.A. and Berry, L.L. (1988), SERVQUAL: a multiple item scale for measuring consumer perceptions of service quality, *Journal of Retailing*, Vol. 64, No. 1, pp 12 -40.

Perrin, J. (1988), *Resource Management In The NHS*, H.M.S.O., London.

Peters, T. *Liberation Management: Necessary Disorganisation For The Nanosecond Nineties*, Knopf, New York.

Pollard, S. (1969), *The Development Of The British Economy 1914-1967*, Pitman, London.

Porter, M.E. (1985), *Competitive Advantage*, Free Press, London.

Slevin, D.P and Covin, J.G. (1990), Juggling entrepreneurial style and organisational structure - how to get your act together, *Sloane Management Review*, Vol. 43, Winter, pp 31 - 42.

Spekman, R.E. and Johnston, W.J. (1986), Relationship management: managing the selling and buying interface, *Journal of Business Research*, Vol. 14, pp 519 - 531.

Schonberger, R.J. (1990), *Building A Chain Of Customers*, Hutchinson, London.

APPENDIX 1. RESPONSES TO THE SURVEY TO ASSESS ASPECTS OF INTERNAL CUSTOMER MANAGEMENT PROCESSES

A. Internal Customer Orientation

	Mean Agreement Rating 5 Point Scale
(1) I am are rarely too busy to respond to requests from other departments	2.87
(2) My manager rarely decides my group is so busy that we cannot respond to request from other departments	2.51
(3) I am encouraged to develop close working relationships with other departments	3.12
(4) I am encouraged to help other departments solve problems which they may be facing	2.98
(5) I try to put requests from other departments ahead of handling day-to-day problems	3.02
(6) I am encouraged to think of new ways for working more closely with other departments	2.63
(7) I am encouraged to suggest new ideas for helping other departments	2.05
(8) New ideas for helping other departments are approved and progress very rapidly	1.86
Overall Mean Rating Score	2.40

B. Understanding of Internal Customer Needs

	Mean Agreement 5 Point Scale
(1) I fully understand the roles and responsibilitiesof other departments	3.34
(2) I understand the importance of my role in contributing to meeting the needs of other departments	3.28
(3) Information which I receive about the needs ofother departments is accurate and appropriate.	2.57
(4) Information which I receive about the needs of other departments is rarely late in arriving.	2.31
(5) My manager keeps me fully informed about the changing needs of other departments	2.74
(6) I regularly meet with staff from other departments to obtain their views on possible changes in future needs	3.14
Overall Mean Rating Score	2.90

C. Specification and Assessment of Performance

	Mean Agreement 5 Point Scale
(1) I have been given clearly defined performance goals for working with other departments.	3.08
(2) I am encouraged to comment about the practicality of achieving defined performance goals for working with other departments	2.12
(3) I am involved in setting the performance goals for working with other departments	3.06
(4) My manager and I regularly discuss my actual performance in working with other departments	2.77
(5) My work group receives the information needed to review our actual performance in working with other departments.	2.12
(6) My work group regularly meets with our manager to discuss actual performance in working with other departments.	2.64
Overall Mean Rating Score	2.63

D. Capability of Departments to Undertake Assigned Tasks

	Mean Agreement 5 Point Scale
(1) I am provided with the equipment and resources required to fulfil needs of other departments.	3.18
(2) I have a job description which specifies my role in providing output for use by other departments.	3.34
(3) I have the skills needed to develop new ways for helping other departments.	3.93
(4) The structure of my department does not prevent me from being able to help other departments.	3.35
(5) My manager does not try to prevent me from seeking new ways of helping other departments.	3.24
(6) The people in my work group co-operate with each other when helping other departments.	3.83
(7) My work group has the necessary skills work together in seeking new ways of helping other departments.	3.85
(8) My manager has the necessary skills to assist my work group find new ways of helping other departments.	3.07
Overall Mean Rating Score	3.47

E. Communication Between Departments

	Mean Assessment 5 Point Scale
(1) The Unit has formalised systems for managing the flow of information between departments.	3.67
(3) The Unit's formalised systems provides the information I need to work effectively with other departments	2.48
(4) Good news about how I am helped other departments is rapidly communicated through the formalised information systems	2.28
(5) Bad news about my working relationship with other departments does not reach me first through the company "grapevine."	2.26
(6) My manager listens to my concerns about problems encountered in undertaking tasks for other departments.	3.16
(7) My work group receives the information needed to assess our effectiveness in working with other departments	2.62
(8) My work group is encouraged to bring problems about working with other departments to the attention of our manager	2.95
Overall Mean Rating Score	2.43

23 Making Priority Setting A Priority

CHARLES NORMAND

London School of Hygiene and Tropical Medicine

THE CONTEXT OF PRIORITY SETTING

Recent reforms in the provision of health care in many countries have given a new focus to the debate about the problems of scarce resources and the consequent need for rationing. There are many reactions to this. Some attempts to deny the problem (the 'health care is a right' response), or take the view that the process is essentially a political one (Carr-Hill 1991). There is a limited rearguard action in favour of a simplistic version of clinical freedom, and in contrast there are very few explicit attempts to do rationing (such as in the Oregon so called 'experiment', Welch and Larson, 1988). It will be argued in this paper that the issues in moving to better priority setting are in fact quite simple, and have been made to seem complicated mainly by the practical difficulties. It will be further argued that there are great dangers in losing the focus on the need to set priorities on as systematic and scientific a basis as possible. It will be shown how the other papers in this volume relate to the debate, but that they risk diverting attention from the central issue.

Papers in this book are concerned with aspects of rationing and setting priorities. Most accept the ideas of priority setting, but many suggest ways in which this needs to take into account various constraints. Much of this is practical and sensible, and is aimed at obtaining some of the advantages of more systematic attempts to identify and set priorities. However, it is important not to lose sight of the main issues, and especially the cost in terms of effective use of health care resources of a failure to give priority setting a high priority. It will be argued that the practical difficulties alluded to in these papers can obscure the costs of failure.

A FOCUS ON HEALTH GAIN

Many economists have argued for setting priorities according to the contribution made by different interventions to health gain, however this is defined (Normand, 1991). In essence there are three dimensions to the notion of health gain in this context - the improvement in life expectancy, the improvement in health related quality of life and the quality of the experience of being a patient. The dynamic

Setting Priorities in Health Care. Edited by M.Malek
© 1994 John Wiley & Sons Limited

quality of health gain, and the emphasis on improvement should be noted. One affect of this is to make it clear that need for services really only makes sense as capacity to benefit (Matthew, 1971). It is not the extent of the ill health, suffering or premature death *per se* that effects health gain, but rather the capacity of the health sector to improve the situation.

The importance of health gain as a basis for setting priorities is mainly in helping policy makers to concentrate on success rather than worthy effort. Put another way, it is to move health services priority setting onto the basis of evidence. The new strategy for research and development by the National Health Service in England (Department of Health 1991) makes clear the rôle of research as a basis for more effective health care. Whereas few would oppose the aggressive use of evidence in assessing the safety of new treatments, there remains a greater willingness to see ineffective and relatively ineffective practice and priorities. Although much of the currently available evidence for priority setting is poor, the same principles should apply. It is often possible to assemble the current evidence in ways that allows more effective prioritising for health gain (for example Effective Health Care 1992).

Despite the temptation to accommodate other agenda and consideration in setting priorities, it is important to consider the alternatives to prioritising for health gain. Many economists are nervous of the health gain tools (and especially the quality of the QALY), few disagree with the basic agenda. The refusal to prioritise for health gain (Harris 1987) is in principle a decision to allow generally shorter life, and worse health than is implied in a policy of maximising health gain from health care resources. It is in this light that we should assess the possibilities and constraints to using health gain as the main criterion in setting priorities.

A common source of nervousness about using health gain as the criterion for setting priorities is the emphasis on efficiency considerations at the expense of equity. Equity questions have been kept on the agenda by persistent voicing of concerns by some researchers (Mooney 1987). There have been attempts to integrate the equity dimension to health gain measures (Gafni and Birch 1991). Attempts to bring equity considerations into cost-benefit analysis go back at least to the 1960s, with the work of Burton Weisbrod and others (Weisbrod 1968). A large study of countries in Europe and North America has recently published evidence on differences in equity (van Doorslaer *et al.*, 1993). Some arguments for less scientific and more political approaches to priority setting come from considerations of equity.

It is impossible and indeed undesirable, to refute the arguments about equity. There are certainly times when we might choose to allocate available health gain to poorer people, or those with the greatest problems *ceteris paribus*. If there is no sacrifice of total gain, then considerations of this sort may be quite appropriate. Even when there is a net loss of health gain, many people would argue for less in total, distributed to those with the worst problems. Such arguments are entirely reasonable, and are cases when it is sensible to use political criteria. However, if a smaller total gain in health is chosen in order to have a more equal distribution, then this should be a clear and transparent decision. Although economists tend to be keen on economic efficiency (in this case as described in prioritising for health gain), the limitations of the health gain measures, and their lack of weighting for factors such as deprivation, make such choices quite legitimate.

Whereas there can be no objection to arguments for choosing less health gain and more equity, much of the public debate on the rôle of equity is confused. There is a body of evidence that poorer, sicker people have problems in gaining access to health services. Although some of this evidence (Le Grand 1978) has recently been challenged for the United Kingdom, it is probably fair to conclude that this problem exists even in countries with well established national health care systems, and certainly does in countries where no effective insurance mechanism exists.

The opportunity to achieve health gain is generally larger where health problems are larger. For example, successful perinatal medicine leads to more babies surviving, with potentially very large gains in length of life. If a disease is curable, and leads to very great disability, then successful treatment brings large gains. Minor ailments do not offer this possibility. Since capacity to benefit is *generally* greater in poorer, sicker people, the failure to provide appropriate services is an efficiency problem rather than one of equity. For example, it is clear that access for women to cardiac surgery is lower than for men with similar need (Petticrew *et al.*, 1993). The failure to treat women the same as men in this case leads to a loss of health benefits. It is inequitable and unjust. More importantly, it is inefficient. There is no trade-off in this case between efficiency and equity, but rather more efficiency would bring more equity.

POLITICS AND PRACTICE OF PRIORITY SETTING

If we accept the basic principle of prioritising for health gain, then constraints to doing so are practical or political. Practical reasons for failure may be concerned with mechanisms to make it happen or the failure to have satisfactory measures of health gain and the data to support such measures. Political constraints are mainly the interests of health care providers and of those groups who would be losers under a policy of maximising health gain. However, there is also something of a constraint from the pattern of public opinion, where it is far from clear that this favours health gain over other considerations (Bowling *et al.*, 1993). It is interesting to consider whether the enthusiasms for medical technology, the treatment of malignancy and any services for children reflect a belief that these are in fact services which maximise health gain. It is quite possible that some idea of injustice or desert lies behind the lack of enthusiasm for services for people with HIV related diseases, but this is not matched by a similar lack of support for treating disease caused by smoking.

Three papers in this collection are of interest in the debate about involving the public in priority setting. McKeown *et al.*, explicitly argue for rejecting the scientific approach of priorities for health gain. They suggest that this could lead to more openly political and subjective priority setting, in place of the current political and subjective (but dishonest) systems. Donovan and Coast discuss involving the public directly. It is not clear whether it will ever be possible to provide the quality and quantity of data to the public to allow full and effective participation, although this is a more general critique of the democratic process. Frankel *et al.,* suggest what is in effect a simplified version of prioritising for health gain, which may be easier to combine with active participation by the public. They argue for systematic use of evidence, but accept the impossibility of a system that uses this evidence to maximum effect.

In addition to the more obviously political constraints to prioritising for health gain, there are practical and process problems in achieving this. Health services are provided in decentralised ways, with many decision makers, and no simple central control. Setting priorities is effectively about finding a range of administrative and market levers to control use of services. The use of waiting lists for this purpose has problems, as discussed by Edwards. Using optimal market structures or management structures (Harrison) also has drawbacks. Denis, Lemay *et al.,* and Cramp and Carson discuss priority setting in planned health care systems.

The desire of governments to control health sector expenditure has changed the environment within which health services are provided. A greater awareness of the processes of rationing and setting priorities now exists. Denis, Lemay *et al.,* consider the effects of measures to contain costs, and Bruce and Bailey discuss the relationship of health policy goals and funding arrangements.

A major constraint to prioritising for health gain is the lack of data on what are the effects of what interventions for what people. It is easier to argue for the principle than the practice. It is commonly argued that we should await better evidence before changing the use of health services resources. The logic of this argument requires examination. In general we should prefer weak evidence to no evidence. Although there may be many areas of health care that are effective despite the lack of evidence, where some evidence exists this can give a guide. It should be remembered how little of what is done is based on well conducted studies (Smith 1991).

The large gaps in knowledge are reasons for well focused research on outcomes in health care. Szczepura *et al.,* and Oortwijn *et al.,* discuss aspects of health services research, and Freemantle and Watt consider health technology assessment. Moving research and research priorities to meet the needs of health care prioritising has been a slow process. There is a clash between the cultures of laboratory and statistical science of much of traditional medical research, and the more social science based evaluation sciences. Economic evaluations are now often included in clinical trials, but often this is reluctant and superficial. A strategy to run evidence based health services needs good strategies to obtain the evidence. Without this there must be concerns about the effects of rationing, as discussed in the paper by Goddard and Tavakoli.

In addition to the lack of information on which to base priority setting, there is a need for mechanisms to give access to those who are high priority, and deny it to those who are low priority for services. This is particularly important in the common case where health services would be useful to some people, but not sufficiently useful to be a priority. If the price faced by the patient is lower than the cost (which it normally is), then some deterrent to use is needed. Marketing approaches can be used to encourage or discourage use. These approaches are discussed by Scaggs *et al.*, and Mark. Influencing referral is an alternative approach, considered by McColl *et al.* Primary care 'gate keepers' to hospital services are a common feature of national health care systems, but have been under some strain. In some central European countries, such as Romania, there is a collapse in the system of primary care, and this prevents its use for gate keeping. Even in the UK, with a long tradition of primary care, there is a tendency for self-referral to hospital to increase. Discouragement of those whose priority for care is low is a mechanism that deserves more attention. Its ineffectiveness is more often asserted than demonstrated.

SUMMARY

The papers in this volume consider conceptual and practical constraints to prioritising for health gain, and some strategies to overcome these constraints. Few emphasise the importance of trying to priorities for maximum health gain.

Priority setting should be based on health gain, measured by a combination of longer life and better health related quality of life. It may sometimes be important to take account of the experiences of patients, and the distribution of the services. However, there is a need to be quite explicit about the grounds for moving away from health gain as a basis for priorities.

Constraints to prioritising on this basis come mainly from poor evidence, weak policy levers and political opposition. The appropriate response to the first is to carry out well focused research. In time it will become possible to do better. To an extent it is necessary to accommodate the political and policy environment. However, it is argued that the aim should continue to be to achieve priorities based on health gain.

REFERENCES

Bowling Ann, Jacobson B and Southgate L (1993) Health Service Priorities: explorations in consultation of the public and health professional on priority setting in an inner London health district *Social Science and Medicine* 37,7:851-857.

Carr-Hill R A (1991) Allocating resources to health care: is the QALY a technical solution to a political problem? *International Journal of Health Services* 21,3:351-363.

Department of Health (1991) *Research for Health: a research and development strategy for the NHS* London, Department of Health.

Effective Health Care (1992) *The treatment of persistent glue ear in children* Leeds, University of Leeds.

Gafni A and Birch S (1991) Equity considerations in utility based measures of health outcomes in economic appraisals: an adjustment algorithm *Journal of Health Economics* 10:329-342.

Harris J (1987) QUALYfying the value of life *Journal of Medical Ethics* 13:117-123.

Le Grand J (1978) The Distribution of Public Expenditure The case of health care *Economica* 45, 125-142.

Matthew G K (1971) Measuring need and evaluating services in McLachlan G (1971) *Problems and Progress in Medical Care* Oxford, Oxford University Press.

Mooney G (1987) What does equity in health care mean? *World Health Statistics Quarterly* 40.

Normand C (1991) Economics, Health and the Economics of Health *British Medical Journal* 303; 1572-1577.

Petticrew M, McKee M and Jones J (1993) Coronary artery surgery: are women discriminated against? *British Medical Journal* 306: 1164-1166.

Smith R (1991) Where is the wisdom? The poverty of medical evidence *British Medical Journal* 303: 798-799.

Van Doorslaer E, Wagstaff A and Rutten F (1993) *Equity in the finance and delivery of health care: an international perspective* Oxford, Oxford University Press.

Weisbrod B A (1968) Income redistribution effects and benefit-cost analysis in Chase S B *Problems in Public Expenditure Analysis* Brookings Institution, London, George Allen and Unwin Ltd.

Welch H G and Larson E B (1988) Dealing with limited resources: The Oregon decision to curtail funding for organ transplantation *New England Journal of Medicine* 319,3: 171-173.